Systemic Amyloidosis due to Monoclonal Immunoglobulins

Editor

RAYMOND L. COMENZO

HEMATOLOGY/ONCOLOGY CLINICS OF NORTH AMERICA

www.hemonc.theclinics.com

Consulting Editors
GEORGE P. CANELLOS
EDWARD J. BENZ Jr

December 2020 • Volume 34 • Number 6

ELSEVIER

1600 John F. Kennedy Boulevard • Suite 1800 • Philadelphia, Pennsylvania, 19103-2899

http://www.theclinics.com

HEMATOLOGY/ONCOLOGY CLINICS OF NORTH AMERICA Volume 34, Number 6
December 2020 ISSN 0889-8588, ISBN 13: 978-0-323-79165-6

Editor: Stacy Eastman
Developmental Editor: Julia McKenzie

Hematology/Oncology Clinics (ISSN 0889-8588) is published bimonthly by Elsevier Inc., 360 Park Avenue South, New York, NY 10010-1710. Months of issue are February, April, June, August, October, and December. Business and Editorial Offices: 1600 John F. Kennedy Blvd., Ste. 1800, Philadelphia, PA 19103–2899. Customer Service Office: 3251 Riverport Lane, Maryland Heights, MO 63043. Periodicals postage paid at New York, NY and at additional mailing offices. Subscription prices are $443.00 per year (domestic individuals), $876.00 per year (domestic institutions), $100.00 per year (domestic students/residents), $480.00 per year (Canadian individuals), $100.00 per year (Canadian students/residents), $1085.00 per year (Canadian institutions) $547.00 per year (international individuals), $1085.00 per year (international institutions), and $255.00 per year (international students/residents). International air speed delivery is included in all *Clinics* subscription prices. All prices are subject to change without notice. **POSTMASTER:** Send address changes to *Hematology/Oncology Clinics of North America*, Elsevier Health Sciences Division, Subscription Customer Service, 3251 Riverport Lane, Maryland Heights, MO 63043. Customer Service (orders, claims, online, change of address): Elsevier Health Sciences Division, Subscription **Customer Service, 3251 Riverport Lane, Maryland Heights, MO 63043. Tel:** 1-800-654-2452 (U.S. and Canada); 314-447-8871 (outside U.S. and Canada). Fax: 314-447-8029. E-mail: journalscustomerservice-usa@elsevier.com (for print support); journalsonlinesupport-usa@elsevier.com (for online support).

Reprints. For copies of 100 or more, of articles in this publication, please contact the Commercial Reprints Department, Elsevier Inc., 360 Park Avenue South, New York, New York 10010-1710; Tel.: 212-633-3874, Fax: 212-633-3820, E-mail: reprints@elsevier.com.

Hematology/Oncology Clinics of North America is covered in *MEDLINE/PubMed (Index Medicus), EMBASE/Excerpta Medica, and BIOSIS.*

Contributors

CONSULTING EDITORS

GEORGE P. CANELLOS, MD
William Rosenberg Professor of Medicine, Department of Medical Oncology, Dana-Farber Cancer Institute, Boston, Massachusetts, USA

EDWARD J. BENZ Jr, MD
Professor, Pediatrics, Richard and Susan Smith Professor, Medicine, Professor, Genetics, Harvard Medical School, President and CEO Emeritus, Office of the President, Dana-Farber Cancer Institute, Boston, Massachusetts, USA

EDITOR

RAYMOND L. COMENZO, MD
Professor of Medicine, Tufts University School of Medicine, Director, John C Davis Myeloma and Amyloid Program, Tufts Medical Center, Boston, Massachusetts, USA

AUTHORS

SUSAN BAL, MD
Assistant Professor, Division of Hematology and Oncology, O'Neal Comprehensive Cancer Center, The University of Alabama at Birmingham, Birmingham, Alabama, USA

GIADA BIANCHI, MD
Associate Director, Amyloidosis Program, Brigham and Women's Hospital/Dana-Farber Cancer Institute, Instructor in Medicine, Harvard Medical School, Boston, Massachusetts, USA

MACKENZIE BOEDICKER
Founder and President, Mackenzie's Mission, Great Falls, Virginia, USA

RAJ CHAKRABORTY, MD
Assistant Professor of Medicine, Multiple Myeloma and Amyloidosis Service, New York, New York, USA

CHAKRA CHAULAGAIN, MD, FACP
Director of Myeloma and Amyloidosis Program, Department of Hematology and Oncology, Maroone Cancer Center, Cleveland Clinic Florida, Weston, Florida, USA

RAYMOND L. COMENZO, MD
Professor of Medicine, Tufts University School of Medicine, Director, John C Davis Myeloma and Amyloid Program, Tufts Medical Center, Boston, Massachusetts, USA

NAOMI G. DEMPSEY, MD
Hematology/Oncology Fellow, Department of Medicine, Division of Hematology, University of Miami, Sylvester Comprehensive Cancer Center, Miami, Florida, USA

ANGELA DISPENZIERI, MD
Professor of Medicine, Professor of Laboratory Medicine and Pathology, Division of Hematology, Mayo Clinic, Rochester, Minnesota, USA

P. JAMES B. DYCK, MD
Department of Neurology, Mayo Clinic College of Medicine, Rochester, Minnesota, USA

TERESA FOGAREN, AGNP-C
Nurse Practitioner, Division of Hematology/Oncology, Tufts Medical Center, Boston, Massachusetts, USA

MORIE A. GERTZ, MD, MACP
Consultant, Division of Hematology, Mayo Clinic, Rochester, Minnesota, USA

AMANDEEP GODARA, MD
Division of Hematology/Oncology, Tufts Medical Center, Boston, Massachusetts, USA

JAMES E. HOFFMAN, MD
Assistant Professor of Clinical Medicine, Department of Medicine, Division of Hematology, University of Miami, Sylvester Comprehensive Cancer Center, Miami, Florida, USA

SABINE KARAM, MD
Division of Nephrology and Hypertension, Saint George Hospital-Development Program, Saint George Hospital University Medical Center, Beirut, Lebanon

SHAJI KUMAR, MD
Professor of Medicine, Chair, Myeloma, Amyloidosis, Dysproteinemia Group, Mayo Clinic, Rochester, Minnesota, USA

HEATHER J. LANDAU, MD
Associate Attending, Division of Hematologic Oncology, Memorial Sloan Kettering Cancer Center, Associate Professor of Clinical Medicine, Weill Cornell Medical College, New York, New York, USA

SUZANNE LENTZSCH, MD, PhD
Professor of Medicine, Columbia University, Director, Multiple Myeloma and Amyloidosis Service, Herbert Irving Pavillion, New York, New York, USA

NELSON LEUNG, MD
Division of Nephrology and Hypertension, Division of Hematology, Mayo Clinic, Rochester, Minnesota, USA

ISABELLE LOUSADA, MA
President and CEO, Amyloidosis Research Consortium, Newton, Massachusetts, USA

MATHEW S. MAURER, MD
Clinical Cardiovascular Research Laboratory for the Elderly, Columbia University Irving Medical Center, New York, New York, USA

GIAMPAOLO MERLINI, MD
Professor of Laboratory Medicine, Department of Molecular Medicine, University of Pavia, and Amyloidosis Center, Foundation IRCCS Policlinico San Matteo, Pavia, Italy

GARETH J. MORGAN, PhD
Research Assistant Professor, Amyloidosis Center and Section of Hematology and Medical Oncology, Department of Medicine, Boston University School of Medicine, Boston, Massachusetts, USA

GIOVANNI PALLADINI, MD, PhD
Department of Molecular Medicine, Amyloidosis Research and Treatment Center Foundations, "Istituto di Ricovero e Cura a Carattere Scientifico (IRCCS) Policlinico San Matteo," University of Pavia, Pavia, Italy

AYAN R. PATEL, MD
CardioVascular Center, Tufts Medical Center, Boston, Massachusetts, USA

MICHAEL ROSENZWEIG, MD
Assistant Clinical Professor of Hematology and Hematopoietic Cell Transplantation, City of Hope Helford Clinical Research Hospital, City of Hope, Duarte, California, USA

SUNIL E. SAITH, MD, MPH
Clinical Cardiovascular Research Laboratory for the Elderly, Columbia University Irving Medical Center, New York, New York, USA

VAISHALI SANCHORAWALA, MD
Professor of Medicine, Director of Autologous Stem Cell Transplant Program, Director of Amyloidosis Center, Boston University School of Medicine and Boston Medical Center, Boston, Massachusetts, USA

STEFAN SCHONLAND, MD
Department of Internal Medicine V, Division of Hematology/Oncology, Amyloidosis Center, Heidelberg University Hospital, Heidelberg, Germany

PARIWAT THAISETTHAWATKUL, MD
Professor of Neurology, Department of Neurological Sciences, University of Nebraska Medical Center, Omaha, Nebraska, USA

SASCHA A. TUCHMAN, MD, MHS
Associate Professor, Director of Multiple Myeloma and Amyloidosis Program, Lineberger Comprehensive Cancer Center, The University of North Carolina at Chapel Hill, Chapel Hill, North Carolina, USA

CINDY VARGA, MD
Assistant Professor, The John Conant Davis Myeloma and Amyloid Program, Division of Hematology/Oncology, Tufts Medical Center, Boston, Massachusetts, USA

JONATHAN S. WALL, PhD
Professor and Director of Research, Amyloidosis and Cancer Theranostics Program, Preclinical and Diagnostic Molecular Imaging Laboratory, The University of Tennessee Graduate School of Medicine, Knoxville, Tennessee, USA

ASHUTOSH D. WECHALEKAR, MD
National Amyloidosis Centre, University College London, London, United Kingdom

SANDY W. WONG, MD
Assistant Clinical Professor, Hematology/Blood and Marrow Transplantation, Director, Comprehensive Amyloid Program, University of California, San Francisco, California, USA

JEFFREY A. ZONDER, MD
Professor of Oncology, Leader, Multiple Myeloma and Amyloidosis Multidisciplinary Team, Barbara Ann Karmanos Cancer Institute, Wayne State University School of Medicine, Detroit, Michigan, USA

Contents

The spectrum of immunoglobulin paraprotein-associated diseases requiring therapy extends beyond multiple myeloma and AL amyloidosis. Awareness of these is essential in ensuring timely accurate diagnosis and appropriate treatment. As most paraprotein-associated diseases are fairly uncommon, therapeutic decisions must often be made in the absence of data from randomized controlled trials. Treatment is generally directed at the underlying clonal cell population. This review focuses on the spectrum of the less common paraprotein-associated disorders. In most instances, the monoclonal immunoglobulin plays a direct role in the pathophysiology of the disease course; in a select few, the paraprotein may be a disease marker.

Immunoglobulin light chain amyloidosis is the most common systemic amyloidosis. The pathogenetic mechanism is deposition of fibrils of misfolded immunoglobulin free light chains, more often lambda, typically produced by clonal plasma cells. Distinct Ig light chain variable region genotypes underlie most light chain amyloidosis and dictate tissue tropism. Light chain amyloidosis fibrils cause distortion of the histologic architecture and direct cytotoxicity, leading to rapidly progressive organ dysfunction and eventually patient demise. A high index of clinical suspicion with rapid tissue diagnosis and commencement of combinatorial, highly effective cytoreductive therapy is crucial to avoid irreversible organ damage and early mortality.

Lymphoma-related amyloidosis is a rare entity. Systemic AL amyloidosis is generally caused by an underlying plasma cell clone in the bone marrow with an intact monoclonal immunoglobulin G (IgG) or IgA protein. The rarity of the lymphoma-related amyloidosis makes the generation of data in randomized trials and the determination of the optimal treatment almost impossible. Therefore, treatment recommendations discussed here are based on either retrospective or small prospective trials of single centers.

Monoclonal antibodies secreted by clonally expanded plasma cells can form a range of pathologic aggregates including amyloid fibrils. The enormous diversity in the sequences of the involved light chains may be responsible for complexity of the disease. Nevertheless, important common features have been recognized. Two recent high-resolution structures of light chain fibrils show related but distinct conformations. The native structure of the light chains is lost when they are incorporated into the amyloid fibrils. The authors discuss the processes that lead to aggregation and describe how existing and emerging therapies aim to prevent aggregation or remove amyloid fibrils from tissues.

Amyloid light chain amyloidosis (AL) is the most commonly diagnosed systemic form of amyloidosis, resulting from deposition of amyloid fibrils into various organs, such as the heart. Over the past several decades, significant advances in diagnosis and treatment have reduced overall mortality. Short-term survival, however, has not improved, in large part due to cardiovascular mortality from advanced AL cardiac amyloidosis. Early clinical suspicion of cardiac involvement is critical in order to initiate appropriate treatment and referrals for successful management. This review discusses the current challenges in diagnosis as well as available treatment options for different stages of cardiac involvement.

Kidney involvement in immunoglobulin-related amyloidosis (AIg) is common. Although patients with renal-limited AIg tend not to have the high mortality that patients with cardiac amyloidosis have, they do experience significant morbidity and impact on quality of life. The complexity of the pathogenesis remains incompletely understood. Models have been established to prognosticate and assess for the response to therapy. Patients with advanced renal impairment from immunoglobulin light chain amyloidosis still have poor renal prognosis, and better therapy is needed in order to preserve kidney function. Patients who develop end-stage renal disease can undergo renal replacement therapy with kidney transplantation.

Early diagnosis of AL amyloidosis and appreciation of the nutritional and coagulation abnormalities associated with liver and gastrointestinal involvement are critically important in the treatment and management. In cases of severe malabsorption total parenteral nutrition can be extremely helpful as a bridge to organ improvement. Rarely the use of antifibrinolytic agents such as oral aminocaproic acid with transfusion support may control severe bleeding in patients with coagulation abnormalities. It is important to keep in mind that organ improvement should follow in lag phase after the reduction in the pathologic free light chain with treatment. Closely following light chain levels may permit brief holidays from treatment and enable periods of recovery before resuming therapy in patients with prompt early and deep hematologic responses.

Peripheral nervous system involvement in primary systemic amyloidosis is another important organ involvement in the spectrum of this disease entity. Early recognition may lead to an earlier diagnosis and treatment with improvement in prognosis.

Clinical features of soft tissue amyloid light-chain (AL) amyloidosis include macroglossia, arthropathy, muscle pseudohypertrophy, skin plaques, and carpal tunnel syndrome. Vascular manifestations of AL amyloid include periorbital ecchymosis, jaw or limb claudication, and even myocardial infarction caused by occlusion of small vessel coronary arteries. Some of these features, such as macroglossia, periorbital ecchymosis, and the so-called shoulder-pad sign, are pathognomonic for AL amyloidosis. These findings may be the initial presenting features of the disease, and the recognition of these red flag symptoms is very important for the diagnosis and early intervention on the underlying plasma cell disease.

Chemotherapy for amyloid light chain (AL) amyloidosis has evolved over the years. Although high-dose melphalan and stem cell transplantation remain the standard of care for eligible patients, a vast majority of the patients at the time of presentation are not eligible for this approach and require low-intensity but highly effective induction therapy, usually based on bortezomib. Immunomodulatory agents are not well tolerated, particularly by patients with AL amyloidosis cardiomyopathy, and are reserved for second-line or later therapy. Because there currently is no Food Drug and Administration–approved therapy, participation in well-designed clinical trials of high scientific merit should be considered.

Stem cell transplantation was one of the first proven effective regimens for the management of immunoglobulin light-chain amyloidosis. Criteria for patient selection and the mobilization regimen become important features in ensuring a safe outcome. The technique of stem cell transplantation has evolved considerably in parallel with the development of new

treatment; and management of this complex multisystemic disease. Included are descriptions of the most significant AL amyloidosis symptoms as well as addressing burden of disease, including financial concerns, and psychological impact. In 2015 a Patient Focused Drug Development meeting held at the Food and Drug Administration provided valuable data that is shaping the drug development landscape and are reviewed here. The article concludes with a list of useful resources and organizations for patients and caregivers.

Angela Dispenzieri and Giampaolo Merlini

Opportunities and challenges in the field of systemic amyloidosis can be grouped into 4 categories. First, a deeper understanding of the pathogenesis of the disease is required. Second, a greater awareness of the disease, which will lead to an earlier diagnosis, is imperative. Third, end points for interventional trials are required to convey us to our fourth aspirations, which are novel therapies for patients with light chain amyloidosis.

HEMATOLOGY/ONCOLOGY CLINICS OF NORTH AMERICA

FORTHCOMING ISSUES

February 2021
Melanoma
F. Stephen Hodi, *Editor*

April 2021
Myeloproliferative Neoplasms
Ronald Hoffman, Ross Levine, John
Mascarenhas, and Raajit Rampal, *Editors*

June 2021
Bladder Cancer
Guru P. Sonpavde, *Editor*

RECENT ISSUES

October 2020
Mantle Cell Lymphoma
John P. Leonard, *Editor*

August 2020
Follicular Lymphoma
Jonathan W. Friedberg, *Editor*

June 2020
**Blastic Plasmacytoid Dendritic Cell
Neoplasm**
Andrew A. Lane, *Editor*

SERIES OF RELATED INTEREST

Surgical Oncology Clinics of North America
https://www.surgonc.theclinics.com/

THE CLINICS ARE AVAILABLE ONLINE!
Access your subscription at:
www.theclinics.com

Preface

Shedding Tears to Clear the Way

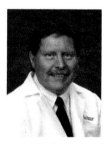

Raymond L. Comenzo, MD
Editor

At 1 AM in mid-February 2002, my phone rang. The covering resident explained that one of my patients, a 45-year-old man with systemic light chain amyloidosis (AL) and heart involvement who was day +2 of stem cell transplant, had experienced a cardiac arrest and died. Stunned, I had the young physician repeat every detail, and I then dressed and walked the 4 blocks down 1st Avenue to the hospital. With the chart in front me, I phoned his wife. They had been high-school sweethearts and were deeply connected. The patient had been well that day, playing the guitar in his room. My dread increased as I punched in each number and, after telling her what had happened, I felt remorseful and profoundly sad as she screamed and sobbed.

For several decades, the majority of the AL patients I tried to help died within a year or two, albeit not as dramatically as this 45-year-old transplant patient. Many, though, were sudden cardiac deaths, in a bathroom or after climbing a flight of stairs, and rarely in the hospital with pulseless electrical activity. In 1998, at an international symposium, I showed a slide with the first names of all the AL patients who had enrolled on my clinical trials and died of AL. It was a busy slide and reflected how the tears of patients and their families sought to clear the way forward. And, over the following 22 years, the way did clear as outcomes changed slightly with patient selection for stem cell transplant, significantly with the application of bortezomib to AL, and dramatically with the effectiveness of daratumumab.

In this issue, the world's experts in AL present the state of the science. I am grateful to my colleagues for their willingness to contribute and for their thoughtful contributions. In this time of great suffering, we cannot minimize the sacrifices that patients with rare fatal diseases like AL, and their families, have made over the decades as they have sought care and understanding. Through and with their tears, the clinical trials that have been conducted in AL have led us to this point. AL is now a treatable illness, especially if recognized early in its course.

Hematol Oncol Clin N Am 34 (2020) xiii–xiv
https://doi.org/10.1016/j.hoc.2020.09.002
0889-8588/20/© 2020 Published by Elsevier Inc.

hemonc.theclinics.com

Let me close by thanking Dr Canellos for the opportunity to edit this issue and to express my gratitude to the *Hematology/Oncology Clinics of North America* staff, particularly Stacy Eastman and Julia McKenzie, for their expert guidance and flawless assistance. Errors and oversights are mine and mine alone. And I must thank my family for giving me space and time to think, work, and write. The love and support of my wife, Sheryl, and my children, Gena, Joe, and Andy, have enabled me to hear the calls and the questions that have come my way, to listen and learn, and it is hoped, to answer with grace and clarity, and to live each day by the abiding and simple dictum: *Age quod agis.*

Raymond L. Comenzo, MD
Tufts University School of Medicine
John C. Davis Myeloma and
Amyloid Program
Tufts Medical Center
Box 826, 800 Washington Street
Boston, MA 02111, USA

E-mail address:
rcomenzo@tuftsmedicalcenter.org

Introduction

After the first description of amyloid infiltration in 1842 by Rokitansky, the chemical composition and pathogenesis of amyloid deposits became a matter of a heated dispute. Extensive evidence of a significant association between "primary" amyloidosis and myeloma-type proteins, particularly Bence Jones proteins, has been provided by the observations of my mentor, Elliott Osserman, in a seminal paper in 1964.[1] The strongest evidence for the immunoglobulin origin of amyloid fibrils has come with the determination of the amino acid sequence of 2 amyloid fibril proteins by George Glenner in 1971.[2] Recognizing "primary amyloidosis" as being a member of plasma cell dyscrasias opened the door to the application of therapies used in multiple myeloma, at that time limited to melphalan and cyclophosphamide. However, late diagnosis and lack of risk stratification led to minimal clinical improvements with these drugs, and for years the disease lagged in a hopeless limbo. The interest in AL amyloidosis rekindled following the advent of high-dose melphalan followed by autologous stem cell transplantation pioneered by Ray Comenzo. This novel approach produced a drastic reduction of the plasma cell clone, and, consequently, of the circulating protein amyloid precursor, which translated into rapid and marked clinical improvement and extended survival, demonstrating that AL amyloidosis was indeed treatable.[3] The introduction of a powerful clonal biomarker, serum-free light chains, and cardiac biomarkers, NT-proBNP and troponin, allowed the development of staging systems for risk assessment,[4,5] and the definition of universal criteria for hematologic and organ response[6] fostering trials with new drugs borrowed from the blooming myeloma field. The development of powerful imaging techniques, from refined echocardiographic evaluation to cardiac MRI and novel amyloid tracers, improved the diagnostic potential and monitoring of cardiac response to therapy.[7]

In this issue, world-leading experts review the most recent advances in AL amyloidosis covering the whole spectrum of the disease, from mechanisms of amyloid fibril formation, to prognosis, to novel-specific therapies and from new small molecules to monoclonal antibodies to, notably, patient voices. In the last decade, the progress in the field has been astonishing, with remarkable survival extension, approaching now a median of 4 to 5 years, and a significant subset, 20% to 30%, of patients who are operationally cured. The magnitude and the power of our diagnostic and therapeutic resources made us optimistic about the future care of AL amyloidosis. However, the main impediment to providing benefits to *all* our patients is represented by late diagnosis and the associated irrecoverable end-organ damage. Early diagnosis depends on awareness, and the collaboration with patient associations is pivotal to spread the knowledge of this rare and challenging, multifaceted disease. Additional aid can come from the applications of artificial intelligence and the deep-learning subtype, in particular, that may facilitate the timely recognition of the disease.[8]

Finally, this issue has been written during the Covid-19 epochal pandemic that swept the world with death and anguish. One of the many radical changes imposed by the virus to our practice is the need to resort to telemedicine to follow our patients. This emergency resource could be exploited to facilitate future clinical trials and will

Hematol Oncol Clin N Am 34 (2020) xv–xvi
https://doi.org/10.1016/j.hoc.2020.08.008
0889-8588/20/© 2020 Elsevier Inc. All rights reserved.

hemonc.theclinics.com

remodel the patient-doctor relationship, particularly in referral centers for rare diseases.

DISCLOSURE

This work was supported by grants from the Italian Ministry of Health (Ricerca Finalizzata, grant RF-2013-02355259 and GR-2018-12368387), the CARIPLO Foundation (grant 2013-0964 and 2018-0257), the Amyloidosis Foundation, the "Associazione Italiana per la Ricerca sul Cancro–Special Program Molecular Clinical Oncology 5 per mille" (grant 9965) and by an Accelerator Award from the Cancer Research UK, the Fundación Científica – Asociación Española Contra el Cáncer and the Associazione Italiana Ricerca sul Cancro.

Giampaolo Merlini, MD
Amyloidosis Center, Foundation IRCCS Policlinico San Matteo, University of Pavia,
Viale Golgi 14, Pavia 27100, Italy

E-mail address:
gmerlini@unipv.it

REFERENCES

1. Osserman EF, Takatsuki K, Talal N. Multiple myeloma I. the pathogenesis of "amyloidosis. Semin Hematol 1964;1:3–85.
2. Glenner GG, Terry W, Harada M, et al. Amyloid fibril proteins: proof of homology with immunoglobulin light chains by sequence analyses. Science 1971;172(988): 1150–1.
3. Comenzo RL, Vosburgh E, Falk RH, et al. Dose-intensive melphalan with blood stem-cell support for the treatment of AL (amyloid light-chain) amyloidosis: Survival and responses in 25 patients. Blood 1998;91(10):3662–70.
4. Dispenzieri A, Gertz MA, Kyle RA, et al. Serum cardiac troponins and N-terminal pro-brain natriuretic peptide: a staging system for primary systemic amyloidosis. J Clin Oncol 2004;22(18):3751–7.
5. Kumar S, Dispenzieri A, Lacy MQ, et al. Revised prognostic staging system for light chain amyloidosis incorporating cardiac biomarkers and serum free light chain measurements. J Clin Oncol 2012;30(9):989–95.
6. Palladini G, Dispenzieri A, Gertz MA, et al. New criteria for response to treatment in immunoglobulin light chain amyloidosis based on free light chain measurement and cardiac biomarkers: impact on survival outcomes. J Clin Oncol 2012;30(36): 4541–9.
7. Dorbala S, Ando Y, Bokhari S, et al. ASNC/AHA/ASE/EANM/HFSA/ISA/SCMR/ SNMMI expert consensus recommendations for multimodality imaging in cardiac amyloidosis: Part 2 of 2-Diagnostic criteria and appropriate utilization. J Nucl Cardiol 2020;27(2):659–73.
8. Topol EJ. High-performance medicine: the convergence of human and artificial intelligence. Nat Med 2019;25(1):44–56.

The Spectrum of Monoclonal Immunoglobulin-Associated Diseases

Sascha A. Tuchman, MD, MHS[a], Jeffrey A. Zonder, MD[b],*

KEYWORDS

- Monoclonal plasma cell diseases • Monoclonal gammopathies
- Nonamyloid diseases

INTRODUCTION AND BACKGROUND

Multiple myeloma and light chain (AL) amyloidosis, two monoclonal plasma cell diseases (PCDs) with life-threatening complications, have a combined incidence of approximately 35,000 cases per year in the United States.[1,2] Both diseases always arise from monoclonal gammopathy of uncertain significance (MGUS),[3,4] which is vastly more common and by definition without symptoms.

It is not uncommon for PCDs to be diagnosed in asymptomatic individuals based on the finding of an elevated protein level on routine bloodwork. An elevated globulin or total protein level should be followed up with serum protein electrophoresis and immunofixation to determine whether there is a monoclonal protein present. Most asymptomatic patients found to have a monoclonal serum protein will have MGUS, but smoldering multiple myeloma (SMM) is another possibility. MGUS and SMM are distinguished from one another based on bone marrow plasmacytosis and the quantity of monoclonal proteins in both blood and urine.[5] PCDs characterized by the production of monoclonal light chains only are more likely to be picked up only if associated with symptoms, because the levels of serum free light chains are generally too low to impact the total protein level. Moreover, serum free light chain measurement is not part of a standard comprehensive metabolic panel and urinalysis registers albuminuria not Bence Jones proteinuria.

Additional findings that should prompt further workup for a PCD that requires therapy include hypogammaglobulinemia affecting 1 or more immunoglobulin subtypes (ie, immunoparesis), unexplained anemia, renal insufficiency without other obvious cause, hypercalcemia, and bone pain, as these are cardinal signs of multiple

[a] Division of Hematology, University of North Carolina – Chapel Hill, Comprehensive Cancer Center, 170 Manning Dr., CB#7305, Chapel Hill, NC 27599, USA; [b] Barbara Ann Karmanos Cancer Institute/Wayne State University School of Medicine, Myeloma and Amyloidosis Team, Barbara Ann Karmanos Cancer Institute, Detroit, MI, USA
* Corresponding author. 4100 John R., Detroit MI, 48201
E-mail address: zonderj@karmanos.org
Twitter: @Amyloid_Planet (J.A.Z.)

Hematol Oncol Clin N Am 34 (2020) 997–1008
https://doi.org/10.1016/j.hoc.2020.07.002
0889-8588/20/© 2020 Elsevier Inc. All rights reserved.

myeloma. Significant albuminuria (even if not nephrotic range), edema, congestive heart failure with a preserved ejection fraction, or unexplained peripheral neuropathy should raise concerns about the possibility of amyloidosis, in a person previously diagnosed as having MGUS or SMM.

It is important to recognize that there are non-PCD conditions associated with monoclonal gammopathy. Waldenstrom macroglobulinemia (lymphoplasmacytic lymphoma) is typically associated with a monoclonal IgM paraprotein that can cause symptoms based on hyperviscosity, sensory neuropathy, or in some cases amyloidosis.[6] Marginal zone non-Hodgkin lymphoma (MZ NHL) is not infrequently associated with a monoclonal paraprotein that is usually either IgG or IgM.[7] One potential consequence of monoclonal gammopathy in MZ NHL is nodular pulmonary amyloidosis.[8] Monoclonal gammopathy, often light chain only, may also accompany chronic lymphocytic leukemia, and has been reported to have possible negative prognostic significance.[9–11] As any of these or other paraprotein-associated lymphoproliferative conditions may require treatment, it is essential to diagnose them in a timely fashion.

The focus of this review is the spectrum of other much less common paraprotein-associated disorders. In most instances, the monoclonal immunoglobulin plays a direct role in the pathophysiology of the disease course, as it does in AL amyloidosis. In a select few, such as Schnitzler syndrome and TEMPI (*Telangiectasias, elevated Erythropoietin, Monoclonal gammopathy, Perinephric fluid collections, and Intrapulmonary shunting*) syndrome, the paraprotein may be a disease marker, as is usually the case in multiple myeloma.

NONAMYLOID, MONOCLONAL GAMMOPATHIES OF RENAL SIGNIFICANCE

Although it has long been recognized that there are patients without multiple myeloma or amyloidosis with various forms of monoclonal immunoglobulin-mediated renal injury, the first known publication referring to such conditions collectively as monoclonal gammopathy of renal significance (MGRS) was in 2012 (**Table 1**).[12] In that article, the International Kidney and Monoclonal Gammopathy Research Group described approximately a dozen noncast nephropathy, nonamyloidosis types of kidney injury, expanding on a previous classification scheme based on the nature (structure and distribution) of the renal protein deposits.[13] Although different subtypes of MGRS are discussed as discrete entities, it is important to

Table 1
Examples of specific forms of monoclonal gammopathy of renal significance

Crystals	Fibrillar	Microtubular	Nonorganized
Cast nephropathy	AL amyloidosis	Types 1 and 2 cryoglobulinemic GN	Monoclonal Ig deposition disease
Light chain proximal tubulopathy[a]	Nonamyloid fibrillary GN	Immunotactoid GN	Proliferative GN with monoclonal Ig
Crystal-storing histiocytosis		GOMMIDD	IgM-mediated mesangiocapillary GN[b]
			C3 glomerulopathy

Abbreviations: GN, glomerulonephritis; GOMMIDD, Glomerulo-nephritis with organized microtubular monoclonal Ig deposits.[12,13]
  [a] With or without Fanconi syndrome.
  [b] Typically in association with Waldenstrom macroglobulinemia.

recognize that in some cases patients may present with more than 1 type of renal lesion simultaneously.[14–16]

Monoclonal Immunoglobulin Deposition Disease

Monoclonal immunoglobulin deposition disease (MIDD) refers to a group of disorders in which injury to the kidneys and, less commonly, other organs is the result of nonfibrillar deposits of monoclonal light chains (usually kappa, termed light chain deposition disease [LCDD]), monoclonal heavy chain deposition disease (HCDD), or a mixture of both light and heavy chain deposition disease (LHCDD).[13] Of these, LCDD is the most common. As was evident even in early descriptions of MIDD, more than half of patients with LCDD may also have multiple myeloma.[17,18] Much less commonly, MIDD can complicate Waldenstrom macroglobulinemia or other lymphoproliferative disorders.[19,20] Clinically, MIDD may be difficult to distinguish from AL amyloidosis. Renal involvement is often initially recognized due to the development of nephrotic range albuminuria, although in MIDD silent tubular injury often precedes clinically significant glomerular dysfunction. On renal biopsy, essentially all patients with MIDD will have smooth linear peritubular deposits that do not demonstrate Congo red birefringence.[21] The most common glomerular abnormality in MIDD is nodular glomerulosclerosis, and immunofluorescent staining generally reveals monotypic immunoglobulin deposition both in the glomerular basement membrane and the nodules themselves.[13] In most cases of LCDD, the monotypic light chain is kappa, whereas in AL amyloidosis lambda predominates. Electron microscopy further distinguishes between MIDD and AL, revealing granular deposits in the former, and fibrillar ones in the latter. Although cast nephropathy occurring concurrently with MIDD has been described as "rare," at least one large series noted approximately a quarter of patients with LCDD had tubular casts.[13,21]

Treatment of MIDD, like that of AL amyloidosis as well as less common forms of MGRS, typically focuses on suppressing the underlying clonal plasma cell or lymphoproliferative disorder. There are two general goals of therapy:

- In patients with preserved (or acutely worsening) renal function, reduction of the pathogenic free light chain or immunoglobulin to prevent permanent or progressive organ injury.
- In patients with irreversible end-stage renal injury, induction of a complete disease remission is generally required to be considered for organ transplantation. Renal transplantation in the setting of persisting gammopathy is associated with a higher risk of MGRS recurrence in the transplanted kidney.

Bortezomib-containing and/or alkylator-containing chemotherapy regimens predominate as first-line options, with immunomodulatory drugs used less frequently.[21] Modern regimens appear to be more effective than older ones,[18] although the advent of commercially available serum free light chain monitoring has likely contributed to more appropriate decision-making related to switching therapy regimens and overall duration of therapy. High-dose melphalan with autologous stem cell transplantation (ASCT) is a viable and often effective option in select patients.[22] Renal dysfunction is a common reason clinicians opt for non-ASCT induction therapy, but even patients with end-stage renal failure may be treated in this fashion (often with reductions in the dose of melphalan used) at centers of excellence.[23] Daratumumab, an anti-CD38 antibody, has been shown to have remarkable single-agent activity in relapsed LCDD, making it a useful consideration for patients with markedly impaired renal function.[24] Hematologic response in MIDD, using the same criteria as for AL amyloidosis,[25] is the initial goal of therapy. High-quality hematologic response (reduction in the difference between the involved and uninvolved free light chain to $\leq$ 4 mg/dL) appears to be predictive of recovery or stabilization of renal function.[22,24]

Other Forms of Monoclonal Gammopathy of Renal Significance

Of the other described types of MGRS, herein we limit discussion to light chain proximal tubulopathy, immunotactoid glomerulonephritis (GN), and proliferative GN with monoclonal immunoglobulin deposits. Types I and II cryoglobulinemic GN are discussed in the section on monoclonal gammopathies of cutaneous significance.

Light chain proximal tubulopathy (LCPT), although less common than other forms of paraprotein-mediated renal injury, is important for the clinician to recognize. Clinical presentation is highly variable with only subsets of patients showing decreased glomerular filtration rate, proteinuria, and/or acquired Fanconi syndrome. Patients with Fanconi syndrome have type 2 renal tubular acidosis with generalized proximal tubular dysfunction, resulting in impaired absorption of bicarbonate, phosphate, glucose, uric acid, and amino acids.[26] In a review of approximately 10,000 archived renal biopsies, there were only 13 cases of LCPT (compared with 157 cases of AL and 49 cases of LCDD).[27] On biopsy, proximal tubular cells typically show cytoplasmic swelling with apical blebbing. Three of 13 specimens showed rhomboid intracytoplasmic crystals derived from the variable region of endocytosed light chains. Electron microscopy demonstrates increased lysosomes and mitochondrial swelling.[27] In contrast to AL, LCDD, and immunotactoid GN, it is not uncommon for the renal injury to occur in the absence of a prior diagnosis of systemic plasma cell disorder, although workup will subsequently identify one.[28] There are no large prospective trials evaluating therapy of LCPT, but there are numerous case reports of patients treated with antimyeloma therapies. Renal outcomes with antiplasma cell therapies have varied, although a subset of patients will have recovery of renal function.

Immunotactoid GN (IGN) typically presents with nephrotic range proteinuria with or without reduced glomerular filtration. Hypocomplementemia is common.[29] IGN often presents in the context of an underlying lymphoproliferative disease.[30] There may a be a race-associated difference in the prevalence of immunotactoid GN, with a larger percentage of cases noted among White nephrotic patients compared with Black patients.[31] IGN may appear morphologically identical to cryoglobulinemia GN on biopsy.[32] Immunofluorescent staining confirms monoclonal immunoglobulin and C3 staining involving the glomerular basement membrane, and electron microscopy reveals the deposits are organized in microtubular fibrils with an average diameter greater than 30 nm.[30] This is in contrast to amyloid fibrils that have a more mesangial predominance and an average diameter of 7 to 13 nm. There are numerous reports of cases of IGN being treated with steroids or immunosuppressive therapy, including rituximab.[33–35] There is also at least one published case report in which a patient was successfully treated with ASCT.[36] Although IGN is typically associated with a monoclonal gammopathy, therapeutic "response" in the published literature generally has focused on resolution of proteinuria or hypocomplementemia, rather than improvement in the pathogenic immunoglobulin as in AL or LCDD.

Membranoproliferative glomerulonephritis (MPGN), although most commonly seen in the setting of chronic viral hepatitis or autoimmune disease, is now also known to be a monoclonal gammopathy–associated condition.[37] Indeed, 28 of 68 hepatitis-negative patients with MPGN at Mayo Clinic had a detectable monoclonal immunoglobulin in the serum or urine.[38] Most patients in this series had albuminuria, and approximately a third had hypocomplementemia. In almost all cases, a concurrent bone marrow biopsy demonstrated MGUS or (less commonly) a low-grade lymphoproliferative disorder such as Waldenstrom, other low-grade non-Hodgkin lymphoma, or chronic lymphocytic leukemia. Identification of a concurrent plasma cell or lymphoproliferative disease was less frequent in other published series.[39] Renal biopsy typically shows an expanded mesangium with focal global glomerulosclerosis, subendothelial deposits in the capillary loops, and variable degrees of tubulointerstitial injury. Immunofluorescent stains confirmed concordance between the material in the renal deposits and the serum/urine monoclonal immunoglobulin. Although reports of therapy include the use of immunosuppressive agents, treatment directed at the associated underlying monoclonal hematologic process is often pursued.[39]

NONAMYLOID, MONOCLONAL GAMMOPATHY OF NEUROLOGIC SIGNIFICANCE

Many nonamyloid diseases associated with a monoclonal gammopathy can manifest with some component of neuropathy, usually either peripheral and/or autonomic. In addition, disease-related neuropathies can be complicated by therapy-related neuropathy, which is common with many agents used to treat plasma cell and lymphoid disorders such as bortezomib, vincristine, and thalidomide. Careful attention to a patient's neurologic status is critical for accurate diagnosis and successful management of these disorders.

Peripheral Neuropathies Associated with an Immunoglobulin M Monoclonal Gammopathy

The phenotype of neurologic disorders associated with a monoclonal gammopathy is variably associated with immunoglobulin class. For decades, the relationship between peripheral neuropathy and IgM monoclonal gammopathies has been strong, well-recognized, and somewhat mapped out pathophysiologically, whereas the association between neuropathy and non-IgM monoclonal gammopathies even now, decades after the initial reports of an association, remains weak and poorly defined. Specifically, up to 50% of patients with IgM MGUS have peripheral neuropathy, whereas a smaller minority of patients non-IgM MGUS are affected with neuropathy.[40]

Whereas non-IgM monoclonal proteins are usually produced by terminally differentiated plasma cells, IgM proteins are typically produced by lymphoplasmacytic B-cell clones, either at lower levels (ie, IgM MGUS) or higher levels, as is usually associated with the diagnosis of lymphoplasmacytic lymphoma/Waldenstrom macroglobulinemia. Although the question commonly arises as to whether the relationship of monoclonal gammopathy plus peripheral neuropathy is purely associative or actually causal, in the case of many demyelinating peripheral neuropathies associated with IgM, laboratory models convincingly demonstrate the IgM to be the direct agent of nerve damage.[41]

The arguably best-characterized disorder among IgM-associated neuropathies involves IgM proteins that bind and form deposits at sites of myelin-associated glycoprotein (MAG) along peripheral nerves. Much like MGUS in general, anti-MAG neuropathy is more common as one ages and in men.[42] MAG is present on Schwann cells, and critical to myelin production and therefore function of peripheral nerves. Disruption of MAG by antibodies leads to demyelination and interference with nerve conduction; indeed, anti-MAG antibodies are present in up to 50% of IgM-associated demyelinating neuropathies. The typical clinical pattern is that of initially distal progressive loss of sensation accompanied by tremor, and demyelination without conduction block on electrophysiological testing, a clinical entity sometimes referred to as distal acquired demyelinating sensory (DADS) neuropathy. DADS is viewed by some as a variant of chronic inflammatory demyelinating polyneuropathy

(CIDP), although controversy surrounds this taxonomy due to distinct differences between DADS and CIDP that suggest that DADS may be a completely different entity. CIDP more often presents with distal or proximal motor weakness as opposed to the sensory deficits seen with DADS.[43,44] Limited research suggests that approaches that commonly serve well in CIDP, such as corticosteroids and intravenous immune globulins (IVIGs), appear to be less efficacious in anti-MAG neuropathy/DADS. Conversely, small studies meta-analyzed in a Cochrane review suggest that the anti-CD20 monoclonal antibody rituximab may be more efficacious in DADS, with evidence that the drug induces an improvement in disability and function.[45]

In addition to MAG, IgM monoclonal gammopathy is also associated, albeit less commonly, with a variety of other autoantibodies, namely gangliosides including GM1, GD1a, GD1b, GT1b, GM2, GM3, as well as the paragloboside SGPG. An example of clinical disorders that accompany these antibodies is chronic sensory ataxic neuropathy, ophthalmoplegia, IgM paraprotein, cold agglutinins, and disialosyl antibodies (CANOMAD). CANOMAD tends to be relapsing-remitting, up to the degree that in one series, multiple patients experienced a transient need for mechanical ventilation due to reversible, CANOMAD-induced respiratory failure. Primarily sensory, particularly proprioceptive, deficits result in what can be profound upper or lower extremity ataxia with relative preservation in motor function. In roughly half of patients in one series, their IgM also functioned as a cold agglutinin. Electrophysiological studies can reveal both axonal and/or demyelinating patterns of nerve injury.[46] Anecdotally, rituximab and/or IVIG may be of use in this disorder.[47]

Another example of an IgM-associated neurologic disorder with an identifiable autoantibody is multifocal motor neuropathy with conduction block (MMNCB), which is associated with the presence of anti-GM1 in at least 40% of affected patients. Like in anti-MAG peripheral neuropathy, in MMNCB again the Schwann cell appears to be the target of the pathologic IgM monoclonal gammopathy, but in this case, the insult is thought to result in nerve conduction block and abnormalities in nerve depolarization that cause dysfunction. Patients often present with asymmetric, upper extremity mononeuropathies, and fasciculations and cramps. Sensory deficits are typically very mild if not absent, and the disorder is often exacerbated by exposure to cold temperatures. The median and ulnar nerves are most commonly impacted, and much like in other IgM disorders, immuno-suppression and -modulation in the form of corticosteroids, chemotherapy, and/or CD20-directed therapies such as rituximab are reported anecdotally to be helpful in mitigating the disease course.[48] A Cochrane review from 2005 endorsed IVIG as the most potent therapy available for MMNCB.[49]

The preceding disorders primarily refer to low-level IgM monoclonal gammopathies and small B-cell clones, that is, monoclonal gammopathies of neurologic significance, referring to disorders that would be characterized as pure MGUS if one ignored the neuropathic component. Conversely, when one examines Waldenstrom macroglobulinemia, the most common true malignancy associated with production of IgM monoclonal gammopathy, one notes that nearly half of patients with Waldenstrom have clinically significant neuropathy of some form, often peripheral neuropathy with primarily sensory deficits, although many other forms have been reported.[50,51]

Peripheral Neuropathies Associated with a Non–immunoglobulin M Monoclonal Gammopathy

The link between neuropathy and non-IgM monoclonal gammopathies (primarily IgG and IgA) is weaker and of less clear clinical significance. Di Troia and colleagues[52] reported decades ago on a series of patients with IgG MGUS and neuropathy and noted that roughly half clinically had CIDP, whereas the other half had a primarily sensory or mixed axonal peripheral neuropathy, that is, no specific pattern. A separate report that provided some of the first data characterizing IgM-associated peripheral neuropathy as a unique entity, showed no significant patterns among IgG-associated and IgA-associated peripheral neuropathies.[40] Lastly, Dyck and colleagues[53] showed that IgG-related or IgA-related demyelinating disorders respond well similarly to the common CIDP therapy of plasma exchange, whereas IgM-associated demyelinating disorders (such as those described previously) respond poorly to exchange. Taken together, neuropathy associated with non-IgM monoclonal gammopathy is a heterogeneous entity with respect to clinical presentation, and particularly the demyelinating forms may be CIDP variants in which the presence or absence of a monoclonal gammopathy itself does not inform clinical management.

Polyneuropathy, Organomegaly, Endocrinopathy, Monoclonal Gammopathy and Skin Changes Syndrome

Polyneuropathy, Organomegaly, Endocrinopathy, Monoclonal Gammopathy and Skin Changes (POEMS) syndrome is best conceived as a unique variant of multiple myeloma that involves a primarily demyelinating, often profoundly disabling peripheral neuropathy and lambda-restricted monoclonal gammopathy, sclerotic bone lesions, and elevation in blood vascular endothelial growth factor (VEGF) levels, occasionally overlapping with Castleman disease. Many patients also experience some combination of organomegaly (usually spleen, liver, and/or lymph nodes), extravascular fluid retention, endocrinopathy (eg, pituitary, adrenal, and/or sex hormones), skin changes (eg, hyperpigmentation, plethora), papilledema, and elevation in hemoglobin and/or platelet counts. The pathophysiology of this rare disorder is not well understood, but appears to involve a plasma cell–driven paraneoplastic overabundance of circulating cytokines.[54] It makes sense that supraphysiologic levels of VEGF drive vascular permeability and hence extravascular volume expansion, but it remains unclear how the disease process drives the multitude of other changes. Further, how and why POEMS can occur with the distinct entity of Castleman disease is also unknown. Diagnosing POEMS is a true internist's quest in that it encompasses a thorough history and physical, plus additional testing as appropriate, to investigate the various organ systems that POEMS can impact. Simply put, however, this disorder is usually referred to the hematologist's clinic for "myeloma workup" with some clinical finding that resulted in testing for a monoclonal gammopathy, such as peripheral neuropathy or sclerotic bone lesions. Findings such as these or others from the preceding list should serve as red flags for the astute hematologist/oncologist that this is not "just myeloma" nor MGUS.[5,55] Therapy for POEMS is extrapolated from standard multiple myeloma, modified in recognition of the often profound peripheral neuropathy that accompanies this disorder and leading to the avoidance of neurotoxic medications. Immunomodulatory agents and high-dose melphalan with ASCT are the best studied approaches and often induce deep responses and neurologic recovery in many patients. Prognosis and specifically survival tend to be superior in POEMS compared with standard multiple myeloma, stemming from the fact that the underlying plasma cell clone is often relatively indolent and slowly proliferative.[56,57]

NONAMYLOID, MONOCLONAL GAMMOPATHY OF CUTANEOUS SIGNIFICANCE

Monoclonal plasma cell disorders infrequently involve the skin in a fascinating spectrum of disorders, as summarized by Lipsker.[58] In some, monoclonal protein deposits directly in the skin that can be visualized using histologic techniques. Examples of these include the subtypes of cryoglobulinemia (CG) derived from monoclonal proteins, such as type 2 (mixed) cryoglobulinemia, in which monoclonal proteins form immune complexes that can deposit in tissues. Type 1 cryoglobulinemia, conversely, results in cold-dependent intravascular precipitation of proteins resulting in thrombotic vascular obstruction resulting in cutaneous ischemia and painful ulcers. In both types of cryoglobulinemia, deposition in other organs is also common, resulting in, for instance, peripheral neuropathy and vasculitic nephropathy. Up to a quarter of patients with cryoglobulinemia have renal involvement, and most such cases occur in the setting of chronic hepatitis C. Renal biopsy in patients with type 1 or 2 CG typically shows membranoproliferative GN and hyaline capillary thrombi, revealed by electron microscopy to have a microtubular structure with a diameter of 20 to 30 nm.[59] In contrast, the fibrils in AL amyloidosis typically measure 7 to 13 nm in diameter. Clinically, cryoglobulinemic nephropathy may present as nephrotic or sub-nephrotic proteinuria, hematuria, gradually progressive chronic kidney injury, or hypertension. Necrobiotic xanthogranulomatosis is a separate, quite rare disorder thought to stem from monoclonal protein-seeded immune complexes that associate with lipoproteins and deposit cutaneously.

In other forms of monoclonal gammopathy of cutaneous significance, however, skin changes are often grossly evident but biopsies do not reveal monoclonal protein, indicating that direct deposition of the monoclonal gammopathy in skin is not driving disease pathogenesis. One such condition is Schnitzler syndrome, a disorder in which excess interleukin-1 (IL-1) secretion drives an inflammatory cascade resulting in an urticarial rash, fevers, and bone pain. Schnitzler syndrome is often associated with a monoclonal IgM protein, but whether that IgM somehow causes Schnitzler syndrome or is simply a byproduct of a dysregulated immune system is poorly understood. IL-1 inhibition generally works well to ameliorate disease-related symptoms. Another example is TEMPI syndrome.[60] It is unknown how often patients present with some but not all of the pentad of symptoms, but it is plausible that this could be the case. In contrast to Schnitzler syndrome, the fact that antiplasma cell therapy has resulted in improvement or resolution of symptoms in several cases suggests the underlying clonal process is causative in TEMPI.[61–63]

SUMMARY

Monoclonal gammopathies derived from monoclonal plasma cells or B-cell clones encompass a broad and fascinating spectrum of disorders from the often completely benign, such as MGUS, to the acutely life-threatening, such as multiple myeloma or plasma cell leukemia. Amyloidosis is one unique disease entity on that spectrum, in which the monoclonal protein happens to be structured in a way such that it aggregates into the classic beta-pleated sheets that underlie the formation of amyloid deposition in organs and the clinical entity of amyloidosis that comprises the focus of this issue. However, amyloidosis is only one of numerous disease entities on this spectrum. Also along that spectrum are the multiple disorders in which monoclonal proteins do not form amyloid but nonetheless induce often severe organ injury either through direct tissue deposition (light chain deposition disease or cryoglobulinemia) or indirect activity, that is, "paraneoplastically," through pathologic pathways that are poorly understood to date (TEMPI). Understanding the relationship between the clinical syndrome complexes and the underlying plasma cell and lymphoid biology is not only challenging and intriguing but also critical to successfully managing patients with these disorders.

CLINICS CARE POINTS

- The spectrum of immunoglobulin paraprotein-associated diseases requiring therapy extends beyond multiple myeloma and AL amyloidosis. Awareness of these is essential in ensuring timely accurate diagnosis and appropriate treatment.
- As most paraprotein-associated diseases are fairly uncommon, therapeutic decisions must often be made in the absence of data from randomized controlled trials. Treatment is generally directed at the underlying clonal cell population.

REFERENCES

1. Kazandjian D. Multiple myeloma epidemiology and survival: a unique malignancy. Semin Oncol 2016;43(6):676–81.
2. Quock TP, Yan T, Chang E, et al. Epidemiology of AL amyloidosis: a real-world study using US claims data. Blood Adv 2018;2(10):1046–53.
3. Weiss BM, Abadie J, Verma P, et al. A monoclonal gammopathy precedes multiple myeloma in most patients. Blood 2009;113(22):5418–22.
4. Weiss BM, Hebreo J, Cordaro DV, et al. Monoclonal gammopathy of undetermined significance (MGUS) precedes the diagnosis of AL amyloidosis by up to 14 years. Blood 2011;118(21):1827.
5. Rajkumar SV, Dimopoulos MA, Palumbo A, et al. International Myeloma Working Group updated criteria for the diagnosis of multiple myeloma. Lancet Oncol 2014;15(12):e538–48.
6. Gertz MA. Waldenström macroglobulinemia: 2019 update on diagnosis, risk stratification, and management. Am J Hematol 2019;94(2):266–76.
7. Asatiani E, Cohen P, Ozdemirli M, et al. Monoclonal gammopathy in extranodal marginal zone lymphoma (ENMZL) correlates with advanced disease and bone marrow involvement. Am J Hematol 2004;77(2):144–6.
8. Telio D, Bailey D, Chen C, et al. Two distinct syndromes of lymphoma-associated AL amyloidosis: a case series and review of the literature. Am J Hematol 2010; 85(10):805–8.
9. Pezzoli A, Pascali E. Monoclonal Bence Jones proteinuria in chronic lymphocytic leukaemia. Scand J Haematol 1986;36(1):18–24.
10. Xu W, Wang YH, Fan L, et al. Prognostic significance of serum immunoglobulin paraprotein in patients with chronic lymphocytic leukemia. Leuk Res 2011; 35(8):1060–5.
11. Maurer MJ, Cerhan JR, Katzmann JA, et al. Monoclonal and polyclonal serum free light chains and clinical outcome in chronic lymphocytic leukemia. Blood 2011;118(10):2821–6.
12. Leung N, Bridoux F, Hutchison CA, et al. Monoclonal gammopathy of renal significance: when MGUS is no longer undetermined or insignificant. Blood 2012; 120(22):4292–5.
13. Preud'homme JL, Aucouturier P, Touchard G, et al. Monoclonal immunoglobulin deposition disease (Randall type). Relationship with structural abnormalities of immunoglobulin chains. Kidney Int 1994;46(4):965–72.
14. Drieux F, Loron MC, Francois A, et al. Light chain deposition disease and proximal tubulopathy in two successive kidney allografts. Clin Nephrol 2015;83(6): 351–6.
15. Koratala A, Ejaz AA, Hiser WM, et al. Trifecta of light chain cast nephropathy, monoclonal plasma cell infiltrates, and light chain proximal tubulopathy. Kidney Int 2017;92(6):1559.

16. Wu CK, Yang AH, Lai HC, et al. Combined proximal tubulopathy, crystal-storing histiocytosis, and cast nephropathy in a patient with light chain multiple myeloma. BMC Nephrol 2017;18(1):170.

17. Randall RE, Williamson WC, Mullinax F, et al. Manifestations of systemic light chain deposition. Am J Med 1976;60(2):293–9.

18. Pozzi C, Fogazzi GB, Banfi G, et al. Renal disease and patient survival in light chain deposition disease. Clin Nephrol 1995;43(5):281–7.

19. Vos JM, Gustine J, Rennke HG, et al. Renal disease related to Waldenström macroglobulinaemia: incidence, pathology and clinical outcomes. Br J Haematol 2016;175(4):623–30.

20. Went P, Ascani S, Strøm E, et al. Nodal marginal-zone lymphoma associated with monoclonal light-chain and heavy-chain deposition disease. Lancet Oncol 2004; 5(6):381–3.

21. Joly F, Cohen C, Javaugue V, et al. Randall-type monoclonal immunoglobulin deposition disease: novel insights from a nationwide cohort study. Blood 2019; 133(6):576–87.

22. Kourelis TV, Nasr SH, Dispenzieri A, et al. Outcomes of patients with renal monoclonal immunoglobulin deposition disease. Am J Hematol 2016;91(11):1123–8.

23. Batalini F, Econimo L, Quillen K, et al. High-dose melphalan and stem cell transplantation in patients on dialysis due to immunoglobulin light-chain amyloidosis and monoclonal immunoglobulin deposition disease. Biol Blood Marrow Transplant 2018;24(1):127–32.

24. Milani P, Basset M, Curci P, et al. Daratumumab in light chain deposition disease: rapid and profound hematologic response preserves kidney function. Blood Adv 2020;4(7):1321–4.

25. Palladini G, Dispenzieri A, Gertz MA, et al. New criteria for response to treatment in immunoglobulin light chain amyloidosis based on free light chain measurement and cardiac biomarkers: impact on survival outcomes. J Clin Oncol 2012;30(36): 4541–9.

26. Maldonado JE, Velosa JA, Kyle RA, et al. Fanconi syndrome in adults. A manifestation of a latent form of myeloma. Am J Med 1975;58(3):354–64.

27. Larsen CP, Bell JM, Harris AA, et al. The morphologic spectrum and clinical significance of light chain proximal tubulopathy with and without crystal formation. Mod Pathol 2011;24(11):1462–9.

28. Kapur U, Barton K, Fresco R, et al. Expanding the pathologic spectrum of immunoglobulin light chain proximal tubulopathy. Arch Pathol Lab Med 2007;131(9): 1368–72.

29. Rosenstock JL, Markowitz GS, Valeri AM, et al. Fibrillary and immunotactoid glomerulonephritis: distinct entities with different clinical and pathologic features. Kidney Int 2003;63(4):1450–61.

30. Fogo A, Qureshi N, Horn RG. Morphologic and clinical features of fibrillary glomerulonephritis versus immunotactoid glomerulopathy. Am J Kidney Dis 1993;22(3):367–77.

31. Korbet SM, Genchi RM, Borok RZ, et al. The racial prevalence of glomerular lesions in nephrotic adults. Am J Kidney Dis 1996;27(5):647–51.

32. Fogo AB, Lusco MA, Najafian B, et al. AJKD atlas of renal pathology: immunotactoid glomerulopathy. Am J Kidney Dis 2015;66(4):e29–30.

33. Ohashi A, Kumagai J, Nagahama K, et al. Case of immunotactoid glomerulopathy showing high responsiveness to steroids therapy despite severe pathological features. BMJ Case Rep 2019;12(7):e229751.

34. Kinomura M, Maeshima Y, Kodera R, et al. A case of immunotactoid glomerulopathy exhibiting nephrotic syndrome successfully treated with corticosteroids and antihypertensive therapy. Clin Exp Nephrol 2009;13(4):378–84.

35. Sathyan S, Khan FN, Ranga KV. A case of recurrent immunotactoid glomerulopathy in an allograft treated with rituximab. Transplant Proc 2009;41(9):3953–5.

36. Witzens-Harig M, Waldherr R, Beimler J, et al. Long-term remission of paraprotein-induced immunotactoid glomerulopathy after high-dose therapy and autologous blood stem cell transplantation. Ann Hematol 2007;86(12):927–30.

37. Sethi S, Fervenza FC. Membranoproliferative glomerulonephritis: pathogenetic heterogeneity and proposal for a new classification. Semin Nephrol 2011;31(4):341–8.

38. Sethi S, Zand L, Leung N, et al. Membranoproliferative glomerulonephritis secondary to monoclonal gammopathy. Clin J Am Soc Nephrol 2010;5(5):770–82.

39. Gumber R, Cohen JB, Palmer MB, et al. A clone-directed approach may improve diagnosis and treatment of proliferative glomerulonephritis with monoclonal immunoglobulin deposits. Kidney Int 2018;94(1):199–205.

40. Gosselin S, Kyle RA, Dyck PJ. Neuropathy associated with monoclonal gammopathies of undetermined significance. Ann Neurol 1991;30(1):54–61.

41. Willison HJ, Chancellor AM, Paterson G, et al. Antiglycolipid antibodies, immunoglobulins and paraproteins in motor neuron disease: a population based case-control study. J Neurol Sci 1993;114(2):209–15.

42. Nobile-Orazio E, Meucci N, Baldini L, et al. Long-term prognosis of neuropathy associated with anti-MAG IgM M-proteins and its relationship to immune therapies. Brain 2000;123(Pt 4):710–7.

43. Nobile-Orazio E, Manfredini E, Carpo M, et al. Frequency and clinical correlates of anti-neural IgM antibodies in neuropathy associated with IgM monoclonal gammopathy. Ann Neurol 1994;36(3):416–24.

44. Katz JS, Saperstein DS, Gronseth G, et al. Distal acquired demyelinating symmetric neuropathy. Neurology 2000;54(3):615–20.

45. Lunn MP, Nobile-Orazio E. Immunotherapy for IgM anti-myelin-associated glycoprotein paraprotein-associated peripheral neuropathies. Cochrane Database Syst Rev 2016;(10):CD002827.

46. Willison HJ, O'Leary CP, Veitch J, et al. The clinical and laboratory features of chronic sensory ataxic neuropathy with anti-disialosyl IgM antibodies. Brain 2001;124(Pt 10):1968–77.

47. Löscher WN, Woertz A, Wallnöfer M, et al. Successful treatment of CANOMAD with IVIg and rituximab. J Neurol 2013;260(4):1168–70.

48. Yeh WZ, Dyck PJ, van den Berg LH, et al. Multifocal motor neuropathy: controversies and priorities. J Neurol Neurosurg Psychiatry 2020;91(2):140–8.

49. Umapathi T, Hughes RA, Nobile-Orazio E, et al. Immunosuppressant and immunomodulatory treatments for multifocal motor neuropathy. Cochrane Database Syst Rev 2015;(3):CD003217.

50. Baehring JM, Hochberg EP, Raje N, et al. Neurological manifestations of Waldenström macroglobulinemia. Nat Clin Pract Neurol 2008;4(10):547–56.

51. Vaxman I, Gertz M. Waldenstrom's macroglobulinemia in the era of immunotherapy. Leuk Lymphoma 2020;61(6):1–13.

52. Di Troia A, Carpo M, Meucci N, et al. Clinical features and anti-neural reactivity in neuropathy associated with IgG monoclonal gammopathy of undetermined significance. J Neurol Sci 1999;164(1):64–71.

53. Dyck PJ, Low PA, Windebank AJ, et al. Plasma exchange in polyneuropathy associated with monoclonal gammopathy of undetermined significance. N Engl J Med 1991;325(21):1482–6.

54. Gherardi RK, Bélec L, Soubrier M, et al. Overproduction of proinflammatory cytokines imbalanced by their antagonists in POEMS syndrome. Blood 1996;87(4): 1458–65.

55. Dispenzieri A. POEMS syndrome: 2017 Update on diagnosis, risk stratification, and management. Am J Hematol 2017;92(8):814–29.

56. Dispenzieri A, Moreno-Aspitia A, Suarez GA, et al. Peripheral blood stem cell transplantation in 16 patients with POEMS syndrome, and a review of the literature. Blood 2004;104(10):3400–7.

57. Royer B, Merlusca L, Abraham J, et al. Efficacy of lenalidomide in POEMS syndrome: a retrospective study of 20 patients. Am J Hematol 2013;88(3):207–12.

58. Lipsker D. Monoclonal gammopathy of cutaneous significance: review of a relevant concept. J Eur Acad Dermatol Venereol 2017;31(1):45–52.

59. Motwani SS, Herlitz L, Monga D, et al. Paraprotein-related kidney disease: glomerular diseases associated with paraproteinemias. Clin J Am Soc Nephrol 2016;11(12):2260–72.

60. Sykes DB, Schroyens W, O'Connell C. The TEMPI syndrome–a novel multisystem disease. N Engl J Med 2011;365(5):475–7.

61. Kwok M, Korde N, Landgren O. Bortezomib to treat the TEMPI syndrome. N Engl J Med 2012;366(19):1843–5.

62. Kenderian SS, Rosado FG, Sykes DB, et al. Long-term complete clinical and hematological responses of the TEMPI syndrome after autologous stem cell transplantation. Leukemia 2015;29(12):2414–6.

63. Sykes DB, Schroyens W. Complete responses in the TEMPI syndrome after treatment with daratumumab. N Engl J Med 2018;378(23):2240–2.

Systemic Amyloidosis Due to Clonal Plasma Cell Diseases

Giada Bianchi, MD[a], Shaji Kumar, MD[b],*

KEYWORDS

- AL amyloidosis • Plasma cell disorders • MGUS • Amyloid fibrils • Multiple myeloma

KEY POINTS

- Light chain amyloidosis is caused by deposition in target organs of misfolded immunoglobulin free light chains, typically produced by clonal plasma cells.
- Distinct Ig light chain variable region genotypes underlie most light chain amyloidosis and dictate tissue tropism.
- Free light chain N-glycosylation contributes to amyloidogenicity and is a biomarker present years before onset of symptoms.
- Light chain amyloidosis is a progressive disease and early diagnosis is critical to avoid irreversible organ damage and patient demise.
- Rapid and deep free light chain reduction via effective plasma cell-directed therapy is necessary to ensure long-term survival and functional recovery of affected organs.

INTRODUCTION

Immunoglobulin light chain (AL) amyloidosis is the most frequent type of systemic amyloidosis, a heterogenous family of multi-system diseases characterized by deposition of a misfolded precursor protein organized in repetitive cross β-fibers strands.[1] Systemic amyloidoses are further classified based on the identity of the precursor protein, which in turns dictate organ tropism and therapy.[2] In AL amyloidosis, misfolded immunoglobulin free light chain (FLC) is the precursor amyloidogenic protein, typically produced by clonal plasma cells (PC), less often by a less mature B-cell neoplasm. In this article, we focus on the etiology, pathogenesis, and clinicopathologic features, as well as the differential diagnosis of AL amyloidosis secondary to PC disorders. We touch briefly on clinical presentation, diagnosis, and treatment because these topics are addressed in detail by our colleagues elsewhere in this issue.

---

[a] Division of Hematology, Department of Medicine, Brigham and Women's Hospital, Harvard Medical School, Boston, MA, 02115, USA; [b] Myeloma, Amyloidosis, Dysproteinemia Group, Mayo Clinic, First Street Southwest, Rochester, MN 55904, USA
* Corresponding author.
E-mail address: Kumar.Shaji@Mayo.edu

Hematol Oncol Clin N Am 34 (2020) 1009–1026
https://doi.org/10.1016/j.hoc.2020.08.001
0889-8588/20/© 2020 Elsevier Inc. All rights reserved.

ETIOLOGY

AL amyloidosis is typically classified as a PC disorder as cases secondary to non-Hodgkin's lymphoma, most often Waldenström's macroglobulinemia, are rare (2%) (see Ashutosh D. Wechalekar and colleagues' article, "Systemic Amyloidosis due to Low-Grade Lymphoma," in this issue).[3,4] Similar to multiple myeloma (MM), the culprit cell leading to development of AL amyloidosis is thought to be a long-lived PC that acquires a primary genetic aberration during the process of isotype switch and somatic hypermutation in the germinal center.[5] It is estimated that about 3% to 5% of patients with a known precursor PC disorder such as monoclonal gammopathy of unknown significance (MGUS) will progress to AL amyloidosis. The determinants of the progression of MGUS to AL amyloidosis versus MM versus other lymphoproliferative disorders are not completely understood; however, AL amyloidosis patients are enriched for λ FLC production (approximately 75% of cases) and t(11;14) (50%–60% of cases) (**Fig. 1**). Furthermore, a limited pool of Ig light chain variable region genotypes are responsible for the production of amyloidogenic FLC, consistent with a biased selection.[6,7] Strikingly, specific Ig light chain variable region correlates with organ tropism (**Table 1**) and somatic mutations in these regions contribute to the kinetic instability of FLC, facilitating extracellular endoproteolysis and generation of amyloidogenic FLC fragments.[8]

PATHOGENESIS

AL amyloidosis is the prototypic proteotoxicity hematologic disorder. The primary pathogenetic event is the misfolding of a circulating, clonal FLC, or its fragments owing to intrinsic folding instability, often related to somatic mutations of the variable chain, and/or saturation or disfunction of extracellular chaperone mechanisms.[9,10] Nucleation of FLC occurs after a variable lag time, depending on the concentration and the intrinsic folding instability of the FLC, and acts as a rapid catalyzer for aggregation of more unstable FLC into oligomeric β sheets. Facilitated by local factors, such as glycosaminoglycans and metal ions, oligomeric β sheets serve as a scaffold for the rapid formation of regularly organized amyloid protofilaments that associate in groups of 4 to 6 to form the pathognomonic 8 to 10 μm, nonbranching amyloid fibril (**Fig. 2**).[11] The Congo red dye intercalates between the protofilaments and confers the typical apple green birefringence under polarized light microscopy. The deposition of insoluble amyloid fibrils in target organs cause distortion of histologic architecture and compromises the normal function of tissues (**Fig. 3**). However, in vitro studies showed that soluble, amyloidogenic FLC themselves induce oxidative stress and apoptosis in cardiomyocytes via activation of p38 pathway.[12] As p38 induces transcription of brain natriuretic peptide (BNP) and N-terminus proBNP (NT-proBNP), this model provides a direct link between amyloid-related cardiac dysfunction and BNP/NT-proBNP levels.

EPIDEMIOLOGY

Epidemiologic studies suggest that, rather than being rare, AL amyloidosis is under-diagnosed.[13,14] The vague nature of early symptoms and variable pattern of disease presentation contribute to diagnostic delay, potentially causing irreversible cardiac damage and sudden cardiac death before diagnosis. Two distinct population-based studies showed AL amyloidosis incidence of 12.0 to 12.5 per million persons per year.[15,16] However, 1 of the studies included exclusively white patients who are twice less likely to have MGUS or a related PC disorders, compared with patients of African descent, suggesting this figure may be an underestimate.[17] The median age of AL

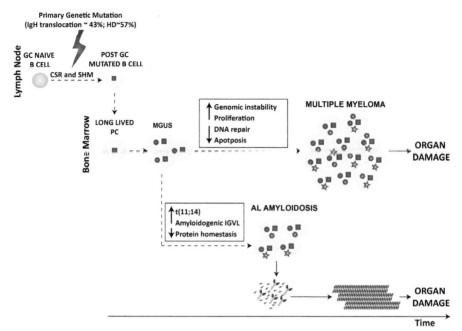

Fig. 1. Pathogenesis of AL amyloidosis. The initial genetic mutation (*small red square*) of AL amyloidosis precursor cell takes place in the lymph node during the maturation of a naïve B cell (*orange circle*) into a mature, post–germinal center (GC) B cell (*yellow circle*) through the process of somatic hypermutation (SHM) and immunoglobulin class switch recombination (CSR) elicited by antigenic encounter. The mutated clone homes to the bone marrow where it completes differentiation in long lived PC, the precursor cell in PC disorders. Contained expansion and accrual of further genetic mutations (*small red circle*) lead to MGUS. Over time, MGUS can progress to MM by becoming more proliferative and genomically unstable and resistant to apoptosis. MM is characterized by an expanded bone marrow population of clonal and subclonal, malignant PC that are directly responsible for organ damage. Progression to AL amyloidosis occurs through poorly defined molecular mechanisms likely impacted by presence of t(11;14), occurrence of distinct Ig light chain variable region resulting in amyloidogenic FLC and dysfunction or exhaustion of intracellular and extracellular protein homeostasis mechanisms. The AL amyloidosis PC clone is typically smaller compared with MM, characterized by reduced clonal heterogeneity and not directly virulent. Rather, the pathogenetic entity in AL amyloidosis is the formation and deposition of fibrillary aggregates of FLC in target organs. Amyloid formation and deposition occur with variable lag time depending on both FLC intrinsic and extrinsic factors.

amyloidosis patients at diagnosis is 63 years and there is a slight male predominance (55%).[13] It is thought that the current prevalence of AL amyloidosis is about 12,000 patients in the United States. Data regarding impact of race on AL amyloidosis are lacking.

RISK FACTORS

The only recognized risk factors for AL amyloidosis are a preexisting diagnosis of MGUS and the presence of specific single nucleotide polymorphisms. In a seminal risk population study, the relative risk of AL amyloidosis was 8.8 in patients with MGUS as compared with healthy controls.[18] Although the risk of transformation to

Table 1
Light chain variable (Ig light chain variable region) regions associated with AL amyloidosis and their distinct organ tropism

Ig Variable Region Genotype	Organ Tropism	Other Characteristics
LV6-57	Kidney	Associated with t(11;14)
LV3-01	Reduced kidney or advanced heart involvement	
LV2-14	Peripheral nervous system	Associated with production of intact Ig M spike and lower difference in FLC. Associated with localized GI AL amyloidosis
LV1-44	Heart	Associated with decreased incidence of hyperdiploid karyotype
KV1-33	Liver Less likely peripheral nervous system	Associated with higher difference in FLC
KV1-05	Heart	Associated with inferior OS when matched for cardiac stage
LV3-21	Decreased renal involvement	Associated with monosomy 13q
KV3-15 and KV3-20	N/A	Associated with localized AL amyloidosis

Abbreviations: GI, gastrointestinal; OS, overall survival.

MM was significantly higher (relative risk, 23.8), it is imperative that patients with MGUS are carefully monitored not just for signs and symptoms of MM, but also for evolution into AL amyloidosis. Further, at the time of diagnosis, approximately 15% of patients with MM are concomitantly diagnosed with AL amyloidosis and an further 1% will be diagnosed with AL amyloidosis during the course of MM care.

The high-risk G allele at cyclin D1 donor spicing site (rs9944), resulting in transcription of full-length cyclin D1 isoform, is among 10 distinct single nucleotide polymorphisms significantly associated with AL amyloidosis.[19] This single nucleotide polymorphism was enriched in a significant manner in patients carrying t(11;14) and may underlie the functional consequences of cyclin D1 overexpression in this patient subgroup. Of note, 5 single nucleotide polymorphisms were found to be specifically associated with AL amyloidosis, but not MM, suggesting an intrinsically different biology.

IMMUNOGLOBULIN LIGHT CHAIN AMYLOIDOSIS GENETICS AND BIOLOGY

AL amyloidosis has been often regarded as a variant of MM with a poor outcome or as an MGUS with a bad protein. However genetic, functional, and natural history data suggest that AL amyloidosis is an entity of its own. Cytogenetic abnormalities are detected in approximately 80% of patients via cytoplasmic immunoglobulin staining-enriched fluorescent in situ hybridization (**Table 2**).[20] The presence of any fluorescent in situ hybridization abnormality in newly diagnosed AL amyloidosis patients is associated with an increased risk of death. Translocation t(11;14), juxtaposing CCND1 to the immunoglobulin heavy chain locus, is the most frequent cytogenetic abnormality in AL amyloidosis, being present in 40% to 60% of patients, versus 15% of

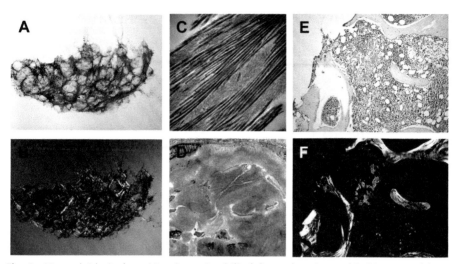

Fig. 2. AL amyloidosis deposition in periumbilical fat pad aspirate, skin biopsy and bone marrow biopsy. (A) Fat pad aspirate stained with Congo red and visualized under direct light microscopy. (B) The same specimen observed under polarized light show pathognomonic apple green birefringence. (C) EM at 25,000× magnification of periumbilical fat punch biopsy showing deposition of nonorganized, nonbranching, 8 to 10 nm fibrils (small, light–grey streaks) interspersed between organized, larger collagen fibers (straight, cylindrical fascicles with cross-striations). (D) In the same specimen, large clumps of abundant amyloid fibrils are visible at 8000× magnification, in the proximity of blood vessels. (E) Bone marrow biopsy of a patient with AL amyloidosis showing foci of Congo red deposition under direct light microscopy (original magnification ×20). (F) Same specimen observed under polarized light show the apple green birefringence of Congo red stained deposits, consistent with amyloid. (Courtesy of [A, B] Edmund S. Cibas MD, Boston, MA; [C, D] Helmut G. Rennke MD, Boston, MA; [E, F] Gabriel K. Griffin MD, Boston, MA.)

patients with MM. Unlike in MM, t(11;14) is an adverse prognostic factor in AL amyloidosis, impacting the hematologic response rate and overall survival, as well as a predictive factor of poor response to bortezomib.[21] The molecular bases for the diverse biological impact of t(11;14) in MM versus AL amyloidosis are unknown. Interestingly, overexpression of CCND1 associates with increased expression of genes involved in endoplasmic reticulum quality control and protein homeostasis, suggesting lower baseline proteotoxicity as a mechanism of bortezomib resistance.[22–24] The remainder of translocations involving the immunoglobulin heavy chain locus, t(4;14), t(6;14), t(14;16), and t(14;20), each account for 1% to 3% of cytogenetic abnormalities and do not seem to impact bortezomib response. Consistent with primary genetic events, hyperdiploid status is mutually exclusive with immunoglobulin heavy chain translocation and accounts for approximately 10% of cytogenetic abnormalities.[25] Del(17p) is a rare finding in AL amyloidosis, accounting for 2% to 6% of cases and associates with a higher bone marrow PC burden (median, 22%) and almost universally present cardiac involvement, with stage III diagnosed in approximately 50% of patients.[26] Similar to MM, gain(1q) retains adverse prognostic significance in AL amyloidosis.[27]

AL amyloidosis samples have a comparable number of exonic, nonsynonymous mutations to MM (39 vs 35; $P = .4$), but higher than in MGUS (n = 20; $P = .002$) and more than 90% of mutated genes are shared with either MM or MGUS.[21] However, compared with MGUS/MM, AL amyloidosis shows less clonal heterogeneity with

KIDNEY   HEART

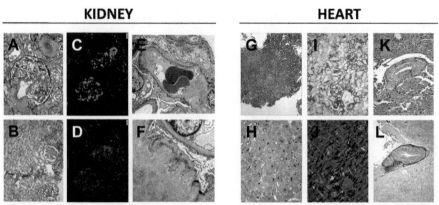

Fig. 3. AL amyloidosis deposition in the heart and kidney. (*A*) Hematoxylin eosin (H&E) staining of a kidney biopsy showing abundant deposition of amorphous, eosinophilic material in the glomeruli and mesangium. In the right upper field, it is a visible an arteriole whose lumen is obliterated owing to deposition of eosinophilic material in the vessel wall (*B*) Congo red staining observed under direct light showing staining of eosinophilic material. Immunofluorescent staining for λ (*C*) and κ (*D*) light chain showing bright positive and background signal in the glomeruli, respectively. (*E*) Electron microscopy of a renal arteriole showing mesangial and subendothelial electron-dense deposits. (*F*) EM images at higher magnification of same specimen showing abundant, nonbranching fibrils, approximately 10 nm in diameter. (Images courtesy of Dr. Rennke). (*G*). Low power H&E staining of an endomyocardial biopsy showing diffuse extracellular deposition of a pale pink material. (*H*) At a higher power, the amorphic, eosinophilic material is seen wrapping around individual cardiomyocytes. (*I*) Congo red staining of endomyocardial biopsy specimen demonstrating positive staining rimming individual cardiac myocytes (*J*). Congo red stain of same specimen observed under polarized light showing apple green birefringence of amyloid deposits (*K*). H&E staining of endomyocardial biopsy showing an intramyocardial arteriole with amyloid deposition leading to wall thickening and stenosis. (*L*) Sulfated Alcian blue staining of endomyocardial arteriole outlining the amyloid in blue green. (*Courtesy of* Robert F. Padera Jr., MD, PhD, Boston, MA.)

subclones identified in 37% of samples as compared with 51% of non-AL PC disorder samples (*P*<.001).[28] This difference is driven by the high frequency of t(11;14) in AL amyloidosis, which suppresses subclonal evolution.

At the gene expression level, AL amyloidosis PC reverses many transcriptomic changes occurring in MM cells and tends to resemble more closely normal PC.[29] In particular, a group of 12 genes, including SDF-1 or CXCL12, the ligand of CXCR4 and CD27, could distinguish AL and MM cells with 92% accuracy. Strikingly, compared with MM PC, pathway analysis showed widespread downregulation of factors involved in protein homeostasis, pointing toward an intrinsic defect in protein quality control systems. In line with these intrinsic differences, single cell RNAseq successfully segregated AL amyloidosis PC from normal, MGUS and MM PC, although interindividual variability was significant and related to distinct genetic abnormalities.[30]

The bone marrow microenvironment of AL amyloidosis patients also seems to be distinct from that of patients with other PC disorders. In fact, AL amyloidosis bone marrow niche was characterized by a higher infiltration with myeloid and "innate-like" T-cell subsets and by expansion of M2 polarized, repairing macrophages, possibly representing a compensatory response to the deposition of amyloid.[31,32]

Table 2		
Common genetic abnormalities in AL amyloidosis and their clinical impact		
	Incidence	Clinical Impact
t(11;14)	40%–60%	Adverse prognostic factor. Predictive factor of poor response to bortezomib-based therapy. Melphalan treatment may abrogate unfavorable prognosis
t(14;16) and t(4;14)	3%–4% each	Standard risk in patients treated with bortezomib. Associated with adverse outcome after high-dose melphalan and ASCT.
Del(13)/(13q)	30%–40%	-
Del(17p)/17	2%–6%	Associated with higher BM plasmacytosis. Cardiac involvement almost universally present. Approximately 45% with stage III cardiac involvement. Associated with adverse outcome after high dose melphalan and ASCT.
Trisomy of a single chromosome	25%–30%	Shorter OS in patients treated with melphalan.
Gain(1q21)	15%–20%	Standard risk in patients treated with bortezomib.
Hyperdiploid	12%	Standard risk.

Abbreviations: ASCT, autologous stem cell transplantation; BM, bone marrow; OS, overall survival.

Data from Bochtler T, Hegenbart U, Kunz C, et al. Prognostic impact of cytogenetic aberrations in AL amyloidosis patients after high-dose melphalan: a long-term follow-up study. Blood. 2016;128(4):594-602 and Vaxman I, Gertz M. Recent Advances in the Diagnosis, Risk Stratification, and Management of Systemic Light-Chain Amyloidosis. Acta haematologica. 2019;141(2):93-106.

LIGHT CHAIN AMYLOIDOSIS PLASMA CELLS IMMUNOPHENOTYPE

AL amyloidosis PC are immunophenotypically indistinguishable from MGUS or MM PC. AL amyloidosis PC are large, ellipsoid-shaped with an eccentric nucleus and coarsely clumped chromatin, along with abundant basophilic cytoplasm with a visible Golgi apparatus as a perinuclear hof. Under electron microscopy, the cytoplasm of AL amyloidosis cells is largely filled with endoplasmic reticulum. Immunophenotypically, AL cells are strongly positive for CD138 (syndecan-1), CD38, BCMA, and monotypic light chain (either κ or λ).[33] Different from normal PC, AL amyloidosis cells are CD19 and CD45 negative and CD56 positive and these differences can be used in multiparametric flow to assess minimal residual disease.[34]

When compared with MM, the PC clone of AL amyloidosis patients is typically smaller, around 10% cellularity, and patients would typically be classified as MGUS if it was not for the virulent nature of the secreted FLC. The standard of care for precursor conditions MGUS and smoldering MM is observation, a careful review of systems and physical examination together with a high index of clinical suspicion is critical to early identification of patients with AL amyloidosis and prompt commencement of treatment (**Table 3**).

CLINICAL PRESENTATION

When AL amyloidosis is suspected, rapid tissue diagnosis and typing of precursor protein via liquid chromatography and mass spectrometry or immunoelectron microscopy is key to start combinatorial, highly effective PC-directed cytoreductive therapy

Table 3
A comparison of diagnostic criteria and distinctive features for PC disorders

	M Protein		BM PC		End-Organ Damage Mediated by PC	End-Organ Damage Directly Mediated by FLC/Ig
MGUS	<3 g/dL (serum)	AND	<10%	AND	No	No[a]
SMM	≥3 g/dL (serum) or ≥500 mg/24 h (urine)	OR	10%–60%	AND	No	No[a]
MM	Any concentration on SPEP/UPEP or abnormal FLC	AND	≥10% or plasmacytoma	AND	Always[b]	Occasionally (cast nephropathy, hyperviscosity and MM/AL overlap)
MGRS	<3 g/dL (serum)	AND	<10%	AND	No	Always. Organized or nonorganized FLC/Ig deposition in the kidneys.[c]
AL Amyloidosis	Absent/present FLC are typically abnormal	AND	Typically present, approximately 10%	AND	No	Always, by FLC organized in amyloid fibrils. Congo red positive.

Abbreviations: BM, bone marrow invasion by monoclonal malignant PCs; M, monoclonal; MGUS, monoclonal gammopathy of undetermined significance; MGRS, Monoclonal Gammopathy of Renal Significance; SMM, smoldering multiple myeloma; SPEP, serum protein electrophoresis; UPEP, urine protein electrophoresis.

[a] Occasionally, MGUS/SMM may present clinical manifestations directly related to FLC/Ig pathogenicity. The term monoclonal gammopathy of clinical significance (MGCS) has been proposed to classify these conditions.[62]

[b] A myeloma defining event must be present according to Rajkumar et al.[63]

[c] Congo red staining must be negative to exclude AL amyloidosis.

to avoid irreversible organ damage and reduce risk of early mortality. With the exclusion of the central nervous system, deposition of AL amyloidosis fibrils can affect every organ and system in the body and thus clinical presentation varies and may mimic several other conditions, often leading to diagnostic delay and making AL amyloidosis a great imitator (**Table 4**).

Early AL amyloidosis symptoms, such as fatigue and weight loss, are rather nonspecific and diagnostic delay exceeding 1 year is common, even in the presence of symptoms and signs consistent with heart failure.[35,36] Presence of periorbital purpura and macroglossia is specific for AL amyloidosis, but rather nonsensitive, being present only in approximately 10% to 20% of patients. Cardiac and/or renal involvement is almost universally present and 75% of patients present with involvement of both. NT-proBNP and albuminuria are biomarkers with 100% sensitivity to detect heart and kidney involvement by amyloidosis, respectively, and should be used routinely to screen patients with MGUS and smoldering MM for progression to AL amyloidosis. Importantly, a diagnosis of amyloidosis in a patient with MGUS does not automatically equal AL amyloidosis as other amyloidosis, particularly transthyretin, can often coexist with MGUS.[37,38] Clinical heart failure with imaging studies consistent with hypertrophic cardiomyopathy with preserved left ventricular ejection fraction; nephrotic syndrome; peripheral neuropathy, mostly sensory; and autonomic dysfunction or carpal tunnel (especially if bilateral) should prompt investigations to rule out AL amyloidosis, particularly if present in patients with preexisting diagnosis of MGUS or smoldering MM.

DIAGNOSIS

A conclusive diagnosis of AL amyloidosis requires fulfillment of 4 criteria: (1) presence of a syndrome compatible with AL amyloidosis, (2) evidence of a PC disorder based on bone marrow aspirate or biopsy and serologic parameters, (3) histopathologic proof of amyloidosis deposition in fat pad or affected organ, and (4) amyloidosis typing for definitive identification of Ig light chain via liquid chromatography and mass spectrometry or immunoelectron microscopy (**Table 5**). Because AL amyloidosis PC are indistinguishable from MGUS, and considering that standard of care for MGUS is observation, a careful review of systems and physical examination together with a high index of clinical suspicion is critical to early identification of patients with AL amyloidosis and prompt commencement of treatment. The pathognomonic feature of amyloidosis deposition is a positive Congo red stain showing apple green birefringence under polarized light. When properly stained and read, Congo red stain has a 100% specificity for amyloidosis, although the sensitivity varies depending on site of tissue biopsy. For instance, a fat pad aspirate biopsy is positive in about 70% to 75% of patients with AL amyloidosis. Sixty-five percent of patients with AL amyloidosis have Congo red positivity on bone marrow biopsy and this can clue be the first to a diagnosis of systemic amyloidosis in about one-third of patients.[39,40] It is worth pointing out that the presence of amyloid in the bone marrow per se is not sufficient to conclusively diagnose AL amyloidosis, because it can be present in both patients with serum amyloid A amyloidosis and patients with transthyretin amyloidosis. However, amyloid deposition in stroma, as opposed to periosteal or in the vessel wall, is exclusively detected in patients with AL amyloidosis, suggesting that spatial distribution is important in guiding the differential diagnosis. Overall, the combination of fat a pad biopsy and a bone marrow biopsy is sufficient for definitive AL amyloidosis diagnosis in more than 80% of patients, thus obviating need for most organ biopsy.[41] In an effort to identify patients with AL amyloidosis before the onset of clinically significant

Table 4
Clinical presentation of AL amyloidosis depending on organ involvement

Organ Involved	Incidence	Typical Clinical Presentation	Diagnostic Findings	Consensus Criteria for Involvement

Heart	60%–75%	Dyspnea on exertion
		Orthopnea
		Paroxysmal nocturnal dyspnea
		Lower extremity edema
		Pleural effusions
		Jugular vein distension
		Arrhythmia
		Syncope
		Angina[a]
			EKG
			  Low QRS voltage
			  Conduction system disease
			  Atrial fibrillation
			  Poor R wave progression in
			    precordial leads
			TTE
			  LV hypertrophy
			  Increased IVSd thickness
			  Diastolic dysfunction with
			    preserved LVEF
			  Reduced GLS
			MRI
			  Late gadolinium enhancement
			RHC
			  Restrictive physiology
				NT-proBNP >332 ng/L[b] or mean
				IVSd >12 mm in the absence of
				other etiology.

Kidney	50%–70%	Lower extremity edema Anasarca Uremia	Proteinuria (albuminuria, typically nephrotic range) Acute kidney injury Hypercholesterolemia Hypothyroidism Hypercoagulability	Proteinuria $\geq$0.5 g/24 h, mostly albumin.

Liver	20%	Right upper quadrant tenderness
		Early satiety
		Weight loss
			Hepatomegaly
			Isolated increase in alkaline
			  phosphatase
			Coagulopathy owing to
			  coagulation factor deficiency[c]
				Liver span >15 cm[d] or alkaline
				phosphatase elevation >1.5
				times upper limit of normal.

Gastrointestinal tract	10%	Diarrhea Weight loss Malabsorption Hematochezia or melena		Direct biopsy verification

Organ	Incidence	Presenting symptoms/signs	Diagnostic findings	Diagnosis
Lung	30%–90%[f]	Shortness of breath Dry cough Recurrent pleural effusions	Pleural effusions Interstitial pulmonary nodules	Direct biopsy verification.
Peripheral nervous system	10%–20%	Distal sensorimotor PN	EMG: symmetric, axonal sensorimotor polyneuropathy	Clinical diagnosis.
Autonomic nervous system	10%–20%	Orthostatic hypotension Early satiety High (pseudo-obstruction, vomiting), or low (constipation alternating with diarrhea) intestinal dysmotility Erectile dysfunction Voiding dysfunction	Delayed gastric emptying Positive tilt test	Clinical diagnosis.
Soft tissue	10%–20%	Periorbital (or upper body) purpura Macroglossia Arthropathy Myopathy Ecchymotic bullae Jaw or buttock claudication[e] Carpal tunnel (often bilateral)		Clinical diagnosis.

The table illustrates the most common presenting symptoms/signs, incidence and diagnostic findings of AL amyloidosis depending on organ involvement. Consensus criteria for organ involvement diagnosis are reported.

Abbreviations: EKG, electrocardiogram; EMG, electromyography; GLS, global longitudinal strain; IVSd, interventricular septal end diastole; LV, left ventricular; LVEF, left ventricular ejection fraction; MRI, magnetic resonance imaging; PN, peripheral neuropathy; RHC, right heart catheterization; TTE, transthoracic echocardiogram.

a Typical of patients with amyloid deposition in the vessel wall, mimicking coronary artery disease in the absence of large vessel disease.
b In the absence of renal failure or atrial fibrillation.
c Factor X deficiency can occur independent of liver involvement owing to direct absorption of factor X by amyloid fibrils.
d In the absence of congestive hepatopathy secondary to heart failure.
e Presumed related to vascular deposition of amyloid.
f Depending on single institution series, often asymptomatic and detected post mortem.
Data from Refs.[61,64,65]

Table 5
Accuracy and availability of diverse methods for amyloidosis typing

	IHC/IF	Immunoelectron Microscopy	Liquid Chromatography and Mass Spectrometry
Sensitivity	75%–80%	75%–80%	95%
Specificity	80%	100%	100%
Comments	Requires high expertise Highly operator dependent Available in most centers	Not available in most centers	Not available in most centers

Abbreviation: IHC/IF, immunohistochemistry/immunofluorescence.

symptoms, novel diagnostic modalities are currently under investigation. Nanobody enrichment followed by liquid chromatography and mass spectrometry for the detection of clonal Ig and FLC has been investigated for screening, diagnosis, and disease response monitoring, including minimal residual disease, in patients with PC disorders. Liquid chromatography and mass spectrometry for the detection of clonal Ig and FLC is significantly more sensitive and specific than serum protein electrophoresis, with a limit of detection as little as 0.1 mg/dL in samples otherwise negative on serum protein electrophoresis, immunofluorescence, and FLC testing.[42] Liquid chromatography and mass spectrometry for the detection of clonal Ig and FLC is a powerful technology to study Ig/FLC posttranslational modifications with clinical impact.[43] Particularly, FLC from patients with AL amyloidosis are 5 times more likely to be N-glycosylated as compared with other PC disorders, a figure that increases to 13 times, if restricting analysis to κ FLC.[44,45] This abnormal pattern precedes clinically overt manifestations by years and nuclear magnetic resonance spectroscopy analysis suggest that glycosylation contributes to FLC proteotoxicity, thus representing an intrinsic property of amyloidogenic FLC.[44] An exciting effort to boost early AL amyloidosis diagnosis is the SAVE study, enrolling patients with MGUS and smoldering MM harboring high-risk λ Ig light chain variable region genotypes to assess FLC amyloidogenicity via a high-throughput competition assay to guide the diagnostic workup.[46,47] Further, peripheral blood MASS-IFX is being investigated as a tool to assess minimal residual disease without the need for a bone marrow biopsy.[48]

STAGING AND PROGNOSTIC FACTORS

The diagnostic and staging studies recommended for patients with suspected/confirmed AL amyloidosis are outlined in **Table 6**. Staging systems have been developed to aid in the prognostication of patients with newly diagnosed AL amyloidosis and all reflect the major impact that advanced cardiac involvement has in determining early mortality.[49–51] A concurrent diagnosis of MM based on presence of CRAB criteria (Calcium elevation, Renal dysfunction, Anemia, and Bone disease) or bone marrow PC cellularity exceeding 10% equally portend an adverse prognosis when normalized for cardiac staging.[52] As mentioned elsewhere in this article, the presence of cytogenetic abnormalities is an adverse prognostic factor. After diagnosis and initiation of therapy, depth of organ response, especially cardiac, is a strong predictor of survival.[53]

TREATMENT CONSIDERATIONS

There is no treatment for AL amyloidosis that has been approved by the US Food and Drug Administration; however, multidrug chemotherapy targeting PC and/or

Table 6
Diagnostic studies for suspected AL amyloidosis

	Test/Procedure
Serum/blood testing	CBC with manual differential
	Basic metabolic panel
	Liver function tests
	SPEP + IFE
	FLC
	LDH
	β2 microglobulin
	Albumin
	High-sensitivity troponin
	NT-proBNP
	TSH and free T4
	Cholesterol panel
	PT and PTT[a]
	Transthyretin (TTR) gene sequencing[b]
Urine analysis	Albumin/creatinine ratio
	UPEP + IFE
Imaging and special studies	Bone survey inclusive of long bones and skull and/or PET/CT
	EKG
	TTE
	Cardiac MRI
	Chest radiograph/CT scan of the chest[c]
	Abdominal imaging[c]
	EMG[c]
	GI transit[c]
	Upper and lower endoscopies[c]
Pathologic specimens	Unilateral bone marrow aspirate and biopsy for IHC, Congo red stain, flow cytometry, cytogenetics and FISH
	Biopsy of plasmacytoma, if present
	Fat pad, minor salivary gland or rectum aspirate, for Congo red stain, immunofluorescence and possibly EM
	Typing of amyloid needs to be performed to confirm light chain identity[d]

Abbreviations: CBC, complete blood count; CT, computed tomography scan; EKG, electrocardiogram; EM, electron microscopy; EMG, electromyogram; FISH, fluorescent in situ hybridization; GI, gastrointestinal; IFE, immunofixation; IHC: immunohistochemistry; LDH, lactate dehydrogenase; PT, prothrombin time; PTT, partial thromboplastin time; SPEP, serum protein electrophoresis; TSH, thyroid-stimulating hormone; UPEP, urine protein electrophoresis.
[a] Factor X absorption onto amyloidosis can lead to PTT prolongation and bleeding diathesis.
[b] as clinically indicated in patients where familial TTR amyloidosis is in the differential diagnosis.
[c] As needed depending on clinical presentation.
[d] If negative, biopsy of the target organ should be pursued.

autologous stem cell transplantation are the standard of care and can elicit deep and durable hematologic responses.[54–56] Chemotherapy does not directly target the deposited amyloid fibrils; however, it halts progressive organ disfunction by abating FLC secretion and thus amyloid deposition. Deep and sustained hematologic remission is necessary for organ response because amyloid removal occurs over time, once circulating FLC has been abated.[57] The causes of the inefficient amyloid removal remain poorly understood, and investigational monoclonal antibodies targeting directly amyloid fibrils are currently being evaluated in clinical trials.[58,59] Both hematologic remission and organ remission, particularly cardiac, impact long-term survival;

however, early mortality is a function of advanced cardiac involvement. Thus, there is a need to raise awareness about AL amyloidosis and improve early diagnosis.[60]

DISCUSSION

This is an exciting time for the AL amyloidosis community; coordinated efforts from patient advocacy groups, academia, pharma, and regulatory agencies are increasing awareness of this devastating disease and provide the opportunity to impact patient survival.

Delayed diagnosis remains a major hurdle in the care of AL amyloidosis patients because this complex disease is often overlooked, resulting in one-third of patients being diagnosed with advanced cardiac disease, a major predictor of early mortality. Clinical trials exploring the combined use of antifibril antibodies and highly active multidrug chemotherapy could profoundly impact the natural history of this incurable illness and impact both early and long-term mortality, at last.

SUMMARY

AL amyloidosis is a PC disorder presenting as a complex, progressive disease with variable clinical presentation, related to the deposition of fibrils of misfolded immunoglobulin FLC. Diagnostic delay is frequent and may result in potentially irreversible cardiac damage, a major determinant of early mortality. The presence of heart failure with preserved left ventricular ejection fraction in the setting of hypertrophic cardiomyopathy; nephrotic syndrome with predominant albuminuria; bilateral carpal tunnel; and autonomic dysfunction or bilateral, symmetric sensorimotor peripheral neuropathy should raise suspicion for AL amyloidosis, particularly in patients with preexisting MGUS. Rapid tissue diagnosis with amyloid typing is critical to avoid irreversible organ damage and early mortality.

CLINICS CARE POINTS

- AL amyloidosis is often under-recognized owing to the vague nature of early symptoms and signs, and its variable clinical presentation.
- The presence of nephrotic syndrome and heart failure with preserved left ventricular function should prompt a workup for AL amyloidosis, particularly in patients with preexisting MGUS.
- NT-proBNP and albuminuria are 100% sensitive biomarkers to detect heart and kidney involvement by AL amyloidosis and should be considered for screening of high-risk patients.

DISCLOSURE

Dr G. Bianchi: Advisory board participation (with personal payment): Pfizer; Dr S. Kumar: Consulting/Advisory Board participation: (with no personal payments) Celgene, Takeda, Janssen, Abbvie, Genentech, Amgen, Molecular Partners and (with personal payment) Oncopeptides, Genecentrix, Cellectar.

REFERENCES

1. Dispenzieri A, Merlini G. Immunoglobulin light chain systemic amyloidosis. Cancer Treat Res 2016;169:273–318.
2. Comenzo RL. Plasma cell neoplasms, their precursor States, and their prediction of organ damage. J Clin Oncol 2014;32(25):2679–82.

3. Gertz MA, Kyle RA, Noel P. Primary systemic amyloidosis: a rare complication of immunoglobulin M monoclonal gammopathies and Waldenstrom's macroglobulinemia. J Clin Oncol 1993;11(5):914–20.
4. Cohen AD, Zhou P, Xiao Q, et al. Systemic AL amyloidosis due to non-Hodgkin's lymphoma: an unusual clinicopathologic association. Br J Haematol 2004;124(3): 309–14.
5. Hauser AE, Muehlinghaus G, Manz RA, et al. Long-lived plasma cells in immunity and inflammation. Ann N Y Acad Sci 2003;987:266–9.
6. Kourelis TV, Dasari S, Theis JD, et al. Clarifying immunoglobulin gene usage in systemic and localized immunoglobulin light-chain amyloidosis by mass spectrometry. Blood 2017;129(3):299–306.
7. Comenzo RL, Zhang Y, Martinez C, et al. The tropism of organ involvement in primary systemic amyloidosis: contributions of Ig V(L) germ line gene use and clonal plasma cell burden. Blood 2001;98(3):714–20.
8. Morgan GJ, Kelly JW. The kinetic stability of a full-length antibody light chain dimer determines whether endoproteolysis can release amyloidogenic variable domains. J Mol Biol 2016;428(21):4280–97.
9. Blancas-Mejia LM, Tischer A, Thompson JR, et al. Kinetic control in protein folding for light chain amyloidosis and the differential effects of somatic mutations. J Mol Biol 2014;426(2):347–61.
10. Wyatt AR, Yerbury JJ, Dabbs RA, et al. Roles of extracellular chaperones in amyloidosis. J Mol Biol 2012;421(4–5):499–516.
11. Merlini G, Bellotti V. Molecular mechanisms of amyloidosis. N Engl J Med 2003; 349(6):583–96.
12. Shi J, Guan J, Jiang B, et al. Amyloidogenic light chains induce cardiomyocyte contractile dysfunction and apoptosis via a non-canonical p38alpha MAPK pathway. Proc Natl Acad Sci U S A 2010;107(9):4188–93.
13. Quock TP, Yan T, Chang E, et al. Epidemiology of AL amyloidosis: a real-world study using US claims data. Blood Adv 2018;2(10):1046–53.
14. Alexander KM, Orav J, Singh A, et al. Geographic disparities in reported US amyloidosis mortality from 1979 to 2015: potential underdetection of cardiac amyloidosis. JAMA Cardiol 2018;3(9):865–70.
15. Kyle RA, Larson DR, Kurtin PJ, et al. Incidence of AL amyloidosis in Olmsted County, Minnesota, 1990 through 2015. Mayo Clin Proc 2019;94(3):465–71.
16. Duhamel S, Mohty D, Magne J, et al. Incidence and prevalence of light chain amyloidosis: a population-based study. Blood 2017;130(Supplement 1):5577.
17. Landgren O, Graubard BI, Katzmann JA, et al. Racial disparities in the prevalence of monoclonal gammopathies: a population-based study of 12,482 persons from the National Health and Nutritional Examination Survey. Leukemia 2014; 28(7):1537–42.
18. Kyle RA, Larson DR, Therneau TM, et al. Long-term follow-up of monoclonal gammopathy of undetermined significance. N Engl J Med 2018;378(3):241–9.
19. da Silva Filho MI, Forsti A, Weinhold N, et al. Genome-wide association study of immunoglobulin light chain amyloidosis in three patient cohorts: comparison with myeloma. Leukemia 2017;31(8):1735–42.
20. Warsame R, Kumar SK, Gertz MA, et al. Abnormal FISH in patients with immunoglobulin light chain amyloidosis is a risk factor for cardiac involvement and for death. Blood Cancer J 2015;5:e310.
21. Bochtler T, Hegenbart U, Kunz C, et al. Translocation t(11;14) is associated with adverse outcome in patients with newly diagnosed AL amyloidosis when treated with bortezomib-based regimens. J Clin Oncol 2015;33(12):1371–8.

22. Zhou P, Hoffman J, Landau H, et al. Clonal plasma cell pathophysiology and clinical features of disease are linked to clonal plasma cell expression of cyclin D1 in systemic light-chain amyloidosis. Clin Lymphoma Myeloma Leuk 2012;12(1): 49–58.

23. Bianchi G, Oliva L, Cascio P, et al. The proteasome load versus capacity balance determines apoptotic sensitivity of multiple myeloma cells to proteasome inhibition. Blood 2009;113(13):3040–9.

24. Oliva L, Orfanelli U, Resnati M, et al. The amyloidogenic light chain is a stressor that sensitizes plasma cells to proteasome inhibitor toxicity. Blood 2017;129(15): 2132–42.

25. Bianchi G, Munshi NC. Pathogenesis beyond the cancer clone(s) in multiple myeloma. Blood 2015;125(20):3049–58.

26. Wong SW, Hegenbart U, Palladini G, et al. Outcome of patients with newly diagnosed systemic light-chain amyloidosis associated with deletion of 17p. Clin Lymphoma Myeloma Leuk 2018;18(11):e493–9.

27. Bochtler T, Hegenbart U, Kunz C, et al. Gain of chromosome 1q21 is an independent adverse prognostic factor in light chain amyloidosis patients treated with melphalan/dexamethasone. Amyloid 2014;21(1):9–17.

28. Bochtler T, Merz M, Hielscher T, et al. Cytogenetic intraclonal heterogeneity of plasma cell dyscrasia in AL amyloidosis as compared with multiple myeloma. Blood Adv 2018;2(20):2607–18.

29. Abraham RS, Ballman KV, Dispenzieri A, et al. Functional gene expression analysis of clonal plasma cells identifies a unique molecular profile for light chain amyloidosis. Blood 2005;105(2):794–803.

30. Ledergor G, Weiner A, Zada M, et al. Single cell dissection of plasma cell heterogeneity in symptomatic and asymptomatic myeloma. Nat Med 2018;24(12): 1867–76.

31. Kourelis TV, Villasboas JC, Jessen E, et al. Mass cytometry dissects T cell heterogeneity in the immune tumor microenvironment of common dysproteinemias at diagnosis and after first line therapies. Blood Cancer J 2019;9(9):72.

32. Richey T, Foster JS, Williams AD, et al. Macrophage-mediated phagocytosis and dissolution of amyloid-like fibrils in mice, monitored by optical imaging. Am J Pathol 2019;189(5):989–98.

33. Godara A, Zhou P, Rosenthal B, et al. B-cell maturation antigen (BCMA) in systemic light-chain amyloidosis (AL): association with disease activity and its modulation with gamma-secretase inhibition. Blood 2019;134(Supplement_1):4409.

34. Kastritis E, Kostopoulos IV, Terpos E, et al. Evaluation of minimal residual disease using next-generation flow cytometry in patients with AL amyloidosis. Blood Cancer J 2018;8(5):46.

35. Lousada I, Comenzo RL, Landau H, et al. Light chain amyloidosis: patient experience survey from the amyloidosis research consortium. Adv Ther 2015;32(10): 920–8.

36. Hester LL, Gifkins DM, Bellew KM, et al. Diagnostic delay and characterization of the clinical prodrome in AL amyloidosis: data from 1,313 US commercially insured patients between 2006-2018. Blood 2019;134(Supplement 1):5517.

37. Geller HI, Singh A, Mirto TM, et al. Prevalence of monoclonal gammopathy in wild-type transthyretin amyloidosis. Mayo Clin Proc 2017;92(12):1800–5.

38. Connors LH, Prokaeva T, Lim A, et al. Cardiac amyloidosis in African Americans: comparison of clinical and laboratory features of transthyretin V122I amyloidosis and immunoglobulin light chain amyloidosis. Am Heart J 2009;158(4):607–14.

39. Cowan AJ, Seldin DC, Skinner M, et al. Amyloid deposits in the bone marrow of patients with immunoglobulin light chain amyloidosis do not impact stem cell mobilization or engraftment. Biol Blood Marrow Transplant 2012;18(12):1935–8.

40. Javidiparsijani S, Picken MM. Should the reporting of bone marrow positivity for amyloid be revised? a critical assessment based on 66 biopsies from a single institution. Arch Pathol Lab Med 2020. https://doi.org/10.5858/arpa.2019-0324-OA.

41. Muchtar E, Dispenzieri A, Lacy MQ, et al. Overuse of organ biopsies in immunoglobulin light chain amyloidosis (AL): the consequence of failure of early recognition. Ann Med 2017;49(7):545–51.

42. Barnidge DR, Tschumper RC, Theis JD, et al. Monitoring M-proteins in patients with multiple myeloma using heavy-chain variable region clonotypic peptides and LC-MS/MS. J Proteome Res 2014;13(4):1905–10.

43. Kumar S, Murray D, Dasari S, et al. Assay to rapidly screen for immunoglobulin light chain glycosylation: a potential path to earlier AL diagnosis for a subset of patients. Leukemia 2019;33(1):254–7.

44. Kourelis T, Murray DL, Dasari S, et al. MASS-FIX may allow identification of patients at risk for light chain amyloidosis before the onset of symptoms. Am J Hematol 2018;93(11):E368–70.

45. Milani P, Murray DL, Barnidge DR, et al. The utility of MASS-FIX to detect and monitor monoclonal proteins in the clinic. Am J Hematol 2017;92(8):772–9.

46. Martin EB, Williams AD, Heidel RE, et al. A functional assay to identify amyloidogenic light chains. Amyloid 2018;25(2):93–100.

47. Zhou P, Kugelmass A, Toskic D, et al. Seeking AL amyloidosis very early: the SAVE trial — identifying clonal lambda light chain genes in patients with MGUS or smoldering multiple myeloma. Blood 2018;132(Supplement 1):1903.

48. Dispenzieri A, Arendt B, Dasari S, et al. Blood mass spectrometry detects residual disease better than standard techniques in light-chain amyloidosis. Blood Cancer J 2020;10(2):20.

49. Dispenzieri A, Gertz MA, Kyle RA, et al. Serum cardiac troponins and N-terminal pro-brain natriuretic peptide: a staging system for primary systemic amyloidosis. J Clin Oncol 2004;22(18):3751–7.

50. Wechalekar AD, Schonland SO, Kastritis E, et al. A European collaborative study of treatment outcomes in 346 patients with cardiac stage III AL amyloidosis. Blood 2013;121(17):3420–7.

51. Kumar S, Dispenzieri A, Lacy MQ, et al. Revised prognostic staging system for light chain amyloidosis incorporating cardiac biomarkers and serum free light chain measurements. J Clin Oncol 2012;30(9):989–95.

52. Kourelis TV, Kumar SK, Gertz MA, et al. Coexistent multiple myeloma or increased bone marrow plasma cells define equally high-risk populations in patients with immunoglobulin light chain amyloidosis. J Clin Oncol 2013;31(34):4319–24.

53. Muchtar E, Gertz MA, Kumar SK, et al. Improved outcomes for newly diagnosed AL amyloidosis between 2000 and 2014: cracking the glass ceiling of early death. Blood 2017;129(15):2111–9.

54. Venner CP, Lane T, Foard D, et al. Cyclophosphamide, bortezomib, and dexamethasone therapy in AL amyloidosis is associated with high clonal response rates and prolonged progression-free survival. Blood 2012;119(19):4387–90.

55. Mikhael JR, Schuster SR, Jimenez-Zepeda VH, et al. Cyclophosphamide-bortezomib-dexamethasone (CyBorD) produces rapid and complete hematologic response in patients with AL amyloidosis. Blood 2012;119(19):4391–4.

56. Comenzo RL, Gertz MA. Autologous stem cell transplantation for primary systemic amyloidosis. Blood 2002;99(12):4276–82.
57. van G II, van Rijswijk MH, Bijzet J, et al. Histological regression of amyloid in AL amyloidosis is exclusively seen after normalization of serum free light chain. Haematologica 2009;94(8):1094–100.
58. Edwards CV, Bhutani D, Mapara M, et al. One year follow up analysis of the phase 1a/b study of chimeric fibril-reactive monoclonal antibody 11-1F4 in patients with AL amyloidosis. Amyloid 2019;26(sup1):115–6.
59. Gertz MA, Cohen AD, Comenzo RL, et al. Results of the Phase 3 VITAL Study of NEOD001 (Birtamimab) plus standard of care in patients with light chain (AL) amyloidosis suggest survival benefit for mayo stage IV patients. Blood 2019; 134(Supplement_1):3166.
60. Palladini G, Dispenzieri A, Gertz MA, et al. New criteria for response to treatment in immunoglobulin light chain amyloidosis based on free light chain measurement and cardiac biomarkers: impact on survival outcomes. J Clin Oncol 2012;30(36): 4541–9.
61. Vaxman I, Gertz M. Recent advances in the diagnosis, risk stratification, and management of systemic light-chain amyloidosis. Acta Haematol 2019;141(2): 93–106.
62. Fermand JP, Bridoux F, Dispenzieri A, et al. Monoclonal gammopathy of clinical significance: a novel concept with therapeutic implications. Blood 2018; 132(14):1478–85.
63. Rajkumar SV, Dimopoulos MA, Palumbo A, et al. International Myeloma Working Group updated criteria for the diagnosis of multiple myeloma. Lancet Oncol 2014;15(12):e538–48.
64. Gertz MA, Comenzo R, Falk RH, et al. Definition of organ involvement and treatment response in immunoglobulin light chain amyloidosis (AL): a consensus opinion from the 10th International Symposium on Amyloid and Amyloidosis, Tours, France, 18-22 April 2004. Am J Hematol 2005;79(4):319–28.
65. Milani P, Basset M, Russo F, et al. The lung in amyloidosis. Eur Respir Rev 2017; 26(145).

Systemic Amyloidosis due to Low-Grade Lymphoma

Ashutosh D. Wechalekar, MD[a], Raj Chakraborty, MD[b], Suzanne Lentzsch, MD, PhD[b],*

KEYWORDS

- Lymphoma-related AL amyloidosis • IgM amyloidosis • Rituximab
- Waldenstrom macroglobulinemia

KEY POINTS

- Lymphoma-related AL amyloidosis should be considered in any patient with systemic AL amyloidosis and IgM monoclonal protein, localized amyloid deposits, or underlying history of SS
- Bone marrow (or tissue biopsy) should be assessed for underlying lymphoproliferative disorder including MYD-88 testing.
- The goal of treatment is the induction of deepest remission (CR/VGPR), which translates into longer OS and better organ response
- Determine the underlying pathology to choose the optimal treatment
  - LPL: rituxan, bendamustine, velcade, dexamethasone
  - PPCN: daratumumab along with cyclophosphamide, bortezomib and dexamethasone
- Induction followed by ASCT achieves best results
- Consider always ASCT, as this translates in HRR and ORR
- Condition regimen for ASCT should be selected based on pathology
  - LPL: BEAM
  - PPCN: melphalan
- Role of maintenance is unclear.

INTRODUCTION

Lymphoma-related amyloidosis is a rare entity. Systemic AL amyloidosis is generally caused by an underlying plasma cell clone in the bone marrow[1] with an intact monoclonal immunoglobulin G (IgG) or IgA protein identified in 45% to 55% of cases. IgM-associated amyloidosis accounts for around 5% to 7% of all cases and is typically associated with an underlying lymphoplasmacytic lymphoma

[a] National Amyloidosis Centre, University College London (Royal Free Campus), Rowland Hill Street, London NW3 2PF, UK; [b] Multiple Myeloma and Amyloidosis Service, Herbert Irving Pavillion, R 953, 161 Fort Washington Avenue, New York, NY 10032, USA
* Corresponding author.
E-mail address: sl3440@columbia.edu

Hematol Oncol Clin N Am 34 (2020) 1027–1039
https://doi.org/10.1016/j.hoc.2020.08.016
0889-8588/20/© 2020 Elsevier Inc. All rights reserved.

(LPL); it is usually light chain (AL) but rarely can be heavy chain (AH) or a combination of both.[2–5] Other low-grade non-Hodgkin lymphomas (NHLs) are a rare cause of amyloidosis.

Lymphoma-related amyloidosis is a distinct clinical entity with several distinguishing clinical features from AL amyloidosis in general.[6,7] IgM-associated AL amyloidosis, the commonest type, follows systemic AL amyloidosis in terms of presentation. Other types may present with amyloid deposition at specific localized sites, including the lacrimal gland, breast, lung, stomach, and lymph nodes. These cases often lack a clearly detectable circulating monoclonal protein or abnormal serum free light chains. In general, the patients with IgM-associated AL have a lower light chain burden but also poorer hematologic response rates to treatment reflecting very often a more resistant underlying LPL clone. Those clones biologically behave similarly to Waldenstrom disease, which is characterized by a slower progression and higher chemotherapy resistance. In comparison to non-IgM types, fewer patients with IgM-associated AL achieve a complete response (CR) with an uninvolved free light chain (dFLC) less than 10 mg/L or an involved free light chain (iFLC) less than 20 mg/L.

The rarity of the lymphoma-related amyloidosis makes the generation of data in randomized trials and the determination of the optimal treatment almost impossible. Therefore, treatment recommendations discussed here are based on either retrospective or small prospective trials of single centers. The treatment paradigms designed for non-IgM AL have been used in IgM-associated amyloidosis with limited efficacy and, regimens designed for low-grade NHL are needed to treat these cases.

CLINICAL FEATURES OF LYMPHOMA-RELATED AMYLOIDOSIS

Amyloidosis due to low-grade lymphoma can be broadly classified into 3 main categories: IgM-associated, Sjogren syndrome (SS)-associated, and localized lymphoma-related amyloidosis. There can be a significant overlap between the latter 2 categories especially when the diagnosis of SS is not clear.

Immunoglobulin M–Related AL Amyloidosis

Systemic AL amyloidosis with the presence of an IgM monoclonal protein is the commonest type of lymphoma-associated AL amyloidosis. This entity was originally described by the Mayo clinic group in a series of 50 patients with IgM gammopathy presenting with AL amyloidosis.[3] The presentation was cardiac, renal, hepatic, and pulmonary amyloid seen in 44%, 32%, 14%, and 10% of patients, respectively. Despite this, the organ involvement in IgM-AL seems to be distinct with greater propensity for nerve, lymph node, and lung involvement with less frequent cardiac involvement at presentation.[5,7] A European collaborative series reported 250 patients with IgM AL amyloidosis showing that these patients had a median IgM monoclonal paraprotein level of 10 g/L, lower presenting serum free light chains (difference between the involved and uninvolved light chain >50 mg/L in <two-thirds of all patients) and less frequent lambda light chain isotype (**Fig. 1**A).[8] Cardiac involvement was less common in just less than half of all patients with more frequent lymph node (20%) and neuropathic (28%) involvement compared with non-IgM AL. Cardiac involvement, advanced Mayo disease stage, neuropathic involvement, and liver involvement were independent factors that had an impact on survival. Sidana and colleagues[9] from the Mayo Clinic provided a comprehensive evaluation of outcomes of patients with IgM AL with either LPL or pure plasma cell neoplasm (PPCNs) as an underlying clone. They analyzed bone marrow biopsies of 70 patients with IgM AL and found that 23% (16/70

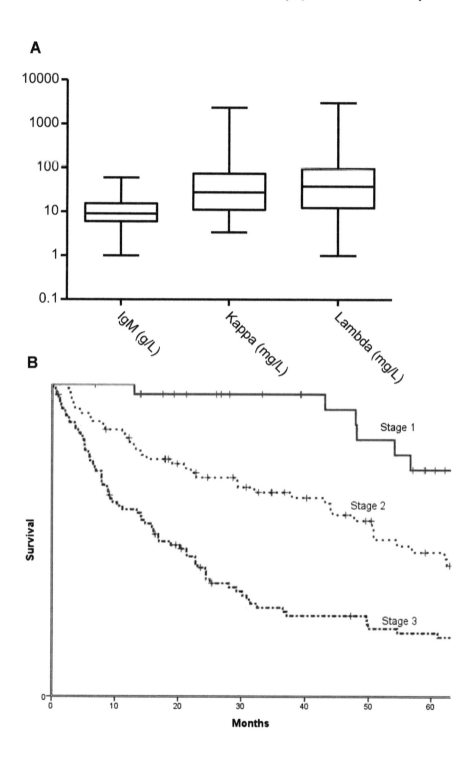

patients) of patients had a PPCN clone and 63% (44/70 patients) had an LPL clone, which included a characteristic *LPL* in 39% (27/70) of patients and a low-grade B-cell lymphoma with plasmacytic differentiation, not further classifiable in 24% (17/70) of patients. In the remaining patients, no other diagnosis could be made, or there were too few cells.[9]

The prognosis of IgM-related AL amyloidosis remains poorer than AL in general due to lack of treatments that can achieve deep clonal responses.[8] Cardiac involvement remains the major determinant of outcomes with worsening outcomes with progressive Mayo 2004 disease stage (stage 1—median 73 months vs stage 2—24 months vs stage 3—10 months). Overall survival (OS) was shorter in IgM AL compared with AL in general (when stratified by Mayo 2012 stage; stage 1/2 [59 vs 125.9 months, $P = .003$] and stage 3/4 [6.5 vs 12.9 months, $P = .075$]) likely due to lower hematologic response rates (6 months: 39% vs 59%, $P = .008$). Because of the unique characteristics of the disease, liver involvement and neuropathy are additional independent prognostic factors. Combining abnormal N-terminal pro-brain natriuretic peptide and troponin T with liver involvement and the presence of neuropathy gives IgM-AL–specific risk stratification model: median OS of patients with none, 1, or 2 or more abnormal factors was 90, 33, and 16 months, respectively (**Fig. 1**B).[8]

Sjogren Syndrome–Related AL Amyloidosis

The association of SS with low-grade NHL is well recognized[10] with a 1000-fold higher incidence of marginal zone and mucosa-associated lymphoid tissue (MALT) lymphomas.[11] Amyloidosis associated with SS has been frequently reported, and data are limited to as individual case reports and very small retrospective series. The sites of amyloidosis track the common sites of lymphoma in SS and include skin, lung, breast, salivary glands, and vocal cords. Deposits can be seen at more than one site. The amyloid deposits are likely to be due to local production of amyloidogenic light chains by the MALT/marginal zone NHL. However, in a significant proportion of cases with amyloidosis in SS, the clonal infiltrate can be difficult to identify clearly due to the extensive amyloid infiltration dispersing the clonal lymphoid cells. The amyloid deposits in skin, breast, and salivary glands usually present as localized nodular deposits or glandular enlargement, respectively. The breast deposits are often identified during screening for breast malignancies due to presence of breast nodules and can be bilateral.[12] Pulmonary amyloidosis is the most challenging of the manifestations, as there is significant overlap with lymphoid interstitial pneumonitis (LIP). Patients may present with single or multiple lung nodules presenting as hemoptysis or progressive cough and shortness of breath. However, they can progress to interstitial amyloid deposition and cystic lung changes, which can lead to irreversible debilitating

---

Fig. 1. (*A*) Monoclonal IgM component and serum free light chains at presentation in IgM AL amyloidosis. (*B*) Staging system for IgM AL amyloidosis using abnormal NTproBNP, abnormal troponin-T, liver involvement, and neuropathy: stage 1—one present, stage 2—two present, stage 3—three or more present. ([*A*] *From* Wechalekar AD, Lachmann HJ, Goodman HJ, et al. AL amyloidosis associated with IgM paraproteinemia: clinical profile and treatment outcome. Blood. 2008;112(10):4009-16; and [*B*] Sachchithanantham S, Roussel M, Palladini G, et al. European Collaborative Study Defining Clinical Profile Outcomes and Novel Prognostic Criteria in Monoclonal Immunoglobulin M-Related Light Chain Amyloidosis. J Clin Onc: official journal of the American Society of Clinical Oncology 2016;34(17):2037-45.)

pulmonary symptoms.[13] LIP is a close differential diagnosis and often difficult to distinguish.

The history of SS predates the amyloid diagnosis variably between 1 to 20 years and most of the patients have hypergammaglobulinemia and positive autoantibodies (rheumatoid factor or anti-Ro/SSA or anti La/SSB antibodies).[14] Distinction of systemic AL amyloidosis causing sicca syndrome from the localized amyloidosis caused by SS is important. The localized amyloid deposits in SS rarely progress to systemic amyloidosis. SS is commoner in women and amyloidosis due to SS is also commoner in women. The localized amyloid deposits are always AL type. Rare patients with systemic AA amyloidosis have been described but they almost always have an overlap rheumatological disorder and present with renal involvement.

Other lymphoma-related amyloidosis
Amyloidosis due to lymphoma (other than IgM-related AL or AH and SS-associated AL) is rare. Most such cases are localized amyloid deposits in the skin, conjunctiva, orbits, lung, or lymph nodes commonly associated with marginal zone/MALT lymphoma.[15] The deposits are almost always at one single site (apart from lymph node amyloid deposits), rarely associated with circulation monoclonal protein, typically indolent or slowly progressive, and very often do not require any systemic intervention.[16] Rare cases of systemic AL amyloidosis have been reported with chronic lymphocytic leukemia[17] and follicular lymphoma.[18] In most cases of lymphoma-associated amyloidosis, there is plasmacytic differentiation of the lymphoid malignancy. Wider use of MYD-88 testing as well as presence of IgH translocations may help to differentiate from LPL or true plasma cell clones.

Diagnostic workup for lymphoma-related AL amyloidosis
The diagnosis and assessments of lymphoma-related AL remain similar to those with systemic AL amyloidosis in general. A tissue biopsy is required to confirm the diagnosis of amyloidosis followed by confirmation of amyloid fibril type. Confirmation of fibril type in IgM-related AL amyloidosis seems to be more challenging on immunohistochemistry, and laser capture followed by mass spectrometry is often required for confirmation.[19,20] Accurate identification of the underlying low-grade NHL and its type is important to planning management. Detailed review of any biopsy material by a hematopathologist is crucial. Assessment of MYD-88 and IgH translocations on bone marrow samples is helpful to differentiate between LPL and neoplastic plasma cell clone.[21,22]

Most patients with lymphoma-related amyloidosis (especially patients with localized amyloid deposits) require whole-body cross-sectional imaging to identify lymph node enlargement and other disease sites that may affect management decisions. PET with fludeoxyglucose F 18 (^{18}F-FDG-PET) scanning is useful in some cases to identify areas of amyloid deposition in patients with localized NHL-related amyloidosis.[23] FDG uptake is typically low grade. The reason for FDG positivity is likely to be a combination of the local NHL clone or tissue macrophage reaction to amyloid deposits.[23] FGD-PET almost never show uptake in visceral organ affected by amyloid deposition. Newer PET tracers such as 18F-Florbetaben are interesting for systemic amyloid imaging[24] but await further evaluation. Cardiac evaluation by echocardiography including global 2-dimensional strain measurements as well as cardiac MRI is required at baseline.[25] Assessment of liver involvement including liver size by ultrasound or computed tomographic scanning, ^{123}I-labeled serum amyloid P component scintigraphy (where available), and liver function tests is important.[26,27]

Factor X levels and clotting factor assessments are required based on presentation with bleeding symptoms.

Treatment of lymphoma-related AL amyloidosis

Patients with lymphoma-related AL are rarely treated with regimens that showed efficacy in the treatment of non-IgM AL amyloidosis. But given that the different underlying monoclonal clones consist in most cases of a LPL, regimens targeting Waldenstrom disease should be considered. Furthermore, a better understanding of the role of genetic abnormalities such as CXCR4[WHIM] or MYD88[LL265P] mutations in the pathogenesis of IgM AL will help to better tailor treatments according to the underlying biology of the light chain producing clone.

Furthermore, the fact that patients with IgM AL do not respond well to a plasma cell–directed regimen is not a surprise, as, in those cases, an NHL is treated with myeloma-directed therapy. Based on the fundamental biological differences in patients with LR-AL versus PPCN IgM AL, patients should be treated according to their underlying clone to ensure a tailored treatment of either LPL or PPCN. Patients with SS-related AL or other lymphoma-related AL follow the paradigm described for the patients with IgM-related AL with caveat that nonprogressive local lesions may not require chemotherapy treatment and individual lesions, at amenable sites, can be considered for treatment with local radiotherapy.

TREATMENT OF IMMUNOGLOBULIN M–RELATED AL AMYLOIDOSIS

There are no prospective randomized studies on IgM amyloidosis, and the published treatment regimens are very heterogeneous. In a large European collaborative study of patients with IgM-related AL amyloidosis, 172 had available data on hematologic response. The hematologic response rate was 57% with 43% partial response (PR), 9% very good partial response (VGPR), and 5% CR. The median OS was not reached for patients achieving VGPR/CR, 64 months for PR, and 28 months for nonresponders ($P<.001$). Organ response rates were poor, with renal and cardiac response rates of 18% and 5%.[8]

A retrospective study from the Boston Amyloidosis Center analyzed the treatment responses for 46 patients after 2003.[28] They chose the regimens based on the bone marrow pathology and patient-specific factors. The hematologic overall response rate (ORR) and VGPR/CR were as follows: high-dose melphalan/stem cell transplant 100% and 80%, Bortezomib 82% and 27%, Rituximab 80% and 27%, immunomodulatory derivatives (IMiDs) 75% and 0%, and standard-dose alkylating agents (melphalan or cyclophosphamide) 63% and 19%. Overall, the 5-year survival rates were significantly higher in patients with a hematologic response: $79.2 \pm 8.5\%$ versus $41 \pm 14.9\%$ in nonresponders, which is more favorable than typically expected in AL amyloidosis.[28]

Both retrospective studies from amyloid centers reflect the relatively low rate of deep remission, translating into low organ responses and subsequent poorer outcomes.

Autologous Stem Cell Transplantation

Although the role of autologous stem cell transplantation (ASCT) in Waldenstrom is not well established and only recommended in selected cases, several studies have shown that ASCT is a very effective therapy for patients with IgM AL. In a retrospective analysis, Sidiqi and colleagues[2] from the Mayo Clinic reported 38 patients receiving ASCT for IgM AL between May 1999 and June 2018. The ORR was 92%. Three-quarters of patients achieved at least a VGPR. The median

OS was 106 months and the progression-free survival (PFS) 48 months. Organ response predicted an improved PFS and OS (median PFS 93 months for organ response vs 16 months for no organ response, P = .0006 and median OS 123 months for organ response vs 41 months for no organ response, P = .02). The 100-day transplant-related mortality was 5% (2 patients). The investigators reported that the conditioning regimen has changed over time. Although the preferred regimen was high-dose melphalan in earlier years, in recent years, they have moved toward carmustine, etoposide, cytarabine, and melphalan (BEAM) conditioning in patients with the lymphoplasmacytic disease. Specifically, 84% (n = 32) of patients received high-dose melphalan (200 mg/m^2 in 63% n = 24 and 140 mg/m^2 in 21% n = 8). Six patients received conditioning with BEAM. Patients did not receive maintenance. Renal responses were seen in 65% (15/23) (median time 18 months post-ASCT, range 3–52 months) and cardiac responses in 60% (6/10) of patients (median time 12 months postASCT, range 10–35 months).[2]

Those data are very encouraging, but unfortunately, despite the marked decrease in transplant-related mortality to around 5% and the fact that ASCT is an effective therapy in patients with IgM-related AL amyloidosis, only about 20% of patients may be eligible for this modality.

Rituximab-Based Regimens

Patients with IgM AL usually have a lower response compared with those with a non-IgM–related disease. The biological features of the underlying neoplastic clone in patients with IgM-related AL amyloidosis, especially with an LPL phenotype resembling low-grade NHL requires a clone specific treatment, which was not always considered based on the heterogeneous data in the literature. In most of the IgM AL, an LPL clone is the underlying source of the production of FLC requiring regimen used in Waldenstrom disease.

A small study of 10 patients treated with a combination of rituximab, bortezomib, and dexamethasone showed a promising response rate in 7/9 (78%) patients, suggesting that CD20 directed therapy in conjunction with antiplasma cell therapy is a very effective approach.[29] Despite the very promising response rates, the use of bortezomib remains a challenge because of the high frequency of peripheral neuropathy in IgM amyloidosis.

In the large European trial, it was shown that since 2010, the use of rituximab in combination with bortezomib; cyclophosphamide and dexamethasone [R-CD]; rituximab plus cyclophosphamide, vincristine, and prednisolone [R-CVP]; or rituximab plus cyclophosphamide, vincristine, doxorubicin, and prednisolone [R-CHOP] has increased. The rituximab-containing regimens resulted in PR or better responses in 63% of patients.[8]

Bendamustine

Bendamustine is a bifunctional alkylating agent with efficacy in treating several hematologic malignancies, including chronic lymphocytic leukemia, NHL, and multiple myeloma. Bendamustine induces DNA interstrand cross-links leading to cytotoxicity.[30,31] Also bendamustine blocks several mitotic checkpoints, DNA repair, and induces apoptosis via a p53-dependent DNA damage stress response.[32] Based on the encouraging data from using bendamustine in multiple myeloma, Lentzsch and colleagues performed a multicenter phase 2 clinical trial of bendamustine combined with dexamethasone for relapsed or refractory AL. This trial includes all subtypes of AL. Fifty-seven percent of patients achieved a PR or better (11% CR, 18%

VGPR). The organ response was 29%. In this frail patient population, treatment with bendamustine was well tolerated with no grade 5 treatment-related adverse events. The median OS was 18.2 months (95% confidence interval [CI] 11.3 to 43.8 months), and the hematologic response was associated with significantly better survival (P = .0291).[33] Based on the high response rates of bendamustine in multiple myeloma and bendamustine combined with rituximab (BR) in patients with low-grade lymphoma, BR has also been used for patients with IgM AL. Manwani and colleagues[34] reported the outcomes in 27 patients treated with bendamustine (90 mg/m^2) and rituximab (375 mg/m^2). The ORR on an intention-to-treat (ITT) basis was 59%. Hematological responses were as follows: CR in 11% of patients, VGPR in 37%, partial response (PR) in 11%, and no response (NR) in 41% (including 22% deaths). Among the 5 patients treated for refractory AL, 3 achieved a VGPR, and 2 were nonresponders (including one death). On a 6-month landmark analysis of patients who achieved VGPR or better, median OS and PFS were not reached, compared with 34 and 11 months, respectively, in patients who did not. Even though Manwani and colleagues[34] presented a small retrospective study, the data demonstrate an excellent hematological response with 48% VGPR or better on an ITT basis. Even in a relapsed situation, 60% of patients treated with second-line BR achieved a VGPR.

Those data suggest that upfront bendamustine in combination with rituximab leads to long-lasting and high response rates in IgM AL. The regimen is also well tolerated, as bendamustine has an excellent safety profile. It is neither neurotoxic nor cardiotoxic, and dosing is not affected by renal failure, suggesting that BR is an excellent choice for patients with IgM AL. Based on the promising data, this combination should be further studied in larger prospective trials on patients with IgM-related AL amyloidosis.

Other Alkylating Agents

The Boston Amyloidosis Center reported a series of 27 patients treated with melphalan or cyclophosphamide. Sixty-three percent of the patients achieved a PR with 19% CR/VGPR.[28] In a large European collaborative study of patients with IgM-related AL, different combinations of cyclophosphamide in regimens such as CHOP (cyclophosphamide, vincristine, doxorubicin, and prednisolone) and COP (cyclophosphamide, vincristine, and prednisolone) resulted in a PR rate of 62% but none achieved a VGPR or better.[8]

Immunomodulatory Derivatives

Despite the extensive use of IMiDs such as thalidomide, lenalidomide, and pomalidomide in multiple myeloma, few data on the efficacy of IMiDs in IgM AL are available. The European study reported 11 patients treated with thalidomide resulting in a PR or better in 63% and VGPR or better in 9% of patients.[8] The Boston Amyloidosis Center treated only 4 patients with IMiDs, only 3 achieving a partial response to therapy.[28] Based on those data and the lack of efficacy of IMiDs in Waldenström macroglobulinemia (WM), we cannot recommend IMiDs for LPL IgM AL. In patients with PPCN IgM AL, IMiDs might be considered if no other options are available. However, deep hematologic responses are not seen with IMiDs, which is critical for organ response and survival.

Ibrutinib

Bruton's tyrosine kinase (BTK) is a cytoplasmatic tyrosine kinase expressed in B cells. The BTK inhibitor, ibrutinib, is approved for the treatment of several B cell malignancies including WM. Treon and colleagues[35] reported an impressive response rate of 90.5% of patients with relapsed/refractory WM.[36] Based on those data, Pika and colleagues[37] from the Heidelberg Group in Germany retrospectively evaluated the effect of ibrutinib therapy in 8 patients with AL associated with WM or marginal zone lymphoma. The treatment affected neither the free light chains nor the complete M-protein molecules in 5 patients, and one patient even had hematologic progression during the treatment. The therapy was not well tolerated and associated with multiple adverse events, including peripheral edema, especially in patients with cardiac and kidney involvement, and polyneuropathy. Two patients developed atrial fibrillation, and one patient with preexisting atrial fibrillation experienced a transient ischemic attack. The data suggested that although ibrutinib treatment is associated with a high percentage of therapeutic responses in WM, it is not recommended for IgM AL due to a considerable amount of adverse effects translating into poor survival in this small subgroup of pretreated systemic AL.[37]

RESPONSE ASSESSMENT AND GOALS OF TREATMENT

The authors recommend evaluating hematologic response based on the consensus criteria for the difference in iFLC and uninvolved free light chains (dFLC).[38] For patients with a free light chain burden dFLC less than 5 mg/dL, the VGPR assessment with a dFLC less than 4 cannot be used. The CR assessment or decrease in dFLC to less than 1 mg/dL should be used.[39–41] If present, the baseline monoclonal protein of at least 0.5 g/dL should be assessed by criteria for WM response.[42] Both FLC and monoclonal protein should be included in the evaluation of the response, as often only one parameter is elevated.

The goal of the treatment is to achieve the deepest response possible, as it was shown in a study by Sidana and colleagues that the FLC and M-spike CR lead to the best outcome. They showed that dFLC CR resulted in a significantly longer OS (83.4 vs 8.9 months, $P = .006$). Similarly, the achievement of monoclonal protein CR led to a significantly longer OS (83.4 months vs 6.5 months, $P<.001$).[9]

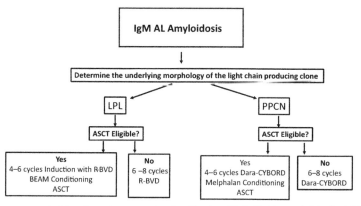

Fig. 2. Recommended treatment approach of patients with IgM AL amyloidosis. ASCT, autologous stem cell transplantation; BEAM, carmustine, etoposide, cytarabine and melphalan; Dara-CYBORD, daratumumab, cyclophosphamid, bortezomib, dexamethasone; LPL, lymphoplasmacytic clone; PPCN, pure plasma cell neoplasia; R-BVD, rituximab, bendamustine, velcade, dexamethasone.

Nevertheless, it is known that the induction of hematologic CR associated with organ response is much more difficult to achieve in IgM AL than in non-IgM AL. Sidana and colleagues reported significantly lower hematologic response rates in the IgM AL compared with non-IgM AL with an ORR of 39% versus 59% ($P = .008$) and a CR/VGPR of 24% versus 41% ($P = .02$) at 6 months. The poorer hematologic response rate (HRR) resulted in lower organ response rates for heart, kidney, and liver in the IgM cohort, with response rates being 35% (6/17), 40% (10/25), and 0% (0/5), respectively compared with non-IgM AL organ responses (heart: 47%, kidney: 48%, and liver: 41%).[9]

SUMMARY

Lymphoma-related amyloidosis is a rare but distinct clinical entity. IgM-related AL amyloidosis due to underlying LPL is the best studied, has a systemic presentation, and is treated with chemotherapy; the AH variant is extremely rare. SS-related AL amyloidosis and other NHL-related AL amyloidoses are typically localized diseases with amyloid deposition at one or more isolated site with rare progression to systemic disease. The treatment paradigm follows that for LPL or other low-grade NHL with rituximab-based regimes. Despite new and improved treatment options, patients with IgM AL have a lower hematologic response to treatment resulting in an inferior outcome compared with patients with non-IgM AL.

Once the exact amyloid producing clone has been identified, therapy needs to aim for the deepest possible remission. The treatment recommendations are summarized in **Fig. 2**. Patients with an LPL morphology should receive an anti-CD20–directed treatment, such as rituximab combined with an alkylating agent such as bendamustine and bortezomib to target both the lymphoid and plasmacytic components of the disease. This recommendation is mainly based on the observation that PR rates of 78% have been observed when patients with IgM AL were treated with rituximab, bortezomib, and dexamethasone and that the combination of rituximab with bendamustine resulted in PR of 59% with impressive CR/VGPP rate of 48%.[29,34] This recommendation is further supported by the results of a phase II study with rituximab, bendamustine, and bortezomib in low-grade B-cell lymphomas. The trials included LPL and mantle cell lymphoma and resulted in high ORRs of 88% to 94%, including CR rates of 53% to 64%.[43,44] Nevertheless, the authors point out that no data investigating this regimen in IgM AL are available. Future trials are needed to support a regimen of rituximab, bendamustine, bortezomib, and dexamethasone for IgM AL. Patient presenting with a neuropathic phenotype should avoid bortezomib.

Patients with a pure plasma cell clonal neoplasm are best treated with a plasma cell–directed treatment regime. The authors recommend treatment with daratumumab, cyclophosphamide, bortezomib, and dexamethasone, given an outstanding ORR of 96% with CR 54% and VGPR 82% in the run-in safety trial of 28 patients. The high hematologic response rates resulted in impressive organ response: 53% cardiac, 83% renal, and 50% liver response.[45]

In contrast to Waldenstrom disease, in which ASCT plays a minor role, ASCT in IgM AL amyloidosis has led to deep and durable response rates. Based on the Boston Amyloidosis Center and the Mayo Clinic's excellent data, reporting an ORR of 100% and 92%, respectively, ASCT needs to be considered in this patient population.[9,28] Unfortunately, only a small fraction of around 20% of IgM AL might be eligible for ASCT. When considering ASCT, the conditioning regimens in patients with LPL morphology should be similar to those used for WM, such as BEAM, and in patients with PPCN morphology similar to myeloma such as melphalan. Treatment should be continued until the deepest remission is achieved.

DISCLOSURE

The authors have nothing to disclose.

REFERENCES

1. Sipe JD, Benson MD, Buxbaum JN, et al. Nomenclature 2014: amyloid fibril proteins and clinical classification of the amyloidosis. Amyloid 2014;21(4):221–4.
2. Sidiqi MH, Buadi FK, Dispenzieri A, et al. Autologous stem cell transplant for IgM-associated amyloid light-chain amyloidosis. Biol Blood Marrow Transplant 2019; 25(3):e108–11.
3. Gertz MA, Kyle RA, Noel P. Primary systemic amyloidosis: a rare complication of immunoglobulin M monoclonal gammopathies and Waldenström's macroglobulinemia. J Clin Oncol 1993;11(5):914–20.
4. Palladini G, Russo P, Bosoni T, et al. AL amyloidosis associated with IgM monoclonal protein: a distinct clinical entity. Clin Lymphoma Myeloma 2009;9(1):80–3.
5. Wechalekar AD, Lachmann HJ, Goodman HJ, et al. AL amyloidosis associated with IgM paraproteinemia: clinical profile and treatment outcome. Blood 2008; 112(10):4009–16.
6. Gertz MA, Kyle RA. Amyloidosis with IgM monoclonal gammopathies. Semin Oncol 2003;30(2):325–8.
7. Terrier B, Jaccard A, Harousseau JL, et al. The clinical spectrum of IgM-related amyloidosis: a French nationwide retrospective study of 72 patients. Medicine 2008;87(2):99–109.
8. Sachchithanantham S, Roussel M, Palladini G, et al. European collaborative study defining clinical profile outcomes and novel prognostic criteria in monoclonal immunoglobulin M-related light chain amyloidosis. J Clin Oncol 2016; 34(17):2037–45.
9. Sidana S, Larson DP, Greipp PT, et al. IgM AL amyloidosis: delineating disease biology and outcomes with clinical, genomic and bone marrow morphological features. Leukemia 2020;34(5):1373–82.
10. Ekstrom Smedby K, Vajdic CM, Falster M, et al. Autoimmune disorders and risk of non-Hodgkin lymphoma subtypes: a pooled analysis within the InterLymph Consortium. Blood 2008;111(8):4029–38.
11. Baimpa E, Dahabreh IJ, Voulgarelis M, et al. Hematologic manifestations and predictors of lymphoma development in primary Sjogren syndrome: clinical and pathophysiologic aspects. Medicine 2009;88(5):284–93.
12. Fernandez-Aguilar S, Sourtzis S, Chaikh A. IgM plasma cell myeloma with amyloidosis presenting as mammary microcalcifications. APMIS 2008;116(9): 846–9.
13. Arrossi AV, Merzianu M, Farver C, et al. Nodular pulmonary light chain deposition disease: an entity associated with Sjogren syndrome or marginal zone lymphoma. J Clin Pathol 2016;69(6):490–6.
14. Hernandez-Molina G, Faz-Munoz D, Astudillo-Angel M, et al. Coexistance of amyloidosis and primary Sjogren's syndrome: an overview. Curr Rheumatol Rev 2018;14(3):231–8.
15. Walsh NM, Lano IM, Green P, et al. Amyloidoma of the skin/subcutis: cutaneous amyloidosis, plasma cell dyscrasia or a manifestation of primary cutaneous marginal zone lymphoma? Am J Surg Pathol 2017;41(8):1069–76.

16. Mahmood S, Bridoux F, Venner CP, et al. Natural history and outcomes in localised immunoglobulin light-chain amyloidosis: a long-term observational study. Lancet Haematol 2015;2(6):e241–50.

17. Kourelis TV, Gertz M, Zent C, et al. Systemic amyloidosis associated with chronic lymphocytic leukemia/small lymphocytic lymphoma. Am J Hematol 2013;88(5): 375–8.

18. Matsumoto Y, Masuda T, Nishimura A, et al. A case of AL amyloidosis associated with follicular lymphoma with plasmacytic differentiation. Int J Hematol 2020; 111(2):317–23.

19. Vrana JA, Theis JD, Dasari S, et al. Clinical diagnosis and typing of systemic amyloidosis in subcutaneous fat aspirates by mass spectrometry-based proteomics. Haematologica 2014;99(7):1239–47.

20. D'Souza A, Theis J, Quint P, et al. Exploring the amyloid proteome in immunoglobulin-derived lymph node amyloidosis using laser microdissection/tandem mass spectrometry. Am J Hematol 2013;88(7):577–80.

21. Leblond V, Kastritis E, Advani R, et al. Treatment recommendations from the Eighth International Workshop on Waldenstrom's Macroglobulinemia. Blood 2016;128(10):1321–8.

22. Treon SP, Hunter ZR, Castillo JJ, et al. Waldenstrom macroglobulinemia. Hematol Oncol Clin North Am 2014;28(5):945–70.

23. Glaudemans AW, Slart RH, Noordzij W, et al. Utility of 18F-FDG PET(/CT) in patients with systemic and localized amyloidosis. Eur J Nucl Med Mol Imaging 2013;40(7):1095–101.

24. Fox TA, Lunn M, Wechalekar A, et al. [(18)F]Florbetaben PET-CT confirms AL amyloidosis in a patient with Waldenstrom's Macroglobulinemia. Haematologica 2018;103(7):e322–4.

25. Dorbala S, Ando Y, Bokhari S, et al. ASNC/AHA/ASE/EANM/HFSA/ISA/SCMR/SNMMI expert consensus recommendations for multimodality imaging in cardiac amyloidosis: part 1 of 2-evidence base and standardized methods of imaging. J Card Fail 2019;25(11):e1–39.

26. Hawkins PN, Lavender JP, Pepys MB. Evaluation of systemic amyloidosis by scintigraphy with 123I-labeled serum amyloid P component. N Engl J Med 1990; 323(8):508–13.

27. Gertz MA, Comenzo R, Falk RH, et al. Definition of organ involvement and treatment response in immunoglobulin light chain amyloidosis (AL): a consensus opinion from the 10th International Symposium on Amyloid and Amyloidosis, Tours, France, 18-22 April 2004. Am J Hematol 2005;79(4):319–28.

28. Sissoko M, Sanchorawala V, Seldin D, et al. Clinical presentation and treatment responses in IgM-related AL amyloidosis. Amyloid 2015;22(4):229–35.

29. Palladini G, Foli A, Russo P, et al. Treatment of IgM-associated AL amyloidosis with the combination of rituximab, bortezomib, and dexamethasone. Clin Lymphoma Myeloma Leuk 2011;11(1):143–5.

30. Cheson BD. Bendamustine: a new therapeutic option for hematologic malignancies. Clin Adv Hematol Oncol 2008;6(9):631–3.

31. Cheson BD, Brugger W, Damaj G, et al. Optimal use of bendamustine in hematologic disorders: TREATMENT recommendations from an international consensus panel - an update. Leuk Lymphoma 2016;57(4):766–82.

32. Leoni LM, Hartley JA. Mechanism of action: the unique pattern of bendamustine-induced cytotoxicity. Semin Hematol 2011;48(Suppl 1):S12–23.

33. Lentzsch S, Lagos GG, Comenzo RL, et al. Bendamustine with dexamethasone in relapsed/refractory systemic light-chain amyloidosis: results of a phase II study. J Clin Oncol 2020;38(13):1455–62.

34. Manwani R, Sachchithanantham S, Mahmood S, et al. Treatment of IgM-associated immunoglobulin light-chain amyloidosis with rituximab-bendamustine. Blood 2018;132(7):761–4.

35. Treon SP, Tripsas CK, Meid K, et al. Ibrutinib in previously treated Waldenstrom's macroglobulinemia. N Engl J Med 2015;372(15):1430–40.

36. Castillo JJ, Palomba ML, Advani R, et al. Ibrutinib in Waldenstrom macroglobulinemia: latest evidence and clinical experience. Ther Adv Hematol 2016;7(4): 179 86

37. Pika T, Hegenbart U, Flodrova P, et al. First report of ibrutinib in IgM-related amyloidosis: few responses, poor tolerability, and short survival. Blood 2018; 131(3):368–71.

38. Palladini G, Dispenzieri A, Gertz MA, et al. New criteria for response to treatment in immunoglobulin light chain amyloidosis based on free light chain measurement and cardiac biomarkers: impact on survival outcomes. J Clin Oncol 2012;30(36): 4541–9.

39. Dittrich T, Bochtler T, Kimmich C, et al. AL amyloidosis patients with low amyloidogenic free light chain levels at first diagnosis have an excellent prognosis. Blood 2017;130(5):632–42.

40. Milani P, Basset M, Russo F, et al. Patients with AL amyloidosis and low free light-chain burden have distinct clinical features and outcome. Amyloid 2017; 24(sup1):64–5.

41. Sidana S, Tandon N, Dispenzieri A, et al. Clinical presentation and outcomes in light chain amyloidosis patients with non-evaluable serum free light chains. Leukemia 2018;32(3):729–35.

42. Owen RG, Kyle RA, Stone MJ, et al. Response assessment in Waldenstrom macroglobulinaemia: update from the VIth International Workshop. Br J Haematol 2013;160(2):171–6.

43. Fowler N, Kahl BS, Lee P, et al. Bortezomib, bendamustine, and rituximab in patients with relapsed or refractory follicular lymphoma: the phase II VERTICAL study. J Clin Oncol 2011;29(25):3389–95.

44. Flinn IW, Thompson DS, Boccia RV, et al. Bendamustine, bortezomib and rituximab produces durable complete remissions in patients with previously untreated, low grade lymphoma. Br J Haematol 2018;180(3):365–73.

45. Palladini G, Kastritis E, Maurer MS, et al. Daratumumab plus CyBorD for patients with newly diagnosed AL amyloidosis: safety run-in results of ANDROMEDA. Blood 2020;136(1):71–80.

The Process of Amyloid Formation due to Monoclonal Immunoglobulins

Gareth J. Morgan, PhD[a],*, Jonathan S. Wall, PhD[b]

KEYWORDS

• Amyloidosis • Amyloid fibrils • Cross-beta • Antibody • Protein aggregation

KEY POINTS

- Amyloid fibrils are nonnative protein aggregates that are associated with organ dysfunction in the systemic amyloidoses.
- Amyloid light-chain (AL) amyloidosis is caused by amyloid derived from a unique, monoclonal immunoglobulin light chain secreted by clonally expanded B cells.
- Many factors contribute to whether a particular light chain can form amyloid, all of which are likely influenced by its unique sequence. Therefore, the structure of the fibrils, the organs affected, and the range of symptoms all vary between patients.
- Suppression of light chain secretion by eradication of the clonal cells is the only successful treatment of AL amyloidosis. Therapies at various stages of development that target the misfolded protein or amyloid fibrils are potentially valuable but have not yet been shown to be clinically efficacious.

INTRODUCTION

Disruption of the structural integrity of proteins causes misfolding and aberrant interactions, which can lead to disease. One manifestation of protein misfolding is the formation of amyloid fibrils, which are long, straight, unbranched protein aggregates that deposit extracellularly (**Fig. 1**). Amyloid fibrils have a "cross-β" molecular structure, where intermolecular hydrogen bonds between backbone amide groups create long β-sheets parallel to the fibril axis.[1] This repeating structure gives rise to the defining histologic property of amyloid fibrils: when stained with Congo red dye, amyloid deposits exhibit an "apple-green" birefringence under cross-polarized illumination.

[a] Amyloidosis Center and Section of Hematology and Medical Oncology, Department of Medicine, Boston University School of Medicine, 72 East Concord Street, Boston, MA 02118, USA; [b] Amyloidosis and Cancer Theranostics Program, Preclinical and Diagnostic Molecular Imaging Laboratory, The University of Tennessee Graduate School of Medicine, 1924 Alcoa Highway, Knoxville, TN 37920, USA
* Corresponding author.
E-mail address: gjmorgan@bu.edu

Hematol Oncol Clin N Am 34 (2020) 1041–1054
https://doi.org/10.1016/j.hoc.2020.07.003

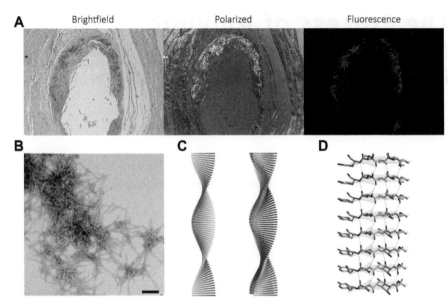

Fig. 1. Amyloid fibrils are nonnative protein aggregates. (*A*) Amyloid deposits from a cardiac biopsy stained with Congo red show a distinctive apple-green birefringence under polarized illumination. Congo red is also fluorescent when bound to amyloid fibrils, but the birefringence is considered diagnostic. (*B*) Electron micrographs of negative-stained amyloid fibrils formed in vitro from recombinant LCs. Fibrils are classically straight, nonbranching, and 10 nm wide. The scale bar represents 200 nm. (*C*) Amyloid fibrils are composed of long cross-β sheets. Multiple sheets may pack together to build up the structure. (*D*) Hydrogen bonding network of cross-β sheets, as observed in a cryoelectron microscopy structure of patient-derived AL amyloid, protein data bank (PDB) entry 6IC3.

Thirty-five different human proteins have been observed to form amyloid fibrils associated with disease.[2] However, regardless of the tertiary structure of the precursor protein, the cross-β configuration in fibrils seems to be a "generic" conformation for polypeptides, defined by peptide backbone interactions and modulated by the pattern of sidechains.[1] Amyloid-like structures are also found in many other contexts including functional assemblies and pathologic intracellular aggregates. Here, the authors focus on pathologic amyloid formed by immunoglobulins: antibodies and their fragments.

Healthy individuals have an immensely diverse repertoire of antibodies in circulation, secreted by long-lived plasma cells, which are terminally differentiated B lymphocytes. Each plasma cell secretes a single heavy chain (HC) and light chain (LC) protein that comprise the antibody. Aberrant proliferation of a single plasma cell clone, however, leads to the domination of the repertoire by a monoclonal antibody, which can be detected in blood.[3] A minority of individuals with such a "monoclonal gammopathy" exhibit amyloid formation or other forms of insoluble protein deposition. Amyloid light-chain (AL) amyloidosis, where the aggregated protein is derived from the LC of the monoclonal antibody, is the most commonly diagnosed form of systemic amyloidosis, with an incidence of 10 per million per year.[4] Systemic amyloidosis occurs when proteins secreted from one tissue deposit as amyloid elsewhere in the body. Amyloid diseases are named according to the protein that forms amyloid fibrils[2]; thus, "AL" strictly refers to the LC protein in its amyloid form but is often used informally as a shorthand for the disease. In AL amyloidosis, LC-derived amyloid fibrils deposit in a variety of tissues, leading to progressive organ failure that is fatal if untreated. Plasma cell proliferation can eventually lead to multiple myeloma, an incurable plasma cell cancer, which can be complicated by amyloidosis. Amyloid heavy chain (AH) amyloidosis, a far rarer condition, is discussed in **Box 1**. How amyloid fibrils damage tissue is not fully understood but may involve simple bulk displacement of tissue. In systemic amyloidosis, prevention of amyloid deposition by suppression of precursor protein production or misfolding has been shown clinically to benefit patients.[5–7] Therefore, identifying how and why some, but not all, LCs aggregate as amyloid fibrils may lead to new therapeutic strategies.

FROM SOLUBLE IMMUNOGLOBULINS TO INSOLUBLE AMYLOID FIBRILS

Antibodies have enormously diverse primary amino acid sequences: each patient with AL-associated amyloidosis or myeloma has an essentially unique monoclonal protein. These diverse proteins can deposit as amyloid fibrils or other deposits in various organs. The factors that determine what type of aggregates are formed and which organs are affected in a particular patient are unknown but are likely driven by the LC primary structure, the extent of denaturation, and ligand interactions. Given this diversity, it is important to remember that there are likely to be multiple mechanisms for the processes involved in disease pathology, and an individual patient's LC may behave in an unexpected or counterintuitive way.

Antibodies are secreted as folded, oligomeric proteins with a discrete structure that is essential for their function (**Fig. 2**). Both the LC and HC components of antibodies are composed of immunoglobulin (Ig) domains. The N-terminal variable domains of both the LC and HC (V_L and V_H, respectively) contain the hypervariable antigen-binding loops (also known as complementarity-determining regions) where most of the sequence and structural differences between individual antibodies are found. The constant (C_L and C_H) domains have scaffolding and effector functions. Plasma cells secrete both mature antibodies such as IgG and "free" LCs (fLCs), without a corresponding HC. The HCs require the help of the LCs to fold, so LCs act as a quality control system for HCs: only correctly assembled LC:HC complexes, or fLCs, can be secreted.[8] Thus, LCs are synthesized in excess of HCs in the plasma cell, and surplus LCs are secreted from plasma cells into the circulation. Approximately half of patients with AL amyloidosis and a sixth of those with myeloma have no intact monoclonal antibody in circulation, apparently due to loss of HC expression in the plasma cells.[9,10] Free LCs have no known function and are excreted by glomerular filtration with a half-life of 2 to 4 hours.[11] Measurement of fLCs in the serum or urine is an important test for diagnosis and management of plasma cell disorders including AL amyloidosis.[6,12] Monoclonal fLCs can be excreted in the urine of individuals with kidney damage associated with multiple myeloma or AL amyloidosis. These urinary fLCs, known as Bence-Jones proteins (BJPs), were some of the first

---

Box 1

Heavy chain amyloidosis

In contrast to diseases where immunoglobulin LCs aggregate, heavy chain (AH) amyloidosis is rare and involves deposition of a nonnative HC, such as a protein that lacks the C_H1 domain that would otherwise prevent its secretion.[84] A retrospective review found 5 cases of AH amyloidosis, 11 with both LC and HC deposition ("AHL amyloidosis"), and 207 with AL amyloidosis.[85] Identification of amyloid formed by both LCs and HCs is challenging and it is possible that AHL amyloidosis is not a separate entity, but rather represents accumulation of HCs within AL amyloid fibrils. Treatment of AH and AHL amyloidosis is similar to that for AL amyloidosis: eradication of the clonal cells by chemotherapy.

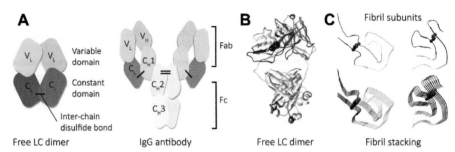

Fig. 2. Native and fibril structures of immunoglobulins. (*A*) The domain organization of mature antibodies and free LCs. The free LC is shown as a dimer. Shapes represent Ig domains, and interchain disulfide bonds are shown as black lines. (*B*) Native structure of a full-length Ig λ-LC (PDB entry 6MG4). The protein backbone is shown in ribbon representation and the disulfide bonds shown as spheres. The residues of the V_L-domain are colored from purple (N-terminus) to red (C-terminal end of the V-region). (*C*) Structures of fibril subunits (top) and their arrangement within amyloid fibrils (bottom), determined by cryoelectron microscopy. The 2 fibril structures (PDB entries 6HUD and 6IC3) are distinct. Colors correspond to the same residues as in B.

immunoglobulins—and indeed the first proteins—to be studied, because they are relatively easily isolated.[13] However, the presence of BJPs in urine does not necessarily correlate with disease.

Antibody LC sequences were identified as the constituents of amyloid fibrils in patients in 1970,[14] but it took almost 50 years for the atomic structures of LC amyloid fibrils to be determined.[15,16] Two λ-LC fibrils were independently isolated from cardiac biopsy samples and characterized by cryoelectron microscopy. In both cases, the native Ig fold has been completely lost, and the proteins are "flattened out" and stacked so that multiple cross-β strands pack against one another, with their hydrogen bonds arranged parallel to the fibril axis (see **Fig. 2**). The 2 AL fibrils are structurally distinct, with different regions forming the cross-β strands and a different configuration of the structured core, despite their 63% sequence identity and the similarity of their native structures. The disulfide bond between the 2 cysteine residues of each domain remains intact, but the orientation of the peptide chains around the disulfide is reversed in the fibrillary state. In both fibrils, only parts of the V_L-domain are observed. The C_L-domains seem to have been cleaved, likely by proteolytic enzymes either before or after fibril formation—this has yet to be resolved. Most patient-derived LC fibrils comprise fragments including V_L-domains, although partial C_L-domain sequences and full-length LCs have also been observed.[14,17–19] Other structural techniques have shown diverse patterns of β-sheet structure in LCs, consistent with alternative packing arrangements of multiple strands.[20–23] These initial structural studies highlight the potential diversity of LC amyloid fibrils and immediately raise questions about which, if any, shared structural features are important in determining the pathologic effects of the fibrils.

How, then, do the circulating full-length, folded LCs that are secreted from plasma cells escape excretion and instead misfold and misassemble into amyloid fibrils, with or without concurrent proteolysis?

SEQUENCE DETERMINANTS OF AMYLOID FORMATION

To identify determinants of amyloidosis, LC sequences from patients with amyloidosis are often compared with those from individuals without amyloid. Amyloid-associated

BJPs are able to form amyloid-like deposits in mice[24] and have different activities in a variety of other model systems.[25–28] A challenge with BJPs, however, is that the precise protein sequence, posttranslational modifications, and 3-dimensional structure are not always known, and they can only be extracted in finite quantities from an individual patient. Recombinant LCs, generated from cDNA cloned from patient plasma cells, provide a renewable, structurally uniform source of study material but may lack disease-relevant modifications such as glycosylation. A recurrent challenge in the field has been replication of observations, generally due to the primary structural heterogeneity: which observations are specific to the individual LC being studied and which can be applied more generally?

Studies of fibril formation by LCs have focused on the behavior of V_L-domains, which form the fibril core and are the site of most sequence differences. Antibody genes are assembled from "germline" gene fragments in B cells, which then undergo rounds of mutation and selection for antigen affinity. Several germline variable genes are highly associated with amyloidosis, most prominently λ1-44, λ1-51, λ2-14, λ3-1, λ6-57, κ1-33, and κ4-1.[29–31] Among LCs from the same germline gene, amyloid-associated V_L-domains are less thermodynamically stable and more prone to form amyloid fibrils in vitro, as compared with those derived from patients with myeloma.[32,33] Specific domain-destabilizing mutations of individual residues from the germline sequence have been associated with the generation of a proamyloidogenic sequence and fibril formation.[33–38]

Aggregation of soluble protein into amyloid fibrils requires favorable interactions in the fibril. These interactions are modulated by the polarity, charge complementarity, and β-sheet propensity of the different amino acids comprising the LC within the fibrils. Packing of individual strands together through complementary interfaces ("steric zippers") stabilizes each strand and helps to build up the macroscopic fibril structure.[39] These interactions are modulated by solvent conditions including pH, temperature, and ionic strength. Aggregation propensity can be modeled and predicted from a protein's amino acid sequence.[40] Fibril formation depends on the concentration-dependent rate of collisions between precursors and their concentration-independent dissociation from the fibril. Therefore, fibrils form at high concentrations, which explains why increased fLC levels drive aggregation.

However, for a folded immunoglobulin, amyloid formation competes with the similar forces that maintain the native fold of the protein. Thus, the concentration of the unfolded or misfolded amyloid precursor conformation is the critical parameter. Unfortunately, it is difficult to measure this parameter, because these precursor conformations are likely present transiently and at low concentration. The ease with which a protein can maintain its native state is called its stability. Stability often refers to the protein's susceptibility to several processes in vitro or in the body, including unfolding, aggregation, or proteolysis. For a V_L-domain, folding and unfolding without reduction of the intramolecular disulfide bond are highly cooperative processes,[41] so different measures of stability are correlated. Because LCs are continually secreted and excreted, the lifetime of the folded state after secretion is a useful measure of "kinetic" stability.[42] A kinetically stable fLC will, on average, be filtered by the kidneys before it has chance to unfold, whereas a kinetically unstable protein will have time to transiently unfold into a protease- or aggregation-susceptible conformation.

There is a strong correlation between V_L-domain global stability and the rate of amyloid formation in vitro.[20,32–34] LC V_L-domains can form native dimers with varying affinity that contribute to the stability of the folded state.[20,43] Therefore, the rate-limiting transition state for aggregation (the conformational ensemble that can self-associate in order to form amyloid) is likely to be monomeric and highly unstructured. This hypothesis is supported by the nonnative structures of AL amyloid fibrils.[15,16] In vitro, aggregation is surprisingly tolerant of mutations designed to disrupt the amyloid structure or unfolded-state interactions.[20,44] Conversely, alterations at the termini of V_L-domains can significantly change their aggregation.[45] These results are consistent with a model where unstructured LCs can form amyloid via alternative pathways, which may correlate with alternative fibril structures.[46]

POSTTRANSLATIONAL FACTORS AFFECTING AMYLOID FORMATION

The effect of LC posttranslational modifications on aggregation is another layer of complexity that is difficult to study in vitro but probably plays an important role in vivo.[47] Many LCs are modified on the C-terminal cysteine that could otherwise form a disulfide bond.[47] Disulfide-linked small molecules or oxidative modification of reactive residues[48,49] could reduce dimerization and thus destabilize the protein. N-glycosylation has been observed in several AL-associated LCs.[47,50,51] A minority of healthy antibody V_L-domains are glycosylated,[52] although all antibodies are also glycosylated in their C_H2 domains. Recently, a study using mass spectrometry identified glycosylation of LCs as a potential risk factor for amyloidosis.[53] This observation is somewhat surprising, because native N-glycosylation is often stabilizing and solubilizing.[54] It is reasonable to assume that a fibril comprising an N-glycosylated V_L-domain will be structurally distinct from the models that have recently been elucidated. A model for such a fibril might be found in the pentameric core of the IgM Fc region, where a short cross-β "tailpiece" formed by the C-termini of each chain contains an array of glycosylated asparagine residues.[55]

The most substantial modification of LCs is loss of the C_L-domain observed in many fibrils, including those for which structures are known. This is presumed to occur via proteolysis after secretion, because full-length LCs are the major species in serum and C_L-domains are observed in some fibrils. Proteolysis of the C_L-domain could occur before or after aggregation. In other systemic amyloidoses, both processes have been observed: proteolysis of serum amyloid A component is required for initiation of AA amyloidosis,[5] whereas transthyretin-derived amyloid fibrils seem to be cleaved after aggregation.[56]

Full-length LCs are generally less prone to aggregate in vitro than their associated V_L-domains.[57,58] Full-length LC dimers may be stabilized by an interchain disulfide bond between the cysteine residues that would form a disulfide with the HC in an antibody. Dimer formation and disulfide bond formation stabilize both domains of the full-length LC: there is a strong cooperativity between the folding of the domains and their interactions.[59] These data are consistent with a model where potentially amyloidogenic V_L-domains are "chaperoned" by their own C_L-domains, both by stabilization of the folded state and reduction of the amyloid propensity of the unfolded state ensemble. Therefore, proteolysis of full-length LC and loss of most, or all, of the C_L-domain would invariably generate amyloidogenic fragments.

INTERACTION WITH OTHER TISSUE COMPONENTS AFFECTS AMYLOID FIBRIL FORMATION

Amyloid deposits contain multiple proteins sequestered from the circulation, the most prominent of which is the serum amyloid P component (SAP). SAP is a pentameric extracellular pentraxin protein that binds tightly to all amyloid fibrils, which may serve to mask the fibrils from immune recognition.[60] Extracellular matrix components such as collagen, proteoglycans, and glycosaminoglycans (GAGs), probably contributed by neighboring cells, are also observed in deposits. Tissue- and LC-specific interactions may play a role in determining organ involvement. Amyloid fibrils can interact with GAGs, which are polymeric sugars decorated with repeating patterns of highly sulfated chemical groups. Interactions between basic amino acid sidechains on the surface of fibrils and anionic sulfated saccharides in GAGs such as heparin sulfate may stabilize the fibrils by neutralizing electrostatic repulsions between repeated charged residues. Accordingly, addition of GAGs to LCs enhances the yield of amyloid fibrils and modifies their structure.[61] The role of GAGs in amyloidosis patients and animal models, other than in AA amyloidosis,[62] has yet to be fully elucidated.

Amyloid formation may be accelerated by preformed aggregates, a process known as seeding or nucleated polymerization.[1] Parallel self-association of amyloid fibrils may stabilize them against dissociation. Both effects may be important in the growth of amyloid fibrils in the body: preexisting amyloid may serve as a template for further deposition. Seeding of aggregates is highly specific because the molecular interactions that stabilize the amyloid fibrils are repeated through the fibril. However, experiments with κ1-33 LCs showed that fibrils formed by the V_L-domains are able to act as seeds for the full-length LCs.[63] Preformed fibrils are able to seed aggregation of patient-derived BJPs, and this process is faster and more efficient with AL-derived BJPs.[26] Seeded aggregation may be important in AL patients who have experienced a hematological response to therapy, a reduction in circulating free LCs, but are at risk of relapse. Reemergence of the clonal plasma cells and circulating fLC may lead to rapid resumption of organ damage because the new LC molecules can be readily recruited by preexisting amyloid.

Template-mediated assembly of amyloid fibrils may also be involved in the propagation of amyloid to different anatomic sites. In extreme cases, this leads to "infectious amyloids" or prions.[64] There have been reports that amyloid can be spread between individuals by surgical procedures.[65] This might be unlikely in AL amyloidosis because the very high specificity of amyloid propagation requires that identical proteins are present in both individuals. That said, evidence from other amyloid disorders suggests that cross-seeding between tissues is possible and may play a role in disease progression.[66–70]

THERAPEUTIC OPTIONS

Clinically, the mechanisms by which proteins aggregate can be targeted for therapy (**Fig. 3**). Reducing the circulating concentration of a precursor protein can suppress its aggregation, as demonstrated by management of the underlying inflammation for AA amyloidosis[5] or silencing of precursor messenger RNA by oligonucleotide therapeutics for transthyretin amyloidosis.[71,72] In plasma cell dyscrasias, LC levels are reduced by chemo- or immunotherapeutic eradication of the plasma cell clone. Regimens developed for myeloma have been adapted for use in AL amyloidosis and other conditions.[73] Reducing the circulating concentration of LC benefits patients with all forms of LC-induced toxicity.

However, many patients are diagnosed after the onset of organ damage. These patients struggle to tolerate chemotherapy and have a poor prognosis. Preexisting amyloid deposits continue to limit organ function even after suppression of LC production. Additional therapies are therefore needed: less toxic ways to prevent amyloid formation, and strategies to remove existing amyloid deposits and regenerate damaged tissue. These strategies could potentially be combined with cytotoxic therapy. Stabilizing the precursor protein can suppress amyloid formation. In the case of transthyretin amyloidosis, binding of a small molecule to the transthyretin tetramer

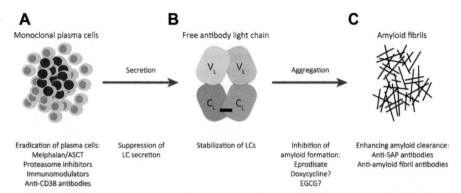

Fig. 3. Therapeutic strategies for AL amyloidosis. Current therapy is directed at eradicating the underlying clonal plasma cells, which decreases the concentration of circulating LCs and thereby prevents further aggregation. Other therapies at varying stages of development include suppression of LC unfolding and aggregation and immunotherapeutic clearance of existing amyloid deposits. Examples of drugs are shown. Note that the mechanisms of doxycycline and EGCG are not fully understood. ASCT, autologous stem cell transplant.

reduces its rate of dissociation and aggregation.[7,74] A similar approach may be possible in AL amyloidosis, although the diversity of involved LCs makes finding a pan-LC stabilizer challenging.[75,76] Several small molecules including doxycycline, an antibiotic, and epigallocatechin gallate (EGCG), a compound found in green tea, have been suggested to interfere with amyloid fibril formation.[77,78] However, identifying a specific mechanism by which these pleiotropic molecules exert their effect has been difficult. The small molecule drug candidate eprosidate was designed to prevent AA amyloidosis by inhibiting interactions between serum amyloid protein A and GAGs, thus preventing amyloid formation. Eprosidate showed some efficacy in a phase II clinical trial[79] but failed to meet its efficacy endpoints in a phase III clinical trial. Another strategy is to suppress secretion of the precursor LC from cells, either by suppressing its translation[80] or by altering the stringency of endoplasmic reticulum quality control.[81]

Inhibition of LC production can lead to regression of amyloid due to clearance mechanisms that are not fully understood. However, most patients retain tissue amyloid deposits after eradication of their clonal plasma cells. Suppression of LC production can also lead to benefits without clearance of amyloid. This benefit may be due to reduction of toxicity associated with soluble amyloidogenic LCs.[25,27] Development of antiamyloid antibodies[82] and anti-SAP antibodies[83] to enhance clearance of tissue amyloid and restore organ function has been a longstanding goal. However, these strategies have yet to show clinical efficacy in phase III trials. The heterogeneity of disease presentation in patients with AL, variable rates of organ recovery, and the difficulty of predicting how individuals will respond after plasma cell–directed therapy make such trials difficult to design and interpret. In addition, in light of the recent LC fibril structure data, it may be difficult to generate a single antibody, raised to a linear epitope, that is capable of recognizing the myriad of potential LC fibrils.

SUMMARY

Igs are highly diverse and the processes by which they form amyloid are similarly complex, which may contribute to the diversity of symptoms and clinical courses experienced by patients with AL amyloidosis. In order to form amyloid fibrils, an LC protein must be sufficiently unstable to populate aggregation-competent unfolded or misfolded conformations. Attaining these conformations may require proteolysis after secretion by a protease that generates a more amyloidogenic fragment. The LC must be secreted by monoclonal plasma cells in sufficient quantity that the aggregation-competent species self-associate in a location where stabilizing interactions with host factors support amyloid formation. Each of these processes may be influenced by the amino acid sequence of the LC and the characteristics of the clonal plasma cells. The complex sequence of events required for fibril formation suggests many processes that may be targeted for therapeutic intervention. However, the simplest approach to prevent amyloid is to kill the cells that produce the LC.

CLINICS CARE POINTS

- Patients each have a unique involved immunoglobulin light chain protein that leads to an unpredictable pattern of organ involvement. Disease severity may be governed by a combination of circulating free light chain level and the propensity of the monoclonal light chain to aggregate.
- Protein aggregation including amyloid fibril formation is related to the circulating concentration of the precursor protein. Therefore, therapies that reduce production of the precursor immunoglobulins by monoclonal plasma cell clones can prevent further aggregation. The goal of current therapies is eradication of the underlying clone.
- Existing amyloid deposits can sometimes resolve if immunoglobulin production is reduced. However, this process is not well understood, and amyloid deposits can continue to affect organ function after a hematological response. Residual amyloid deposits may "seed" renewed amyloid formation if the clonal cells reemerge and free light chain production increases.
- Therapies that aim to prevent misfolding and aggregation of precursor proteins, or to remove existing deposits, are at various stages of development but not yet approved for clinical use.

DISCLOSURE

G.J. Morgan has filed a patent application covering small molecule stabilizers of light chains. J.S. Wall holds patent rights to amyloid reactive peptides and antibodies, is Founder and CSO of Aurora Bio, and has received support from Aurora Bio, Ultragenyx Pharmaceuticals, and Caelum Biosciences.

REFERENCES

1. Chiti F, Dobson CM. Protein Misfolding, Amyloid Formation, and Human Disease: A Summary of Progress Over the Last Decade. Annu Rev Biochem 2017;86: 27–68.
2. Benson MD, Buxbaum JN, Eisenberg DS, et al. Amyloid nomenclature 2018: recommendations by the International Society of Amyloidosis (ISA) nomenclature committee. Amyloid 2018;25(4):215–9.
3. Kyle RA, Therneau TM, Rajkumar SV, et al. A long-term study of prognosis in monoclonal gammopathy of undetermined significance. N Engl J Med 2002; 346(8):564–9.
4. Merlini G, Dispenzieri A, Sanchorawala V, et al. Systemic immunoglobulin light chain amyloidosis. Nat Rev Dis Primers 2018;4(1):38.

5. Westermark GT, Fandrich M, Westermark P. AA amyloidosis: pathogenesis and targeted therapy. Annu Rev Pathol 2015;10:321–44.

6. Palladini G, Dispenzieri A, Gertz MA, et al. New criteria for response to treatment in immunoglobulin light chain amyloidosis based on free light chain measurement and cardiac biomarkers: impact on survival outcomes. J Clin Oncol 2012;30(36): 4541–9.

7. Maurer MS, Schwartz JH, Gundapaneni B, et al. Tafamidis Treatment for Patients with Transthyretin Amyloid Cardiomyopathy. N Engl J Med 2018;379(11): 1007–16.

8. Feige MJ, Groscurth S, Marcinowski M, et al. An unfolded CH1 domain controls the assembly and secretion of IgG antibodies. Mol Cell 2009;34(5):569–79.

9. Bochtler T, Hegenbart U, Heiss C, et al. Hyperdiploidy is less frequent in AL amyloidosis compared with monoclonal gammopathy of undetermined significance and inversely associated with translocation t(11;14). Blood 2011; 117(14):3809–15.

10. Magrangeas F, Cormier ML, Descamps G, et al. Light-chain only multiple myeloma is due to the absence of functional (productive) rearrangement of the IgH gene at the DNA level. Blood 2004;103(10):3869–75.

11. Waldmann TA, Strober W, Mogielnicki RP. The renal handling of low molecular weight proteins. II. Disorders of serum protein catabolism in patients with tubular proteinuria, the nephrotic syndrome, or uremia. J Clin Invest 1972;51(8):2162–74.

12. Bradwell AR, Carr-Smith HD, Mead GP, et al. Serum test for assessment of patients with Bence Jones myeloma. Lancet 2003;361(9356):489–91.

13. Jones HB. On a new substance occurring in the urine of a patient with mollities ossium. Philos Trans R Soc Lond 1848;138:55–62.

14. Glenner GG, Harbaugh J, Ohma JI, et al. An amyloid protein: the amino-terminal variable fragment of an immunoglobulin light chain. Biochem Biophys Res Commun 1970;41(5):1287–9.

15. Radamaker L, Lin YH, Annamalai K, et al. Cryo-EM structure of a light chain-derived amyloid fibril from a patient with systemic AL amyloidosis. Nat Commun 2019;10(1):1103.

16. Swuec P, Lavatelli F, Tasaki M, et al. Cryo-EM structure of cardiac amyloid fibrils from an immunoglobulin light chain AL amyloidosis patient. Nat Commun 2019; 10(1):1269.

17. Lavatelli F, Perlman DH, Spencer B, et al. Amyloidogenic and associated proteins in systemic amyloidosis proteome of adipose tissue. Mol Cell Proteomics 2008; 7(8):1570–83.

18. Olsen KE, Sletten K, Westermark P. Fragments of the constant region of immunoglobulin light chains are constituents of AL-amyloid proteins. Biochem Biophys Res Commun 1998;251(2):642–7.

19. Vrana JA, Gamez JD, Madden BJ, et al. Classification of amyloidosis by laser microdissection and mass spectrometry-based proteomic analysis in clinical biopsy specimens. Blood 2009;114(24):4957–9.

20. Rennella E, Morgan GJ, Yan N, et al. The Role of Protein Thermodynamics and Primary Structure in Fibrillogenesis of Variable Domains from Immunoglobulin Light Chains. J Am Chem Soc 2019;141(34):13562–71.

21. Piehl DW, Blancas-Mejia LM, Wall JS, et al. Immunoglobulin Light Chains Form an Extensive and Highly Ordered Fibril Involving the N- and C-Termini. ACS Omega 2017;2(2):712–20.

22. Hora M, Sarkar R, Morris V, et al. MAK33 antibody light chain amyloid fibrils are similar to oligomeric precursors. PLoS One 2017;12(7):e0181799.

23. Lecoq L, Wiegand T, Rodriguez-Alvarez FJ, et al. A Substantial Structural Conversion of the Native Monomer Leads to in-Register Parallel Amyloid Fibril Formation in Light-Chain Amyloidosis. Chembiochem 2019;20(8):1027–31.
24. Solomon A, Weiss DT, Kattine AA. Nephrotoxic potential of Bence Jones proteins. N Engl J Med 1991;324(26):1845–51.
25. Diomede L, Rognoni P, Lavatelli F, et al. A Caenorhabditis elegans-based assay recognizes immunoglobulin light chains causing heart amyloidosis. Blood 2014; 123(23):3543–52.
26. Martin EB, Williams A, Wooliver C, et al. Recruitment of human light chain proteins by synthetic fibrils is dependent on disease state and may be used to predict amyloidogenic propensity. Amyloid 2017;24(sup1):24–5.
27. Liao R, Jain M, Teller P, et al. Infusion of light chains from patients with cardiac amyloidosis causes diastolic dysfunction in isolated mouse hearts. Circulation 2001;104(14):1594–7.
28. Oberti L, Rognoni P, Barbiroli A, et al. Concurrent structural and biophysical traits link with immunoglobulin light chains amyloid propensity. Sci Rep 2017;7(1): 16809.
29. Bodi K, Prokaeva T, Spencer B, et al. AL-Base: a visual platform analysis tool for the study of amyloidogenic immunoglobulin light chain sequences. Amyloid 2009;16(1):1–8.
30. Kourelis TV, Dasari S, Theis JD, et al. Clarifying immunoglobulin gene usage in systemic and localized immunoglobulin light-chain amyloidosis by mass spectrometry. Blood 2017;129(3):299–306.
31. Garay Sanchez SA, Rodriguez Alvarez FJ, Zavala-Padilla G, et al. Stability and aggregation propensity do not fully account for the association of various germline variable domain gene segments with light chain amyloidosis. Biol Chem 2017;398(4):477–89.
32. Wall J, Schell M, Murphy C, et al. Thermodynamic instability of human λ 6 light chains: correlation with fibrillogenicity. Biochemistry 1999;38(42):14101–8.
33. Hurle MR, Helms LR, Li L, et al. A role for destabilizing amino acid replacements in light-chain amyloidosis. Proc Natl Acad Sci U S A 1994;91(12):5446–50.
34. Baden EM, Randles EG, Aboagye AK, et al. Structural insights into the role of mutations in amyloidogenesis. J Biol Chem 2008;283(45):30950–6.
35. Pokkuluri PR, Raffen R, Dieckman L, et al. Increasing protein stability by polar surface residues: domain-wide consequences of interactions within a loop. Biophys J 2002;82(1 Pt 1):391–8.
36. Raffen R, Dieckman LJ, Szpunar M, et al. Physicochemical consequences of amino acid variations that contribute to fibril formation by immunoglobulin light chains. Protein Sci 1999;8(3):509–17.
37. Myatt EA, Westholm FA, Weiss DT, et al. Pathogenic potential of human monoclonal immunoglobulin light chains: relationship of in vitro aggregation to in vivo organ deposition. Proc Natl Acad Sci U S A 1994;91(8):3034–8.
38. del Pozo Yauner L, Ortiz E, Sanchez R, et al. Influence of the germline sequence on the thermodynamic stability and fibrillogenicity of human lambda 6 light chains. Proteins 2008;72(2):684–92.
39. Nelson R, Sawaya MR, Balbirnie M, et al. Structure of the cross-beta spine of amyloid-like fibrils. Nature 2005;435(7043):773–8.
40. Tsolis AC, Papandreou NC, Iconomidou VA, et al. A consensus method for the prediction of 'aggregation-prone' peptides in globular proteins. PLoS One 2013;8(1):e54175.

41. Goto Y, Azuma T, Hamaguchi K. Refolding of the immunoglobulin light chain. J Biochem 1979;85(6):1427–38.
42. Sanchez-Ruiz JM. Protein kinetic stability. Biophys Chem 2010;148(1–3):1–15.
43. Brumshtein B, Esswein SR, Landau M, et al. Formation of amyloid fibers by monomeric light chain variable domains. J Biol Chem 2014;289(40):27513–25.
44. Brumshtein B, Esswein SR, Sawaya MR, et al. Identification of two principal amyloid-driving segments in variable domains of Ig light chains in systemic light-chain amyloidosis. J Biol Chem 2018;293(51):19659–71.
45. Nokwe CN, Hora M, Zacharias M, et al. The Antibody Light-Chain Linker Is Important for Domain Stability and Amyloid Formation. J Mol Biol 2015;427(22): 3572–86.
46. Eichner T, Radford SE. A diversity of assembly mechanisms of a generic amyloid fold. Mol Cell 2011;43(1):8–18.
47. Connors LH, Jiang Y, Budnik M, et al. Heterogeneity in primary structure, post-translational modifications, and germline gene usage of nine full-length amyloidogenic kappa1 immunoglobulin light chains. Biochemistry 2007;46(49):14259–71.
48. Lu Y, Jiang Y, Prokaeva T, et al. Oxidative Post-Translational Modifications of an Amyloidogenic Immunoglobulin Light Chain Protein. Int J Mass Spectrom 2017; 416:71–9.
49. Zottig X, Laporte Wolwertz M, Golizeh M, et al. Effects of oxidative post-translational modifications on structural stability and self-assembly of lambda6 immunoglobulin light chain. Biophys Chem 2016;219:59–68.
50. Omtvedt LA, Bailey D, Renouf DV, et al. Glycosylation of immunoglobulin light chains associated with amyloidosis. Amyloid 2000;7(4):227–44.
51. Stevens FJ. Four structural risk factors identify most fibril-forming kappa light chains. Amyloid 2000;7(3):200–11.
52. van de Bovenkamp FS, Derksen NIL, Ooijevaar-de Heer P, et al. Adaptive antibody diversification through N-linked glycosylation of the immunoglobulin variable region. Proc Natl Acad Sci U S A 2018;115(8):1901–6.
53. Kumar S, Murray D, Dasari S, et al. Assay to rapidly screen for immunoglobulin light chain glycosylation: a potential path to earlier AL diagnosis for a subset of patients. Leukemia 2019;33(1):254–7.
54. Hanson SR, Culyba EK, Hsu TL, et al. The core trisaccharide of an N-linked glycoprotein intrinsically accelerates folding and enhances stability. Proc Natl Acad Sci U S A 2009;106(9):3131–6.
55. Li Y, Wang G, Li N, et al. Structural insights into immunoglobulin M. Science 2020; 367(6481):1014–7.
56. Schmidt M, Wiese S, Adak V, et al. Cryo-EM structure of a transthyretin-derived amyloid fibril from a patient with hereditary ATTR amyloidosis. Nat Commun 2019;10(1):5008.
57. Blancas-Mejia LM, Horn TJ, Marin-Argany M, et al. Thermodynamic and fibril formation studies of full length immunoglobulin light chain AL-09 and its germline protein using scan rate dependent thermal unfolding. Biophys Chem 2015;207: 13–20.
58. Morgan GJ, Kelly JW. The Kinetic Stability of a Full-Length Antibody Light Chain Dimer Determines whether Endoproteolysis Can Release Amyloidogenic Variable Domains. J Mol Biol 2016;428(21):4280–97.
59. Rennella E, Morgan GJ, Kelly JW, et al. Role of domain interactions in the aggregation of full-length immunoglobulin light chains. Proc Natl Acad Sci U S A 2019; 116(3):854–63.

60. Pepys MB, Booth DR, Hutchinson WL, et al. Amyloid P component. A critical review. Amyloid 1997;4(4):274–95.
61. Ren R, Hong Z, Gong H, et al. Role of glycosaminoglycan sulfation in the formation of immunoglobulin light chain amyloid oligomers and fibrils. J Biol Chem 2010;285(48):37672–82.
62. Li JP, Galvis ML, Gong F, et al. In vivo fragmentation of heparan sulfate by heparanase overexpression renders mice resistant to amyloid protein A amyloidosis. Proc Natl Acad Sci U S A 2005;102(18):6473–7.
63. Blancas-Mejia LM, Ramirez Alvarado M. Recruitment of Light Chains by Homologous and Heterologous Fibrils Shows Distinctive Kinetic and Conformational Specificity. Biochemistry 2016;55(21):2967–78.
64. Jucker M, Walker LC. Propagation and spread of pathogenic protein assemblies in neurodegenerative diseases. Nat Neurosci 2018;21(10):1341–9.
65. Purro SA, Farrow MA, Linehan J, et al. Transmission of amyloid-beta protein pathology from cadaveric pituitary growth hormone. Nature 2018;564(7736):415–9.
66. Friesen M, Meyer-Luehmann M. Abeta Seeding as a Tool to Study Cerebral Amyloidosis and Associated Pathology. Front Mol Neurosci 2019;12:233.
67. Tripathi T, Khan H. Direct Interaction between the beta-Amyloid Core and Tau Facilitates Cross-Seeding: A Novel Target for Therapeutic Intervention. Biochemistry 2020;59(4):341–2.
68. Yan J, Fu X, Ge F, et al. Cross-seeding and cross-competition in mouse apolipoprotein A-II amyloid fibrils and protein A amyloid fibrils. Am J Pathol 2007;171(1):172–80.
69. Lundmark K, Westermark GT, Olsen A, et al. Protein fibrils in nature can enhance amyloid protein A amyloidosis in mice: Cross-seeding as a disease mechanism. Proc Natl Acad Sci U S A 2005;102(17):6098–102.
70. Westermark GT, Fandrich M, Lundmark K, et al. Noncerebral Amyloidoses: Aspects on Seeding, Cross-Seeding, and Transmission. Cold Spring Harb Perspect Med 2018;8(1).
71. Adams D, Gonzalez-Duarte A, O'Riordan WD, et al. Patisiran, an RNAi Therapeutic, for Hereditary Transthyretin Amyloidosis. N Engl J Med 2018;379(1):11–21.
72. Benson MD, Waddington-Cruz M, Berk JL, et al. Inotersen Treatment for Patients with Hereditary Transthyretin Amyloidosis. N Engl J Med 2018;379(1):22–31.
73. Kourelis T, Murray DL, Dasari S, et al. MASS-FIX may allow identification of patients at risk for light chain amyloidosis before the onset of symptoms. Am J Hematol 2018;93(11):E368–70.
74. Bulawa CE, Connelly S, Devit M, et al. Tafamidis, a potent and selective transthyretin kinetic stabilizer that inhibits the amyloid cascade. Proc Natl Acad Sci U S A 2012;109(24):9629–34.
75. Morgan GJ, Yan NL, Mortenson DE, et al. Stabilization of amyloidogenic immunoglobulin light chains by small molecules. Proc Natl Acad Sci U S A 2019;116(17):8360–9.
76. Brumshtein B, Esswein SR, Salwinski L, et al. Inhibition by small-molecule ligands of formation of amyloid fibrils of an immunoglobulin light chain variable domain. Elife 2015;4:e10935.
77. Wechalekar AD, Whelan C. Encouraging impact of doxycycline on early mortality in cardiac light chain (AL) amyloidosis. Blood Cancer J 2017;7(3):e546.
78. Andrich K, Hegenbart U, Kimmich C, et al. Aggregation of Full-length Immunoglobulin Light Chains from Systemic Light Chain Amyloidosis (AL) Patients Is Remodeled by Epigallocatechin-3-gallate. J Biol Chem 2017;292(6):2328–44.

79. Dember LM, Hawkins PN, Hazenberg BP, et al. Eprodisate for the treatment of renal disease in AA amyloidosis. N Engl J Med 2007;356(23):2349–60.

80. Zhou P, Ma X, Iyer L, et al. One siRNA pool targeting the lambda constant region stops lambda light-chain production and causes terminal endoplasmic reticulum stress. Blood 2014;123(22):3440–51.

81. Plate L, Cooley CB, Chen JJ, et al. Small molecule proteostasis regulators that reprogram the ER to reduce extracellular protein aggregation. Elife 2016;5: e15550.

82. Gertz MA, Landau HJ, Weiss BM. Organ response in patients with AL amyloidosis treated with NEOD001, an amyloid-directed monoclonal antibody. Am J Hematol 2016;91(12):E506–8.

83. Richards DB, Cookson LM, Barton SV, et al. Repeat doses of antibody to serum amyloid P component clear amyloid deposits in patients with systemic amyloidosis. Sci Transl Med 2018;10(422):eaan3128.

84. Eulitz M, Weiss DT, Solomon A. Immunoglobulin heavy-chain-associated amyloidosis. Proc Natl Acad Sci U S A 1990;87(17):6542–6.

85. Nasr SH, Said SM, Valeri AM, et al. The diagnosis and characteristics of renal heavy-chain and heavy/light-chain amyloidosis and their comparison with renal light-chain amyloidosis. Kidney Int 2013;83(3):463–70.

Systemic Amyloidosis due to Monoclonal Immunoglobulins: Cardiac Involvement

Sunil E. Saith, MD, MPH[a],*, Mathew S. Maurer, MD[a],
Ayan R. Patel, MD[b]

KEYWORDS

- AL amyloidosis • Cardiac disease • Light chains • Diagnosis

KEY POINTS

- Although overall survival for amyloid light chain (AL) amyloidosis has improved, mortality within 6 months to 12 months of diagnosis remains unchanged, in large part due to delayed diagnosis, with resulting cardiovascular mortality from advanced cardiac involvement.
- Those with primary cardiac involvement report a greater likelihood of being diagnosed after at least 6 months compared with those with primary renal involvement.
- Light chains not only infiltrate into the myocardium but also are directly toxic to cardiomyocytes, resulting in the generation of reactive oxygenation species and subsequent cellular apoptosis.
- AL cardiac amyloidosis requires tissue sampling to establish the diagnosis.
- Laser capture microdissection with tandem mass spectrometry is the gold standard for identifying the amyloid precursor protein, which is essential for guiding selection of the most appropriate treatment.

INTRODUCTION

Cardiac involvement is the major determinant of all-cause mortality in amyloid light chain (AL) amyloidosis. Although overall survival has improved over the past 30 years, mortality within the first 6 months to 12 months after diagnosis has remained virtually unchanged during this same period of time, in large part due to cardiovascular causes

[a] Clinical Cardiovascular Research Laboratory for the Elderly, Columbia University Irving Medical Center, 5141 Broadway 3F-034, New York, NY 10034, USA; [b] CardioVascular Center, Tufts Medical Center, 800 Washington Street, #32, Boston, MA, 02111, USA
* Corresponding author.
E-mail address: ss5286@cumc.columbia.edu
Twitter: @s7saith (S.E.S.)

Hematol Oncol Clin N Am 34 (2020) 1055–1068
https://doi.org/10.1016/j.hoc.2020.07.006
0889-8588/20/© 2020 Elsevier Inc. All rights reserved.

of death.[1] Delayed recognition and diagnosis of AL cardiac amyloidosis are common and attributable to several factors, including masquerading as more common cardiovascular conditions, given the nonspecific signs and symptoms, misconceptions about diagnosis, confusion over the role of biopsy to establish a diagnosis, and the erroneous belief that it is untreatable. In a survey of 341 patients diagnosed with AL amyloidosis, approximately 70% of patients reported being diagnosed at least 6 months after symptom onset, with one-fourth of those reporting seeing at least 6 physicians across multiple disciplines before being diagnosed.[2] Those with primary cardiac involvement report a greater likelihood of being diagnosed after at least 6 months compared with those with primary renal involvement.[2] The importance of a heightened clinical suspicion for cardiac involvement in AL amyloidosis is essential to mitigate the delays in diagnosis, which can be fatal. Previous estimates of cardiac involvement in AL amyloidosis have been reported to range from 30% to 50%. More recent estimates suggest, however, that as many as three-fourths of patients with AL amyloidosis may have cardiac involvement as either an isolated manifestation or as part of multiorgan involvement, with no difference in survival, thus further emphasizing the heart as a determinant in overall outcome.[3] This supports the need for clinicians to suspect AL cardiac amyloidosis in the differential diagnosis to facilitate more timely referral and initiation of treatment.[4]

EPIDEMIOLOGY

The most recent epidemiologic data on AL amyloidosis from the Mayo Clinic suggest an incidence of approximately 10 to 12 per million.[5] This appears to be consistent with previously published data[6] and concordant with data reported from the National Amyloidosis Centre in England, which estimates an approximate incidence of at least 8 per million.[7] The geography and diversity sampled from these populations are limited and the disease actually may be underdiagnosed in areas with less access to specialty care or in more diverse populations.[8] Initial estimates of cardiac involvement in AL amyloidosis suggested a frequency between 30% and 50%.[9] Utilizing laser capture mass spectrometry, cardiac involvement may occur as frequently as 75% in patients with AL amyloidosis.[3] Over time, almost all subjects with AL amyloidosis, if untreated, develop cardiac involvement.[5,6] The widespread use of nuclear scintigraphy, intended to diagnose transthyretin cardiac amyloidosis (ATTR-CA), may lead to an increase in the number of patients diagnosed with AL cardiac amyloidosis and, subsequently, a potential change in the epidemiology.

DELAYED DIAGNOSIS

Timely diagnosis of amyloidosis remains a challenge for both clinician and patient. Although patients are more likely to be initially referred to a cardiologist or nephrologist by their primary care physician, hematologist/oncologists are the most likely subspecialists to diagnose amyloidosis, accounting for a little over one-third of all diagnoses made.[10] Unfortunately, a referral to only 1 subspecialist from a primary care physician rarely is the case for most patients who ultimately are diagnosed with AL amyloidosis. More than 80% report seeing 3 or more physicians, over an average of 3 years, with 70% diagnosed at least 6 months after symptom onset. Cardiac involvement is 43% more likely to be diagnosed at least 6 months after symptom onset than is primary renal involvement.[2] This may be attributed to symptoms that overlap with more common causes of heart failure, such as dyspnea on exertion and fatigue. It is helpful to remember that AL amyloidosis is a systemic disease, characterized by specific signs and symptoms not otherwise associated with heart failure, which otherwise should prompt further investigation (**Box 1**).

PATHOPHYSIOLOGY

Cardiac involvement of AL amyloidosis results in a toxic infiltrative cardiomyopathy. Mutations in the variable chain region alter the kinetics and stability of the tertiary structure of the light chain.[11,12] These conformational changes favor amyloidogenesis via endoproteolytic cleavage of the unstable tertiary structure into fragments, which interact with molecular chaperones, facilitating deposition of fibrils into myocardial tissue.[12] Additionally, light chains are toxic to cardiomyocytes (**Fig. 1**). Light chain toxicity is mediated through the p38 mitogen-activated protein kinase (MAPK) signaling pathway, resulting in the generation of reactive oxygenation species, impairing cardiomyocyte contractility and leading to apoptosis.[13–17] Successful p38 inhibition has demonstrated protection against the development of myocardial cellular dysfunction.[17] Because the p38 MAPK signaling pathway is intimately involved in the transcription of brain natriuretic peptide, a direct link between the degree of light chain toxicity and elevations of the N-terminal fragment of the prohormone brain natriuretic peptide (NT-proBNP) levels has been established.[18] Accordingly, declines in the NT-proBNP follow lowering of the involved toxic light chains by anti–plasma cell therapy[19] and are a valuable biomarker effective in gauging response to treatment and predicting outcomes.[18,20] Serial measurement of NT-proBNP in AL amyloidosis is a valuable biomarker in outcomes. This contrasts with the role of NT-proBNP in decompensated heart failure, where serial changes have not been shown a reliable predictor in outcomes. AL amyloidosis results in a restrictive cardiomyopathy, leading to heart failure with typically preserved ejection fraction and tachyarrhythmias as well as brady-arrhythmias related to underlying conduction disease. In advanced stages of disease, however, left ventricular systolic dysfunction can develop.

Box 1
Red flags associated with amyloid light chain cardiac amyloidosis

- Carpal tunnel syndrome—particularly when bilateral
- Peripheral neuropathy
- Heart failure with preserved ejection fraction, often in the absence of hypertension.
- Intolerance to ACE inhibitors, angiotensin receptor blockers, or β-blockers
- Elevation of NT-proBNP out of proportion to clinical condition
- Elevated troponin T in the absence of angina or acute coronary syndrome
- Presence of macroglossia or periorbital purpura[2]
- Increased wall thickness in the absence of increased voltage on electrocardiogram (low voltage-to-mass ratio)[64,65]
- Nephrotic syndrome with hypoalbuminemia in the absence of diabetes[66]
- Factor X deficiency with bleeding either spontaneously or after procedures[67]
- Postural hypotension
- Apical sparing pattern on strain echocardiography
- Low tissue Doppler velocities

Abbreviations: ACE, Angiotensin-converting enzyme; ECG, Electrocardiogram.
   Data from Refs.[64–67]

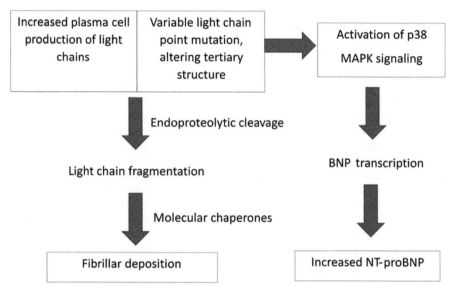

Fig. 1. Light chain disease is mediated through 2 different mechanisms. Increased plasma cell disorder and point mutations favor endoproteolytic cleavage, resulting in light chain fragmentation, which deposit into organs with molecular chaperones. Additionally, light chains activate the p38 MAPK signaling pathway. This results in increased brain natriuretic peptide (BNP) and the prohormone NT-BNP. Elevation and changes in levels have been found to correlate with degree of cardiac involvement and, consequently, overall prognosis and the rate of survival as well as assessing response to treatment.

Organ and tissue tropism in AL amyloidosis is linked with the sequence of the light chain variable region.[21,22] The first identified germline mutation associated with dominant cardiac involvement was IGVL1-44, identified through polymerase chain reaction sequencing of bone marrow plasma cells from a case-control study.[23] Utilization of a proteomics-based approach with liquid chromatography/tandem mass spectroscopy of clinical tissue led to the identification of the LV3-19 and KV1-05 genes exhibiting some cardiac tropism, with KV1-05 having a significantly decreased median survival, appearing to be associated directly to stage of cardiac involvement.[24]

DIAGNOSIS

Although imaging has facilitated the noninvasive diagnosis of ATTR-CA, confirmation of AL cardiac amyloidosis still requires pathologic verification of amyloidosis, with biopsy specimens demonstrating apple-green birefringence on Congo red staining.[25] Additionally, determining the precursor protein responsible for amyloid formation and accurate amyloidosis typing are critical for establishing diagnosis and guiding appropriate therapy.[25] Older methodologies, such as immunohistochemistry and immune-gold labeling, have been supplanted by laser capture microdissection with tandem mass spectrometry as the gold standard for typing the precursor protein.[26] Identification of amyloid fibrils on electron microscopy may be helpful in some cases. Cardiac involvement in AL amyloidosis is established by obtaining tissue through an endomyocardial biopsy (EMB), the gold standard for diagnosis. Several factors, however, limit its utilization; EMB costs may exceed $5000 and rarely can result in complications, such as perforation and resulting cardiac tamponade, associated bleeding, or induction of arrhythmias, all of which can be minimized if performed by an experienced interventionalist with technical expertise, who often is available at cardiac transplant centers.[25,27,28] Cardiac involvement alternatively may be established in the setting of a typical clinical picture, such as increased wall thickness on echocardiography or magnetic resonance imaging in the absence of a known stimulus, such as hypertension or aortic stenosis (see **Box 1**), and the presence of AL amyloidosis on an extracardiac biopsy, typically an abdominal fat pad biopsy. Abdominal fat pad biopsy typically is obtained by fine-needle aspiration, with most recent estimates of its diagnostic sensitivity ranging from 78% to 84%.[27] If clinical suspicion is high for AL amyloidosis, a negative extracardiac biopsy should not dissuade further evaluation with EMB, because it is the definitive test to evaluate for light chain cardiac amyloidosis[11] (**Fig. 2**).

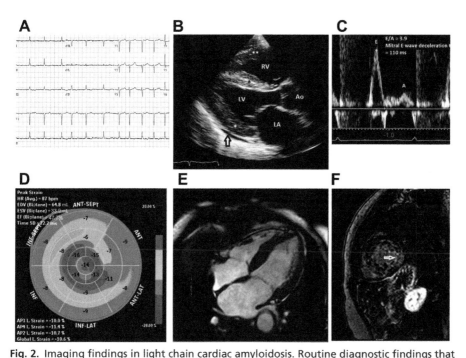

Fig. 2. Imaging findings in light chain cardiac amyloidosis. Routine diagnostic findings that may suggest AL amyloidosis. (*A*) Typical electrocardiogram findings with low limb lead voltages. (*B*) Echocardiographic parasternal long-axis view image, demonstrating findings seen in AL amyloidosis. Increased wall thickness of the interventricular septum (*black asterisk*), left ventricular posterior wall (*white asterisk*), and right ventricular free wall (*double asterisk*) is noted as well as a small posterior pericardial effusion (*arrow*), left atrial enlargement, and bright appearance of the myocardium. (*C*) Echocardiographic mitral inflow pattern showing high E/A ratio (>2) and short mitral E-wave deceleration time consistent with advanced diastolic dysfunction. (*D*) Apical sparing pattern seen on polar map of speckle-tracking 2-dimensional strain imaging. (*E*) Noncontrast CMR demonstrating increased left ventricular wall thickness and atrial enlargement. (*F*) CMR showing diffuse late enhancement pattern consistent with amyloidosis (*arrow*). ANT, Anterior; Ao, aorta; AP, Apical; Avg, Average heart rate; bpm, Beats per minute; E/A, Early (E) to late (A) ventricular filling velocity ratio; EDV, End-diastolic Volume; EF, Ejection Fraction; EKG, Electrocardiogram; ESV, End-systolic volume; HR, Heart Rate; INF, Inferior wall; LAT, Lateral wall; LA, left atrium; LV, left ventricle; RV, right ventricle; SEPT, Septal wall.

Consensus recommendations recently were established to clarify the role of imaging in diagnosis of ATTR-CA.[29,30] It is important to understand that AL amyloidosis must be excluded by assessment of monoclonal proteins for the noninvasive diagnostic algorithm using nuclear scintigraphy to be specific, because one of the common causes of a false-positive scintigraphy is AL cardiac amyloidosis.[29,31] Indeed, 20% to 40%[32] of patients with ATTR-CA can have evidence of a monoclonal protein, necessitating the performance of EMB to distinguish the presence of AL amyloidosis from monoclonal gammopathy of undetermined significance. The feasibility of PET imaging using a monoclonal antibody against amyloid fibrils is an area of active investigation to diagnose AL amyloidosis noninvasively.[33]

STAGING OF DISEASE WITH BIOMARKERS

The prognosis and extent of cardiac involvement in AL amyloidosis can be assessed according to several staging systems, which have been validated in response to anti-plasma cell therapies and stem cell transplantation (SCT). The Mayo staging system was established in 2004 as a 3-point staging system, awarding points based on cardiac biomarkers, using cutoff values of an NT-proBNP 332 ng/L or troponin T of 0.035 μg/L.[34] The initial model has been modified over time to reflect understanding of light chain synthesis in prognosticating long-term outcomes, selecting candidates for STC, and following patients during therapy. The discriminatory value of the original Mayo staging system was enhanced in 2012, by reclassifying cutpoints of NT-proBNP to 1800 ng/L and troponin T to 0.025 μg/L and by adding a free light chain difference of 18 mg/dL.[35] The National Amyloidosis Centre further identified a high-risk subset of the original Mayo stage III criteria,[36] identified now as stage IIIb, based on a combined NT-proBNP greater than 8500 ng/L and systolic blood pressure less than 100 mm Hg. This subset had an overall survival of 4 months compared with a median survival of 7.1 months in stage III.[37] As high-sensitive troponins replace cardiac troponin T in many hospitals, it has been suggested that a high-sensitive troponin value of 75 ng/mL is the correct cutpoint for the Mayo staging system.[38] A cardiac response is defined as a decrease in the NT-proBNP of 300 ng/mL from baseline below an absolute value of 600 ng/mL or a 30% decrease, whichever is greater.[39] Such responses in natriuretic peptides are predicted clinical outcome and survival,[18] and, despite these analyses being limited by their retrospective nature, prospective data have suggested similar predictive capacity.[40]

THE ROLE OF QUALITATIVE ECHOCARDIOGRAPHIC ASSESSMENTS IN PROGNOSIS

Although increased wall thickness on echocardiography suggests cardiac amyloidosis, it is not pathognomonic. Qualitative echocardiographic features can further assist clinicians in differentiating increased wall thickness due to amyloid infiltration from other causes and are recommended by the multisociety position statement on imaging if cardiac amyloidosis is suspected.[29] Strain, myocardial contraction fraction (MCF), and stroke volume index (SVI) all have demonstrated prognostic capacity independent of biomarker staging systems.[41–43] Speckle-tracking echocardiography can help characterize segmental distribution of myocardial strain, measuring changes in myocardial length in response to force. Amyloid involvement typically results in greater impaired longitudinal basal segment contraction with relative apical sparing and can differentiate amyloidosis from other causes of increased left ventricular wall thickness, such as hypertrophic cardiomyopathy, where strain patterns correspond directly to regions with the greatest degree of hypertrophy.[41] The MCF is the ratio of stroke volume to myocardial volume. Although analogous to global ejection fraction, MCF is highly correlated with global longitudinal strain, with an MCF less than 30 demonstrating an increased risk of death.[43] Similarly, SVI less than 33 mL/m^2 also has been identified as an additional cutpoint.[42]

ADVANCED IMAGING APPROACHES

Cardiac magnetic resonance imaging (CMR) with and without gadolinium has demonstrated enhanced ability over echocardiography to characterize chamber function and myocardial tissue characteristics. Amyloid infiltration of the myocardium results in an increase in extracellular volume (ECV). Late gadolinium enhancement can help characterize degree and distribution of ECV gadolinium uptake in the myocardium. The ability to characterize ECV uptake and quantify ECV over time may indicate a response to treatment.[44] The utilization of CMR may be prohibited, however, if a patient has an incompatible pacemaker, claustrophobia, or impaired renal dysfunction, which increases the risk of nephrogenic systemic fibrosis due to gadolinium contrast. Florbetapir, a Food and Drug Administration–approved isotope targeting β-amyloid deposits in Alzheimer disease, may be used in PET imaging for diagnosis of AL amyloidosis and objectively quantified using standardized uptake value ratio.[45]

TREATMENT

The neurohormonal hypothesis of heart failure, which attributes disease progression to activation of the sympathetic and renin-angiotensin-aldosterone system (RAAS), has led to the development of multiple effective therapies for heart failure with a reduced ejection fraction that reduce adverse remodeling and decrease morbidity and mortality. These therapies do not, however, address the unique underlying pathophysiologic processes in AL cardiac amyloidosis related to light chain formation and amyloid deposition in the myocardium. Accordingly, standard heart failure therapy, including angiotensin-converter enzyme (ACE) inhibitors, angiotensin receptor antagonists, and β-blockers, is of no proven benefit in patients with AL cardiac amyloidosis and may be associated with harm. Many patients with AL cardiac amyloidosis have low blood pressure from their reduced stroke volume and cardiac output as well as from concomitant autonomic dysfunction. Accordingly, RAAS antagonism can lower blood pressure further and be poorly tolerated. Additionally, because patients with AL cardiac amyloidosis have low and fixed stroke volumes, they rely on higher heart rates to maintain their cardiac output and β-adrenergic receptor antagonists may exacerbate the low flow state by reducing their compensatory higher heart rate. The goal of amyloid-directed therapy is 2-fold: lowering the concentration of circulating light chains, which can be serially measured to monitor its response,[39] and minimizing the toxicity incurred from light chain formation.[14–17]

For patients who may be candidates for SCT, it is important to understand risk factors associated with significant upfront treatment-related mortality with cardiac involvement, reported in some studies to be as high as 25%.[46–48] Although the role of SCT for AL amyloidosis in the era of modern anti–plasma cell therapy is uncertain, it remains a viable option in carefully selected patients, even among those with cardiac involvement, because, when successful, it can result in long-term survival.[49,50] Candidate selection for SCT requires a comprehensive evaluation of risk factors associated with adverse outcomes. These include age greater than 70 years, New York Heart Association functional class III or class IV, syncope, systolic blood pressure less than 100 mm Hg, low voltage on electrocardiogram, elevated cardiac biomarkers with Mayo stage III, ejection fraction less than 45%, multiorgan involvement (including renal and concomitant autonomic dysfunction reflected by orthostatic hypotension), and reduced pulmonary arterial saturations, indicative of low cardiac output on right heart catheterization. For such patients, induction therapy with bortezomib-based regimens,[51,52] in combination with daratumumab,[53,54] can reduce toxic light chains and result in organ responses, including the heart, allowing patients to become candidates for SCT. For patients with significant cardiac involvement, reducing melphalan from high to intermediate dosing has been employed, given the concern for toxicity.[55] Additional measures during the SCT to reduce treatment-related mortality include telemetry monitoring for treatment of arrhythmias, such as atrial fibrillation, atrial flutter, or ventricular tachycardia, and addressing them promptly. Attention to electrolytes and volume status also is critical.

Daratumumab is a monoclonal antibody to the CD38 antigen on plasma cells, which is found overexpressed in AL amyloidosis[56] and targets these malignant clonal cells for apoptosis with an effective hematological response and minimal toxicity.[57] The phase 3 ANDROMEDA trial demonstrated daratumumab in addition to cyclophosphamide, bortezomib, and dexamethasone was associated with significant cardiac and hematological responses in AL amyloidosis.[58] Subcutaneous daratumumab does not require any administration volume compared with the intravenous route, thus lowering the risk of volume overload. Additionally, significant cardiac toxicity that is observed with other classes of anti–plasma cell therapies is not seen with daratumumab (**Table 1**). Immunomodulatory drugs (IMiDs), such as thalidomide, lenalidomide, and pomalidomide, can cause arterial thrombosis, which can be reduced with concomitant aspirin. Therapy with IMiDs, however, is associated with increases in NT-proBNP levels that confound the interpretation of a biomarker response and should prompt consideration of switching to an alternative treatment class. Proteasome inhibitors may be associated with atrial fibrillation. If there are no contraindications to bleeding, there should be a low threshold to initiate anticoagulation, regardless of the CHA2DS2-Vasc score.

There are several recent trials examining the potential for antiamyloid therapies. NEOD001, a monoclonal antibody against an epitope in AL amyloidosis fibrils that was designed to promote macrophage-mediated clearance of amyloid fibrils from organs, including the heart, was tested in the VITAL trial. The VITAL trial was the first phase 3 randomized controlled trial using an antiamyloid agent in AL amyloidosis. The trial was terminated early, based on findings that NEOD001 did not reduce the combined endpoint of all-cause mortality or cardiovascular hospitalization compared with standard of care, although post hoc subgroup analysis did suggest a potential mortality benefit in Mayo stage IV patients with severe cardiac involvement.[59] The combination of miridesap with dezamizumab, a humanized monoclonal IgG-1 antiserum amyloid protein antibody, demonstrates removal of serum amyloid proteins, both circulating and from tissues, offering a potential treatment modality for cardiac involvement in AL amyloidosis.[60] In early phase 2 trials, however, the risk:-benefit ratio was unfavorable, prompting the sponsor to discontinue its development.[61]

Cardiac transplantation remains a last resort for treatment in carefully selected patients with isolated cardiac AL amyloidosis. Outcomes have improved in the past 10 years, attributed in part to the advent of effective anti–plasma cell therapies, especially proteasome inhibitors, which were used more widely after 2007, and careful selection of candidates for heart tranplantation.[62] Thus, in carefully selected patients with isolated cardiac involvement, outcomes in patients with AL cardiac amyloidosis undergoing cardiac transplantation do not differ significantly from patients undergoing heart transplantation for other causes.[63]

Table 1
Summary of anti–plasma cell therapies, cardiovascular side effects and methods to mitigate in amyloid light chain cardiac amyloidosis

Drug Class	Examples	Cardiovascular Side Effects/Toxicities	Approach to Minimize Side Effects
Steroids	Prednisone Dexamethasone	Volume overload Worsening heart failure	• Reduce dose (eg, dexamethasone <20 mg or lower dose) • Adjust bioavailable loop diuretic concomitant with steroid dosing
IMiDs	Lenalidomide Pomalidomide	Arterial thrombosis Anemia Increased cardiac biomarkers	• Add aspirin to prevent thrombosis • Can exacerbate underlying heart failure; avoid and, if possible, switch to another class • Discordance between cardiac biomarkers and light chain response raises concerns for fluid retention, cardiac toxicity and/or lack of validity of cardiac biomarker response with IMiDs[68]
Proteasome inhibitors	Carfilzomib Bortezomib Ixazomib	Left ventricular dysfunction Neuropathy Low blood pressure Arrhythmias	• Cardiotoxicity and left ventricular dysfunction clearly seen with carfilzomib (approximately 5%–10%)[69,70] • Uncontrolled or worsening hypertension • Gastrointestinal upset can be mistaken for right heart failure • Neuropathy manifesting as autonomic dysfunction can contribute to low blood pressure • Atrial fibrillation—surveillance and low threshold for anticoagulation if present, irrespective of CHA2DS2-Vasc score and no contraindications
Monoclonal antibodies	Daratumumab	Infusion reactions Volume overload	• Require concomitant steroids, see management above • Slow infusion rate, adjust diuretics, and consider subcutaneous administration

Data from Refs.[68–70]

SUMMARY

Although there has been significant improvement in overall survival of AL amyloidosis patients, cardiac involvement remains the determinant factor in overall survival. The time from symptom onset to confirming a diagnosis too often is prolonged due to misdiagnosis. Significant advancements have been made in the past decade, which can assist clinicians, but a heightened index of suspicion is critical to early diagnosis. Although cardiac involvement of AL amyloidosis still requires biopsy to establish a diagnosis, the establishment of novel parameters on echocardiography, adjunct imaging techniques on CMR, and PET-based approaches may facilitate early identification of affected individuals and the ability to follow amyloid load in the myocardium during therapeutic interventions. Laser capture mass spectroscopy has enabled identification of amyloid proteins with greater precision. With evidence-based success of treatment regimens and multiple ongoing trials exploring antiamyloid therapies, the ability to treat cardiac involvement with AL amyloidosis will continue to improve.

DISCLOSURE

Dr M.S. Maurer reports grant support from National Institutes of Health (R01HL139671-01), (R21AG058348), and (K24AG036778); consulting income from Pfizer, GSK, Eidos, Prothena, Akcea, and Alnylam; and Columbia University Irving Medical Center received clinical trial funding from Pfizer, Prothena, Eidos, and Alnylam. Dr A.R. Patel and Dr S.E. Saith have no financial disclosures.

REFERENCES

1. Merlini G. CyBorD: stellar response rates in AL amyloidosis. Blood 2012;119(19): 4343–5.
2. McCausland KL, White MK, Guthrie SD, et al. Light Chain (AL) amyloidosis: the journey to diagnosis. Patient 2018;11(2):207–16.
3. Muchtar E, Gertz MA, Kyle RA, et al. A modern primer on light chain amyloidosis in 592 patients with mass spectrometry-verified typing. Mayo Clin Proc 2019; 94(3):472–83.
4. Quock TP, Yan T, Chang E, et al. Epidemiology of AL amyloidosis: a real-world study using US claims data. Blood Adv 2018;2(10):1046–53.
5. Kyle RA, Larson DR, Kurtin PJ, et al. Incidence of AL Amyloidosis in Olmsted County, Minnesota, 1990 through 2015. Mayo Clin Proc 2019;94(3):465–71.
6. Kyle RA, Linos A, Beard CM, et al. Incidence and natural history of primary systemic amyloidosis in Olmsted County, Minnesota, 1950 through 1989. Blood 1992;79(7):1817–22.
7. Pinney JH, Smith CJ, Taube JB, et al. Systemic amyloidosis in England: an epidemiological study. Br J Haematol 2013;161(4):525–32.
8. Alexander KM, Orav J, Singh A, et al. Geographic disparities in reported US amyloidosis mortality from 1979 to 2015: potential underdetection of cardiac amyloidosis. JAMA Cardiol 2018;3(9):865–70.
9. Dubrey SW, Cha K, Anderson J, et al. The clinical features of immunoglobulin light-chain (AL) amyloidosis with heart involvement. QJM 1998;91(2):141–57.
10. Lousada I, Comenzo RL, Landau H, et al. Light chain amyloidosis: patient experience survey from the amyloidosis research consortium. Adv Ther 2015;32(10): 920–8.
11. Merlini G. AL amyloidosis: from molecular mechanisms to targeted therapies. Hematology Am Soc Hematol Educ Program 2017;2017(1):1–12.

12. Morgan GJ, Kelly JW. The kinetic stability of a full-length antibody light chain dimer determines whether endoproteolysis can release amyloidogenic variable domains. J Mol Biol 2016;428(21):4280–97.
13. Fine NM. Challenges and strategies in the diagnosis of cardiac amyloidosis. Can J Cardiol 2020;36(3):441–3.
14. Brenner DA, Jain M, Pimentel DR, et al. Human amyloidogenic light chains directly impair cardiomyocyte function through an increase in cellular oxidant stress. Circ Res 2004;94(8):1008–10.
15. Liao R, Jain M, Teller P, et al. Infusion of light chains from patients with cardiac amyloidosis causes diastolic dysfunction in isolated mouse hearts. Circulation 2001;104(14):1594–7.
16. Migrino RQ, Hari P, Gutterman DD, et al. Systemic and microvascular oxidative stress induced by light chain amyloidosis. Int J Cardiol 2010;145(1):67–8.
17. Shi J, Guan J, Jiang B, et al. Amyloidogenic light chains induce cardiomyocyte contractile dysfunction and apoptosis via a non-canonical p38alpha MAPK pathway. Proc Natl Acad Sci U S A 2010;107(9):4188–93.
18. Merlini G, Lousada I, Ando Y, et al. Rationale, application and clinical qualification for NT-proBNP as a surrogate end point in pivotal clinical trials in patients with AL amyloidosis. Leukemia 2016;30(10):1979–86.
19. Muchtar E, Dispenzieri A, Leung N, et al. Depth of organ response in AL amyloidosis is associated with improved survival: new proposed organ response criteria. Amyloid 2019;26(sup1):101–2.
20. Palladini G, Barassi A, Klersy C, et al. The combination of high-sensitivity cardiac troponin T (hs-cTnT) at presentation and changes in N-terminal natriuretic peptide type B (NT-proBNP) after chemotherapy best predicts survival in AL amyloidosis. Blood 2010;116(18):3426–30.
21. Comenzo RL, Zhang Y, Martinez C, et al. The tropism of organ involvement in primary systemic amyloidosis: contributions of Ig V(L) germ line gene use and clonal plasma cell burden. Blood 2001;98(3):714–20.
22. Comenzo RL, Wally J, Kica G, et al. Clonal immunoglobulin light chain variable region germline gene use in AL amyloidosis: association with dominant amyloid-related organ involvement and survival after stem cell transplantation. Br J Haematol 1999;106(3):744–51.
23. Perfetti V, Palladini G, Casarini S, et al. The repertoire of lambda light chains causing predominant amyloid heart involvement and identification of a preferentially involved germline gene, IGLV1-44. Blood 2012;119(1):144–50.
24. Kourelis TV, Dasari S, Theis JD, et al. Clarifying immunoglobulin gene usage in systemic and localized immunoglobulin light-chain amyloidosis by mass spectrometry. Blood 2017;129(3):299–306.
25. Gertz MA. Immunoglobulin light chain amyloidosis: 2016 update on diagnosis, prognosis, and treatment. Am J Hematol 2016;91(9):947–56.
26. Vrana JA, Gamez JD, Madden BJ, et al. Classification of amyloidosis by laser microdissection and mass spectrometry-based proteomic analysis in clinical biopsy specimens. Blood 2009;114(24):4957–9.
27. Quarta CC, Gonzalez-Lopez E, Gilbertson JA, et al. Diagnostic sensitivity of abdominal fat aspiration in cardiac amyloidosis. Eur Heart J 2017;38(24):1905–8.
28. Maurer MS. Noninvasive Identification of ATTRwt Cardiac Amyloid: The Re-emergence of Nuclear Cardiology. Am J Med 2015;128(12):1275–80.
29. Dorbala S, Ando Y, Bokhari S, et al. ASNC/AHA/ASE/EANM/HFSA/ISA/SCMR/SNMMI Expert Consensus Recommendations for Multimodality Imaging in

Cardiac Amyloidosis: Part 1 of 2-Evidence Base and Standardized Methods of Imaging. J Card Fail 2019;25(11):e1–39.

30. Dorbala S, Ando Y, Bokhari S, et al. ASNC/AHA/ASE/EANM/HFSA/ISA/SCMR/ SNMMI expert consensus recommendations for multimodality imaging in cardiac amyloidosis: Part 2 of 2-Diagnostic criteria and appropriate utilization. J Nucl Cardiol 2019;25(11):854–65.

31. Dorbala SBS, Miller E, Bullock-Palmer R, et al. ASNC Practice Points: 99mTechnetium-pyrophosphate imaging for transthyretin cardiac amyloidosis. 2019. Available at: https://www.asnc.org/files/19110%20ASNC%20Amyloid%20Practice%20Points%20WEB(2).pdf. Accessed August 24, 2020.

32. Gillmore JD, Maurer MS, Falk RH, et al. Nonbiopsy diagnosis of cardiac transthyretin amyloidosis. Circulation 2016;133(24):2404–12.

33. Fu JBN, Kim J, Castrillon J, et al. Real-Time PET Imaging with Amyloid Fibril-Reactive Antibody CAEL-101 for Personalized AL amyloidosis immunotherapy. Clin Lymphoma Myeloma Leuk 2019;19(10):E314.

34. Dispenzieri A, Gertz MA, Kyle RA, et al. Serum cardiac troponins and N-terminal pro-brain natriuretic peptide: a staging system for primary systemic amyloidosis. J Clin Oncol 2004;22(18):3751–7.

35. Kumar S, Dispenzieri A, Lacy MQ, et al. Revised prognostic staging system for light chain amyloidosis incorporating cardiac biomarkers and serum free light chain measurements. J Clin Oncol 2012;30(9):989–95.

36. Wechalekar AD, Schonland SO, Kastritis E, et al. A European collaborative study of treatment outcomes in 346 patients with cardiac stage III AL amyloidosis. Blood 2013;121(17):3420–7.

37. Manwani R, Foard D, Mahmood S, et al. Rapid hematologic responses improve outcomes in patients with very advanced (stage IIIb) cardiac immunoglobulin light chain amyloidosis. Haematologica 2018;103(4):e165–8.

38. Muchtar E, Kumar SK, Gertz MA, et al. Staging systems use for risk stratification of systemic amyloidosis in the era of high-sensitivity troponin T assay. Blood 2019; 133(7):763–6.

39. Palladini G, Lavatelli F, Russo P, et al. Circulating amyloidogenic free light chains and serum N-terminal natriuretic peptide type B decrease simultaneously in association with improvement of survival in AL. Blood 2006;107(10):3854–8.

40. Palladini G, Dispenzieri A, Gertz MA, et al. New criteria for response to treatment in immunoglobulin light chain amyloidosis based on free light chain measurement and cardiac biomarkers: impact on survival outcomes. J Clin Oncol 2012;30(36): 4541–9.

41. Quarta CC, Solomon SD, Uraizee I, et al. Left ventricular structure and function in transthyretin-related versus light-chain cardiac amyloidosis. Circulation 2014; 129(18):1840–9.

42. Milani P, Dispenzieri A, Scott CG, et al. Independent prognostic value of stroke volume index in patients with immunoglobulin light chain amyloidosis. Circ Cardiovasc Imaging 2018;11(5):e006588.

43. Tendler A, Helmke S, Teruya S, et al. The myocardial contraction fraction is superior to ejection fraction in predicting survival in patients with AL cardiac amyloidosis. Amyloid 2015;22(1):61–6.

44. Banypersad SM. The evolving role of cardiovascular magnetic resonance imaging in the evaluation of systemic amyloidosis. Magn Reson Insights 2019;12. 1178623X19843519.

45. Ehman EC, El-Sady MS, Kijewski MF, et al. Early detection of multiorgan light-chain amyloidosis by whole-body (18)F-florbetapir PET/CT. J Nucl Med 2019; 60(9):1234–9.
46. Muchtar E, Lin G, Grogan M. The challenges in chemotherapy and stem cell transplantation for light-chain amyloidosis. Can J Cardiol 2020;36(3):384–95.
47. Varga C, Comenzo RL. High-dose melphalan and stem cell transplantation in systemic AL amyloidosis in the era of novel anti-plasma cell therapy: a comprehensive review. Bone Marrow Transplant 2019;54(4):508–18.
48. Jaccard A, Moreau P, Leblond V, et al. High-dose melphalan versus melphalan plus dexamethasone for AL amyloidosis. N Engl J Med 2007;357(11).1083–93.
49. Sharpley FA, Petrie A, Mahmood S, et al. A 24-year experience of autologous stem cell transplantation for light chain amyloidosis patients in the United Kingdom. Br J Haematol 2019;187(5):642–52.
50. Sidana S, Sidiqi MH, Dispenzieri A, et al. Fifteen year overall survival rates after autologous stem cell transplantation for AL amyloidosis. Am J Hematol 2019; 94(9):1020–6.
51. Gupta VK, Brauneis D, Shelton AC, et al. Induction therapy with bortezomib and dexamethasone and conditioning with high-dose melphalan and bortezomib followed by autologous stem cell transplantation for immunoglobulin light chain amyloidosis: long-term follow-up analysis. Biol Blood Marrow Transplant 2019; 25(5):e169–73.
52. Landau H, Lahoud O, Devlin S, et al. Pilot study of bortezomib and dexamethasone pre- and post-risk-adapted autologous stem cell transplantation in AL amyloidosis. Biol Blood Marrow Transplant 2020;26(1):204–8.
53. Chung A, Kaufman GP, Sidana S, et al. Organ responses with daratumumab therapy in previously treated AL amyloidosis. Blood Adv 2020;4(3):458–66.
54. Roussel M, Merlini G, Chevret S, et al. A prospective phase II of daratumumab in previously treated systemic light chain amyloidosis (AL) patients. Blood 2020; 135(18):1531.
55. Cohen AD, Zhou P, Chou J, et al. Risk-adapted autologous stem cell transplantation with adjuvant dexamethasone +/- thalidomide for systemic light-chain amyloidosis: results of a phase II trial. Br J Haematol 2007;139(2):224–33.
56. Seckinger A, Hillengass J, Emde M, et al. CD38 as immunotherapeutic target in light chain amyloidosis and multiple myeloma-association with molecular entities, risk, survival, and mechanisms of upfront resistance. Front Immunol 2018;9:1676.
57. Kaufman GP, Schrier SL, Lafayette RA, et al. Daratumumab yields rapid and deep hematologic responses in patients with heavily pretreated AL amyloidosis. Blood 2017;130(7):900–2.
58. Palladini G, Kastritis E, Maurer MS, et al. Daratumumab Plus CyBorD for patients with newly diagnosed AL amyloidosis: safety run-in results of ANDROMEDA. Blood 2020;136(1):71–80.
59. Gertz M, Cohen AD, Comenzo RL, et al. Results of the Phase 3 VITAL Study of NEOD001 (Birtamimab) Plus Standard of Care in Patients with Light Chain (AL) Amyloidosis Suggest Survival Benefit for Mayo Stage IV Patients. Blood 2019; 134:3166.
60. Richards DB, Cookson LM, Barton SV, et al. Repeat doses of antibody to serum amyloid P component clear amyloid deposits in patients with systemic amyloidosis. Sci Transl Med 2018;10(422):eaan3128.
61. Edwards CV, Bhutani D, Mapara M, et al. One year follow up analysis of the phase 1a/b study of chimeric fibril-reactive monoclonal antibody 11-1F4 in patients with AL amyloidosis. Amyloid 2019;26(sup1):115–6.

62. Mehra MR, Canter CE, Hannan MM, et al. The 2016 International Society for Heart Lung Transplantation listing criteria for heart transplantation: A 10-year update. J Heart Lung Transplant 2016;35(1):1–23.

63. Kristen AV, Kreusser MM, Blum P, et al. Improved outcomes after heart transplantation for cardiac amyloidosis in the modern era. J Heart Lung Transplant 2018; 37(5):611–8.

64. Zhao L, Li J, Tian Z, et al. Clinical correlates and prognostic values of pseudoinfarction in cardiac light-chain amyloidosis. J Cardiol 2016;68(5):426–30.

65. Sperry BW, Vranian MN, Hachamovitch R, et al. Are classic predictors of voltage valid in cardiac amyloidosis? A contemporary analysis of electrocardiographic findings. Int J Cardiol 2016;214:477–81.

66. Bever KM, Masha LI, Sun F, et al. Risk factors for venous thromboembolism in immunoglobulin light chain amyloidosis. Haematologica 2016;101(1):86–90.

67. Patel G, Hari P, Szabo A, et al. Acquired factor X deficiency in light-chain (AL) amyloidosis is rare and associated with advanced disease. Hematol Oncol Stem Cell Ther 2019;12(1):10–4.

68. Dispenzieri A, Dingli D, Kumar SK, et al. Discordance between serum cardiac biomarker and immunoglobulin-free light-chain response in patients with immunoglobulin light-chain amyloidosis treated with immune modulatory drugs. Am J Hematol 2010;85(10):757–9.

69. Dimopoulos MA, Roussou M, Gavriatopoulou M, et al. Cardiac and renal complications of carfilzomib in patients with multiple myeloma. Blood Adv 2017;1(7): 449–54.

70. Danhof S, Schreder M, Rasche L, et al. 'Real-life' experience of preapproval carfilzomib-based therapy in myeloma - analysis of cardiac toxicity and predisposing factors. Eur J Haematol 2016;97(1):25–32.

Renal Involvement in Systemic Amyloidosis Caused by Monoclonal Immunoglobulins

Sabine Karam, MD[a], Nelson Leung, MD[b],*

KEYWORDS

- Renal amyloidosis • AL amyloidosis • AH amyloidosis • AH/AL amyloidosis
- Monoclonal immunoglobulins

KEY POINTS

- AL amyloidosis is the most common form of systemic amyloidosis in the western world.
- Kidney is one of the most common organs involved in AL amyloidosis.
- Proteinuria often with full nephrotic syndrome and mild but progressive renal insufficiency are the most common presentation.
- Patients with renal AL amyloidosis are at risk to progress to end stage kidney disease if deep hematologic response is not achieved.

INTRODUCTION

Amyloidosis refers to a group of disorders that stems from the ability of certain proteins to adopt an unstable tertiary structure by misfolding and aggregating. The misfolding and aggregation lead to polymerization into insoluble amyloid fibrils and deposition in the extracellular space of tissues, ultimately causing organ damage and significant morbidity and mortality. The formation of amyloid fibrils follows a complex mechanism that is affected by several factors. Ultimately, it is a deficiency in proteostasis that leads to the accumulation of said proteins.[1] More than 30 precursors of amyloid fibrils have been identified, with many that have been added recently.[2] They range from normal native proteins to ill-produced monoclonal immunoglobulins.[1,2] The most common form of systemic amyloidosis is secondary to monoclonal immunoglobulins.

---

[a] Division of Nephrology and Hypertension, Saint George Hospital University Medical Center, PO Box 166 378 Achrafieh, Beirut 11 00 2807, Lebanon; [b] Division of Nephrology and Hypertension, Division of Hematology, Mayo Clinic, 200 1st Street Southwest, Rochester, MN 55905, USA
* Corresponding author.
E-mail address: leung.nelson@mayo.edu
Twitter: @sabinekaram6 (S.K.)

Hematol Oncol Clin N Am 34 (2020) 1069–1079
https://doi.org/10.1016/j.hoc.2020.08.002
0889-8588/20/© 2020 Elsevier Inc. All rights reserved.

Systemic amyloidosis caused by monoclonal immunoglobulin deposition (Alg) includes immunoglobulin light chain (AL) amyloidosis, immunoglobulin heavy chain (AH) amyloidosis, and immunoglobulin heavy and light chain (AHL) amyloidosis. All 3 types are associated with a plasma cell clonal proliferative disorder that ranges from low tumor burden to full-blown multiple myeloma[3] and can affect all organs except the central nervous system. The 2 most commonly affected organs are the heart and the kidneys, but the liver, nervous system (both autonomic and peripheral), gastrointestinal tract, and others can also be affected.[1,4,5] Patients usually present with a constellation of signs and symptoms that should raise clinical suspicion for amyloidosis.[1] Although cardiac involvement is the primary predictor of mortality, renal involvement does affect quality of life and limits treatment options. Renal involvement is also a major cause of morbidity. Patients with renal amyloidosis often progress to end-stage renal disease (ESRD) and require dialysis if inadequately treated[6,7] This article discusses the specifics of renal involvement in AL, AH, and AHL amyloidosis with regard to epidemiology, clinical and pathologic diagnosis, and prognosis.

EPIDEMIOLOGY

Data concerning epidemiology have been limited because there are no large databases to collect information about the disease.[1] However, studies on the incidence of AL have been conducted both in France and the United States. In the United States, the incidence across various studies ranges from 9 to 12 persons per million per year.[4,8] In France, the incidence was 12.5 persons per million per year over a 5-year period.[1] AL amyloidosis is the most common type of systemic amyloidosis in western countries, and it represents around 85% of Alg amyloidosis but is 5 to 10 times less frequent than multiple myeloma.[3,4] The prevalence of AL amyloidosis increases with age, with those aged more than 65 years having double the prevalence of those between 35 and 54 years.[1,2,5] The average age at diagnosis is 65 years. AL amyloidosis is slightly more common in men than in women, with men making up 55% of the cases. Risk factors for developing AL amyloidosis include the preexistence of monoclonal gammopathy of unknown significance[9] and the existence of particular single nucleotide polymorphisms.[10] Light chains deposit in the kidneys in around 65% to 70% of patients with AL amyloidosis,[2,4] and renal involvement is more frequent for patients with the lambda subtype.[11] In addition, patients with renal involvement tend to be younger than patients without.[12] Renal involvement is more frequent in patients with low free light chain (FLC) burden, often with a difference between involved and uninvolved FLC (dFLC) of less than 50 mg/L.[13,14] AH and AHL amyloidosis represent 15% of the remaining cases of Alg amyloidosis. Similarly to AL amyloidosis, AH and AHL amyloidosis tend to affect older patients and have a male predominance. They are also always associated with some form of plasma cell dyscrasia, which can range from low tumor burden to full-blown multiple myeloma.[3,5] Around 75% of patients with AH and AHL amyloidosis have renal involvement.[5]

PATHOGENESIS

Amyloidosis requires the normally globular and soluble proteins to undergo misfolding and aggregation into insoluble fibrils with a cross-β-sheet quaternary structure that eventually deposit extracellularly in tissues.[1,5] Proteostasis, the process that keeps proteins in adequate concentrations in the right locations, malfunctions in amyloidosis. Several factors contribute to this transformation: an increase in production or a decrease in clearance of a protein, destabilization of the native structure through a mutation, and advanced age contributing to some proteins being more likely to form fibrils.[1] More specifically, AL amyloidosis is caused by overproduction of a lambda or kappa immunoglobulin light chain by clonal plasma cells.[1,2] Around 75% to 80% of cases involve lambda light chain, with a large proportion being λ_{VI} family, specifically IGLV6-57. One factor that allows certain light chains to form fibrils is the formation of an unstable and insoluble fragment after uptake by certain cells.[2,15] Changes in pH may affect the stability of precursor proteins and hence favor fibrillogenesis.[16] The ability of light chain amyloid fibrils to deposit in the kidneys also requires certain interactions.[16] The mechanism that makes certain organs, such as the kidneys, more likely to be involved remains elusive; however, certain structural features related to the germline gene, such as IGLV6-57, may give rise to light chains that are more likely to form amyloid fibrils that interact with mesangial cells of the kidneys.[1,15,16] IGLV6-57 has been shown to be more common in patients with AL amyloidosis and renal involvement.[1] Other factors include interactions with glycosaminoglycans (GAGs), which are found in high concentrations in the glomerular basement membrane and promote fibrillogenesis and amyloid formation. It has been suggested that GAGs might also play a role in protecting the amyloid deposits from proteolysis during formation and after deposition.[16]

CLINICAL PRESENTATION

Renal dysfunction is one of the most common clinical manifestations of Alg amyloidosis.[17,18] Proteinuria is the most common presenting feature, with most patients presenting with nephrotic-range proteinuria (>3 g/24 h).[2,4,12,19] Proteinuria as high as 20 to 30 g/24 h has been reported.[16] The proteinuria consists mostly of albumin, which leads to hypoalbuminemia and full nephrotic syndrome.[2,4,16,19] A decreased glomerular filtration rate is present in 20% to 45% of patients with AL amyloidosis.[17,18,20,21] A creatinine level greater than 2 mg/dL is reported in 18% of patients with AL amyloidosis[20] and in 26% in a series of patients that includes AH and AHL as well.[21] Approximately 10% of patients are already on dialysis at presentation.[17] Most patients progress to ESRD and require dialysis if left untreated or undertreated.[1,7,16,19] The survival of patients with AL amyloidosis on dialysis is significantly inferior compared to dialysis patients without amyloidosis.[22]

Patients with AL amyloidosis with kidney involvement have some distinctive characteristics. Compared with patients with AL-lambda, those with AL-kappa tend to have a higher serum creatinine level (2.2 mg/dL vs 1.7 mg/dL; $P = .001$), higher serum albumin level (2.8 g/dL vs 2.4 g/dL; $P = .01$), and a lower frequency of full nephrotic syndrome (52% vs 72%; $P = .002$).[21] Another observation is that patients with renal-limited AL amyloidosis have lower involved serum FLC levels than patients with cardiac amyloidosis.[23] Patients with renal-limited amyloidosis are also more likely to have higher estimated glomerular filtration rate (eGFR) and 24-hour proteinuria along with higher systolic blood pressure.[12] However, cardiac involvement is significantly less common in patients with AH and AHL amyloidosis compared with renal AL amyloidosis.[5] Amyloid deposition in the kidneys may also lead to kidney enlargement in some cases.[4,16]

Two staging systems have been devised to assess the extent of renal damage and prognosticate the risk of progression to dialysis.[24,25] In 2014, Palladini and colleagues[24] developed a staging system that relied on proteinuria and eGFR. The system has 3 distinct stages, with stage 1 being characterized by proteinuria less than 5 g/24-h urine collection and an eGFR greater than 50 mL/min/1.73 m^2, stage 2 by proteinuria greater than 5 g/24-h urine collection or an eGFR less than 50 mL/min/1.73 m^2, and stage 3 is defined by both proteinuria greater than 5 g/24-h urine collection and an eGFR less than 50 mL/min/1.73 m^2.[1] The risk of progression to dialysis at 2 years was 1%, 12%, and 48% respectively.[1,24] This system is has some shortcomings because its criteria for progression are based solely on eGFR reduction.[26] Kastritis and colleagues[26] proposed a new staging system that is based on the ratio of proteinuria to eGFR and that would allow better monitoring of progression of renal disease.[25] This system also has 3 distinct stages, with stage 1 being characterized by proteinuria/eGFR less than 30 mg/mL/min/1.73 m^2, stage 2 by proteinuria/eGFR between 31 and 99 mg/mL/min/1.73 m^2, and stage 3 by proteinuria/eGFR $\geq$100 mg/mL/min/1.73 m^2.[26] This system is unique in that it allows early identification of effects of treatment on renal function.[25,26] Data showed that those patients who achieved a reduction of this ratio by at least 25%, or who achieved reduction to less than a 100 (if initially higher) at 3 months, had negligible risk of progression to dialysis at 2 years versus a 24% rate of progression to dialysis in those who had no reduction or maintained a ratio greater than 100. Kastritis and colleagues[26] found similar results when applied at 6 months.

DIAGNOSIS AND PATHOLOGY OF RENAL AMYLOIDOSIS
Laboratory Features

Protein electrophoresis with its sensitivity limited to a concentration of 500 mg/L[27] should not be used as a screening modality alone because more than one-third of patients with AL amyloidosis do not have a detectable monoclonal spike in serum.[28] Patients with suspected AL amyloidosis should also be screened instead by immunofixation electrophoresis (IFE) of serum and urine, a modality that is more sensitive (150 mg/L) and allows characterization of the isotype.[1,2] However, the most sensitive technique is nephelometric quantification of the serum FLCs.[28,29] The combination of serum and urine IFE with an FLC assay yields a 97% diagnostic sensitivity for monoclonal protein detection.[28] A 24-hour urine protein measurement is also a part of the initial screening.[17] Acknowledging that a 24-hour urine collection is cumbersome, Palladini and colleagues[24] validated the usage of urinary albumin/creatinine ratio (UACR) instead. For diagnosis of renal involvement, a UACR ratio of 500 mg/g was used to correlate to a 24-hour urinary protein of 0.5 g; the UACR can also be used to predict renal outcome, and possibly to assess renal response in AL amyloidosis.[19]

Pathology

Laboratory features alone cannot confirm the diagnosis of renal amyloidosis given the frequency of monoclonal gammopathies in patients more than 50 years of age.[30] A renal biopsy showing amyloid deposits is ultimately required.[1,4,16] If this is not feasible, histologic evidence from another tissue, such as subcutaneous fat aspirate, lip biopsy, or bone marrow biopsy, with proteinuria exceeding 0.5 g/24-h urine collection is usually enough.[31–33] However, a kidney biopsy provides the highest level of accuracy and allows evaluation of the kidney tissue for prognostic purposes.[5,16] Under light microscopy, amyloid appears as pink deposits that are periodic acid–Schiff negative to weakly positive, trichrome blue or gray, and silver negative.[21] Amyloid deposits give off a specific apple-green birefringence when viewed under polarized light with Congo red stain.[21] Amyloid deposits are seen in the mesangium in 97% and along the glomerular basement membranes in 87% of patients with AL amyloidosis (**Fig. 1**). Deposits are also found in the vasculature in 85% of patients. The distribution of amyloid deposits in the 3 renal compartments (glomeruli, tubulointerstitium, and vessels) is similar between AL and AH/AHL amyloidosis.[4,5,16] Electron microscopy shows

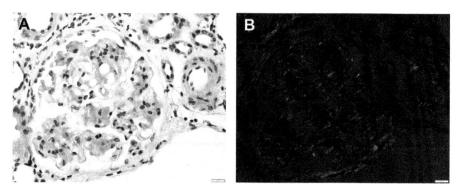

Fig. 1. (*A*) Congo red stain showing congophilic deposits in the glomerulus (mesangium and glomerular basement membranes), interstitium, and the vascular walls. (*B*) Deposits showed a characteristic apple-green birefringence under polarized light. (*Courtesy of* Mariam P Alexander MD, Mayo Clinic, Rochester, MN.)

nonbranching solid fibrils with diameters of 8 to 10 nm that lack any orientation and pattern. After identification of amyloid, typing is of vital importance because it has implications for therapeutic interventions.[34] Typing relies on the demonstration of light chain restriction for AL and AHL amyloidosis and heavy chain restriction for AH amyloidosis on immunofluorescence (IF) microscopy on frozen sections or immunohistochemistry (IHC) on paraffin-embedded tissue sections.[2,4,35] In the diagnosis of AL amyloidosis, IF seems to be more reliable, with a higher rate of successful typing than IHC.[4,36] Local proteolysis of light chain in amyloid deposits may cause partial or complete destruction of the constant domain, which is the target of commercial antibodies, thus antibodies from multiple vendors should be used to increase sensitivity.[4,34] IF studies may be negative for both kappa and lambda light chains in up to 35% of renal AL amyloidosis cases and have been shown to even have a lower sensitivity and specificity for AH and AHL compared with AL amyloidosis.[2,35] This finding has led to development of better tests. Laser microdissection (LMD) followed by mass spectrometry (MS)–based proteomics is currently the most sensitive and specific method of typing amyloid (**Fig. 2**).[37] LMD/MS can identify any protein as long as its proteome is in the database, which is an advantage compared with IF/IHC, which requires a separate test for each protein suspected of forming the amyloid.[34] If the test is not performed on IF/IHC, the protein cannot be identified but LMD/MS compares the proteomic signature with all known protein in the database.[35] In 1 study from 2009, Vrana and colleagues[37] found that LMD/MS was successful in identifying amyloid type in 98% of amyloidosis cases compared with 42% for IHC. A recent study from the Mayo Clinic found IF has a sensitivity of 85% and specificity of 92% when LMD/MS was used as the gold standard.[38] The disadvantage of LMD/MS is the expertise required, which limits its use to a few academic medical centers. Immunoelectron microscopy (IEM) has been in use since at least 1989 and presents a viable alternative to MS.[39,40] It combines IHC and electron microscopy by using gold-labeled secondary antibodies that colocalize the protein within the amyloid fibrils while reducing background staining.[39,40] IEM has been found to be equally sensitive compared with Congo red–based light microscopy (75% vs 80%) but more specific (100% vs 80%); it was able to correctly identify the specific form of amyloidosis in greater than 99% of cases in a prospective study from 2015 that was done on abdominal fat aspirates.[40] IEM of abdominal fat aspirates presents an effective tool in the routine diagnosis of systemic amyloidosis.[40]

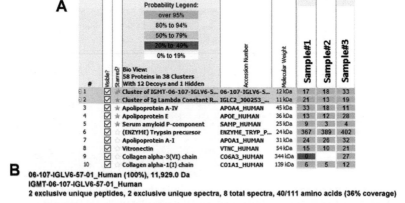

B 06-107-IGLV6-57-01_Human (100%), 11,929.0 Da
IGMT-06-107-IGLV6-57-01_Human
2 exclusive unique peptides, 2 exclusive unique spectra, 8 total spectra, 40/111 amino acids (36% coverage)

```
NFMLTQPHSV  SESPGKTVTI  SCTRSSGNIA  SNYVQWYQQR  PGSAPTTVIY
EDNQRPSGVP  DRFSGSIDSS  SNSASLSISG  LKTEDEADYY  CQSYDSGIFV
VFGGGTKLTV  L
```

Fig. 2. Detection of light chain variable regions from amyloid samples. Congo red–positive amyloid deposits were isolated from biopsy specimens using LMD. Each LMD sample was analyzed using MS and peptides were matched to human proteome augmented with immunoglobulin light chain variable region sequences as described previously (PMID: 19797517,25734799). (A) Protein identification report showing the detection of clonal lambda light chain constant and variable region. Numbers in green boxes represent the number of MS/MS spectra matching to each protein in each sample. Proteins highlighted with yellow stars are generic amyloid markers (PMID: 24747948). Immunoglobulin lambda light chain protein is highlighted with a blue star. Double star highlights the variable region of LV6-57 clonal protein detected in the deposit. (B) Sequence coverage plot of the LV6-57 protein in sample 1. Yellow highlighted portions were detected by the MS method. (Courtesy of Surendra Dasari PhD, Mayo Clinic, Rochester, MN.)

Imaging Methods

The ^{123}I serum amyloid P component (SAP) scintigraphy has been used since the 1980s to detect amyloid deposits in the body.[41] Not only is it useful for diagnosis but it can also be used to assess response to treatment. Although the ^{123}I-SAP is a fairly sensitive and specific nuclear tracer in the kidneys and other organs, 1 deficit is the inability to detect amyloid in the heart.[42,43] SAP scintigraphy is also not approved by the US Food and Drug Administration. Radionuclide imaging methods using 99m-Tc aprotinin or iodinated serum amyloid represent an added tool in the assessment of amyloid deposits.[42,43] In 2003, Schaadt and colleagues[42] sampled 23 patients with known or suspected amyloidosis; they were given 99m-Tc aprotinin intravenous injections and subsequently imaged. Focal accumulations were seen in 22 patients, in whom 20 were confirmed via biopsy or autopsy. Amyloid deposits were also revealed in 5 patients who showed no symptoms at the time but later developed clinical symptoms of amyloidosis.[42] Although found to be useful in detection of a wide range of lesions, including cardiac lesions, 99m-Tc aprotinin scintigraphy is not suitable for renal or bladder assessment because it is excreted through the kidneys.[42,43] More recently, a ^{125}I-labeled peptide named P5+14 has shown high sensitivity of detecting amyloid deposits in all organs by dual energy single-photon emission computed tomography imaging.[44] A clinical trial with P5+14 as an imaging agent is ongoing.

Recent Advances

Growth differentiation factor-15 (GDF-15) is a new biomarker that is released by cardiac myocytes in response to certain stressors and that plays a role in assessment of prognosis and response to therapy in patients with cardiovascular diseases.[45] Kastritis and colleagues[45] explored GDF-15 in 2 independent cohorts of patients from Italy and Greece. They concluded that decrease in GDF-15 level during therapy was associated with better renal outcomes and better survival, whereas a failure in early reduction in levels of GDF-15 less than 4000 pg/mL (either at 3 or 6 months) carried a greater risk for progression to dialysis. GDF-15 level is hence probably the strongest predictor of renal outcomes in patients with AL amyloidosis.[45]

A Mayo Clinic study from 2012 investigated the role of urinary exosomes in patients with AL amyloidosis and concluded that, in patients with no renal response to treatment or in those with worsening renal progression, urinary exosomes contained high-molecular-weight immunoreactive species corresponding with a decamer of light chains.[46] Some patients who were found to have a complete hematologic response but worsening of renal function were also reported to have exosomes with that same decamer. This finding suggests urinary exosomes may play a role in assessment of renal response in patients with Al amyloidosis.[47]

It has been reported that kappa and lambda chains occasionally exist as glycosylated and cysteinylated forms in patients with AL amyloidosis, implying that posttranslational modifications (PTMs) play an important role in amyloidogenicity.[35,48,49] Recently, a study found that patients with AL amyloidosis occasionally have atypical spectra corresponding with PTMs of their kappa light chains consistent with glycosylation by a special MS test called MASS-FIX.[48] This technique may allow clinicians to identify patients at risk of developing amyloidosis.[50]

Treatment

The treatment of renal AL amyloidosis is similar to AL amyloidosis in other organs, which is discussed elsewhere in this issue. However, there are several issues specific to the kidney that should be kept in mind when caring for these patients. First, kidney function should be considered when choosing chemotherapy. Of the chemotherapy available, lenalidomide is the one that is most dependent on renal clearance. Dose reduction of lenalidomide is needed when eGFR decreases to less than 50 mL/min/1.73 m^2.[51] Further reduction is required when eGFR decreases to less than 30 mL/min/1.73 m^2 and again when the patient becomes dialysis dependent.[52] In addition, a small study suggests possible increased nephrotoxicity with lenalidomide in patients with AL amyloidosis.[53] Close monitoring of the kidney function is recommended, especially when starting lenalidomide in patients with impaired kidney function. Another medication that requires dose reduction with renal impairment is ixazomib when the eGFR decreases to less than 30 mL/min/1.73 m^2.[54] Fluid retention with steroids is another concern in patients with severe nephrotic syndrome. Dexamethasone is a glucocorticoid that should not have any sodium retention activity. However, a group of enzymes (11β-hydroxysteroid dehydrogenases) interconverts inactive glucocorticoids to active mineralocorticoids, thus giving dexamethasone mineralocorticoid activity.[55] In patients with volume overload and severe nephrotic syndrome, dexamethasone dose should be reduced until adequate diuresis can be established. In addition, patients with advanced renal involvement may have a short window for renal preservation to occur. In a study from the UK Amyloidosis Centre, patients with advanced renal involvement as defined by an eGFR of less than 20 mL/min/1.73 m^2 required a deep hematologic response (>90% reduction of dFLC) in order to prevent the progression to ESRD.[7] However, the 90% reduction in dFLC was only effective at preventing ESRD if it could be achieved in the first 3 months. Patients who achieved a 90% reduction in dFLC at 12 months still progressed to ESRD. Survival of patients with AL amyloidosis is inferior to those without amyloidosis on dialysis[22]; however, they have good outcomes after kidney transplant. Multiple studies have found excellent graft and patient survival if a deep hematologic response (very good partial response or better) can be achieved before or after kidney transplant.[56–59]

SUMMARY

Kidney involvement in Alg amyloidosis is common. Although patients with renal-limited Alg amyloidosis tend not to have the high mortality that patients with cardiac amyloidosis have, they do experience significant morbidity and impact on quality of life. Despite the discovery of some unique features, such as higher prevalence of light chains from the IGLV6-57 gene family and lower FLC levels than patients with cardiac amyloidosis, the complexity of the pathogenesis remains incompletely understood. Models have been established to prognosticate and assess for the response to therapy, which help guide the development of better treatment. Patients with advanced renal impairment from AL amyloidosis still have poor renal prognosis, and better therapy is needed in order to preserve kidney function. Patients who develop ESRD can undergo renal replacement therapy with kidney transplant.

DISCLOSURE

The authors have nothing to disclose.

REFERENCES

1. Merlini G, Dispenzieri A, Sanchorawala V, et al. Systemic immunoglobulin light chain amyloidosis. Nat Rev Dis Primers 2018;4:38.
2. Rysava R. AL amyloidosis: advances in diagnostics and treatment. Nephrol Dial Transplant 2019;34:1460–6.
3. Picken MM. Non-light-chain immunoglobulin amyloidosis: time to expand or refine the spectrum to include light+heavy chain amyloidosis? Kidney Int 2013; 83:353–6.
4. Desport E, Bridoux F, Sirac C, et al. Al amyloidosis. Orphanet J Rare Dis 2012; 7:54.
5. Nasr SH, Said SM, Valeri AM, et al. The diagnosis and characteristics of renal heavy-chain and heavy/light-chain amyloidosis and their comparison with renal light-chain amyloidosis. Kidney Int 2013;83:463–70.
6. Gertz MA, Leung N, Lacy MQ, et al. Clinical outcome of immunoglobulin light chain amyloidosis affecting the kidney. Nephrol Dial Transplant 2009;24:3132–7.
7. Rezk T, Lachmann HJ, Fontana M, et al. Prolonged renal survival in light chain amyloidosis: speed and magnitude of light chain reduction is the crucial factor. Kidney Int 2017;92:1476–83.
8. Kyle RA, Larson DR, Kurtin PJ, et al. Incidence of AL amyloidosis in Olmsted county, Minnesota, 1990 through 2015. Mayo Clin Proc 2019;94:465–71.
9. Kyle RA, Larson DR, Therneau TM, et al. Long-term follow-up of monoclonal gammopathy of undetermined significance. N Engl J Med 2018;378:241–9.
10. da Silva Filho MI, Forsti A, Weinhold N, et al. Genome-wide association study of immunoglobulin light chain amyloidosis in three patient cohorts: comparison with myeloma. Leukemia 2017;31:1735–42.
11. Sidiqi MH, Aljama MA, Muchtar E, et al. Light chain type predicts organ involvement and survival in AL amyloidosis patients receiving stem cell transplantation. Blood Adv 2018;2:769–76.

12. Muchtar E, Gertz MA, Kyle RA, et al. A modern primer on light chain amyloidosis in 592 patients with mass spectrometry-verified typing. Mayo Clin Proc 2019;94: 472–83.
13. Milani P, Basset M, Russo F, et al. Patients with AL amyloidosis and low free light-chain burden have distinct clinical features and outcome. Amyloid 2017;24:64–5.
14. Nguyen VP, Rosenberg A, Mendelson LM, et al. Outcomes of patients with AL amyloidosis and low serum free light chain levels at diagnosis. Amyloid 2018; 25:156–9.
15. Keeling J, Teng J, Herrera GA. AL-amyloidosis and light-chain deposition disease light chains induce divergent phenotypic transformations of human mesangial cells. Lab Invest 2004;84:1322–38.
16. Dember LM. Amyloidosis-associated kidney disease. J Am Soc Nephrol 2006;17: 3458–71.
17. Pinney JH, Lachmann HJ, Bansi L, et al. Outcome in renal Al amyloidosis after chemotherapy. J Clin Oncol 2011;29:674–81.
18. Kyle RA, Gertz MA. Primary systemic amyloidosis: clinical and laboratory features in 474 cases. Semin Hematol 1995;32:45–59.
19. Milani P, Merlini G, Palladini G. Light chain amyloidosis. Mediterr J Hematol Infect Dis 2018;10:e2018022.
20. Obici L, Perfetti V, Palladini G, et al. Clinical aspects of systemic amyloid diseases. Biochim Biophys Acta 2005;1753:11–22.
21. Said SM, Sethi S, Valeri AM, et al. Renal amyloidosis: origin and clinicopathologic correlations of 474 recent cases. Clin J Am Soc Nephrol 2013;8:1515–23.
22. Tang W, McDonald SP, Hawley CM, et al. End-stage renal failure due to amyloidosis: outcomes in 490 ANZDATA registry cases. Nephrol Dial Transplant 2013;28: 455–61.
23. Sidana S, Tandon N, Gertz MA, et al. Clinical features, laboratory characteristics and outcomes of patients with renal versus cardiac light chain amyloidosis. Br J Haematol 2019;185:701–7.
24. Palladini G, Hegenbart U, Milani P, et al. A staging system for renal outcome and early markers of renal response to chemotherapy in AL amyloidosis. Blood 2014; 124:2325–32.
25. Zhu Z, Yue C, Sun Y, et al. Light-chain amyloidosis with renal involvement: renal outcomes and validation of two renal staging systems in the Chinese population. Amyloid 2019;26:186–91.
26. Kastritis E, Gavriatopoulou M, Roussou M, et al. Renal outcomes in patients with AL amyloidosis: prognostic factors, renal response and the impact of therapy. Am J Hematol 2017;92:632–9.
27. Yadav P, Leung N, Sanders PW, et al. The use of immunoglobulin light chain assays in the diagnosis of paraprotein-related kidney disease. Kidney Int 2015;87: 692–7.
28. Katzmann JA, Kyle RA, Benson J, et al. Screening panels for detection of monoclonal gammopathies. Clin Chem 2009;55:1517–22.
29. Katzmann JA, Abraham RS, Dispenzieri A, et al. Diagnostic performance of quantitative kappa and lambda free light chain assays in clinical practice. Clin Chem 2005;51:878–81.
30. Kyle RA, Therneau TM, Rajkumar SV, et al. Prevalence of monoclonal gammopathy of undetermined significance. N Engl J Med 2006;354:1362–9.
31. Muchtar E, Dispenzieri A, Lacy MQ, et al. Overuse of organ biopsies in immunoglobulin light chain amyloidosis (AL): the consequence of failure of early recognition. Ann Med 2017;49:545–51.

32. Foli A, Palladini G, Caporali R, et al. The role of minor salivary gland biopsy in the diagnosis of systemic amyloidosis: results of a prospective study in 62 patients. Amyloid 2011;18(Suppl 1):80–2.

33. Li T, Huang X, Cheng S, et al. Utility of abdominal skin plus subcutaneous fat and rectal mucosal biopsy in the diagnosis of AL amyloidosis with renal involvement. PLoS One 2017;12:e0185078.

34. Leung N, Nasr SH, Sethi S. How I treat amyloidosis: the importance of accurate diagnosis and amyloid typing. Blood 2012;120:3206–13.

35. Mohamed N, Nasr SH. Renal amyloidosis. Surg Pathol Clin 2014;7:409–25.

36. Picken MM. New insights into systemic amyloidosis: the importance of diagnosis of specific type. Curr Opin Nephrol Hypertens 2007;16:196–203.

37. Vrana JA, Gamez JD, Madden BJ, et al. Classification of amyloidosis by laser microdissection and mass spectrometry-based proteomic analysis in clinical biopsy specimens. Blood 2009;114:4957–9.

38. Gonzalez Suarez ML, Zhang P, Nasr SH, et al. The sensitivity and specificity of the routine kidney biopsy immunofluorescence panel are inferior to diagnosing renal immunoglobulin-derived amyloidosis by mass spectrometry. Kidney Int 2019;96:1005–9.

39. Donini U, Casanova S, Zucchelli P, et al. Immunoelectron microscopic classification of amyloid in renal biopsies. J Histochem Cytochem 1989;37:1101–6.

40. Fernandez de Larrea C, Verga L, Morbini P, et al. A practical approach to the diagnosis of systemic amyloidoses. Blood 2015;125:2239–44.

41. Hawkins PN, Lavender JP, Pepys MB. Evaluation of systemic amyloidosis by scintigraphy with 123I-labeled serum amyloid P component. N Engl J Med 1990;323:508–13.

42. Schaadt BK, Hendel HW, Gimsing P, et al. 99mTc-aprotinin scintigraphy in amyloidosis. J Nucl Med 2003;44:177–83.

43. Minamimoto R, Kubota K, Ishii K, et al. Re-evaluating the potentials and limitations of (99m)Tc-aprotinin scintigraphy for amyloid imaging. Am J Nucl Med Mol Imaging 2013;3:261–71.

44. Martin EB, Williams A, Richey T, et al. Comparative evaluation of p5+14 with SAP and peptide p5 by dual-energy SPECT imaging of mice with AA amyloidosis. Sci Rep 2016;6:22695.

45. Kastritis E, Papassotiriou I, Merlini G, et al. Growth differentiation factor-15 is a new biomarker for survival and renal outcomes in light chain amyloidosis. Blood 2018;131:1568–75.

46. Ramirez-Alvarado M, Ward CJ, Huang BQ, et al. Differences in immunoglobulin light chain species found in urinary exosomes in light chain amyloidosis (Al). PLoS One 2012;7:e38061.

47. Ramirez-Alvarado M, Barnidge DR, Murray DL, et al. Assessment of renal response with urinary exosomes in patients with AL amyloidosis: a proof of concept. Am J Hematol 2017;92:536–41.

48. Kourelis T, Murray DL, Dasari S, et al. MASS-FIX may allow identification of patients at risk for light chain amyloidosis before the onset of symptoms. Am J Hematol 2018;93:E368–70.

49. Baden EM, Sikkink LA, Ramirez-Alvarado M. Light chain amyloidosis - current findings and future prospects. Curr Protein Pept Sci 2009;10:500–8.

50. Dasari S, Theis JD, Vrana JA, et al. Clinical proteome informatics workbench detects pathogenic mutations in hereditary amyloidoses. J Proteome Res 2014;13:2352–8.

51. Chen N, Zhou S, Palmisano M. Clinical pharmacokinetics and pharmacody-namics of lenalidomide. Clin Pharmacokinet 2017;56:139–52.
52. Kastritis E, Roussou M, Gavriatopoulou M, et al. Long-term outcomes of primary systemic light chain (AL) amyloidosis in patients treated upfront with bortezomib or lenalidomide and the importance of risk adapted strategies. Am J Hematol 2015;90:E60–5.
53. Specter R, Sanchorawala V, Seldin DC, et al. Kidney dysfunction during lenalido-mide treatment for AL amyloidosis. Nephrol Dial Transplant 2011;26:881–6.
54. Gupta N, Hanley MJ, Venkatakrishnan K, et al. Effects of strong CYP3A inhibition and induction on the pharmacokinetics of ixazomib, an oral proteasome inhibitor: results of drug-drug interaction studies in patients with advanced solid tumors or lymphoma and a physiologically based pharmacokinetic analysis. J Clin Pharma-col 2018;58:180–92.
55. Raza K, Hardy R, Cooper MS. The 11beta-hydroxysteroid dehydrogenase en-zymes–arbiters of the effects of glucocorticoids in synovium and bone. Rheuma-tology (Oxford) 2010;49:2016–23.
56. Sathick IJ, Rosenbaum CA, Gutgarts V, et al. Kidney transplantation in AL Amyloidosis: is it time to maximize access? Br J Haematol 2020;188:e1–4.
57. Pinney JH, Lachmann HJ, Sattianayagam PT, et al. Renal transplantation in sys-temic amyloidosis-importance of amyloid fibril type and precursor protein abun-dance. Am J Transplant 2013;13:433–41.
58. Herrmann SM, Gertz MA, Stegall MD, et al. Long-term outcomes of patients with light chain amyloidosis (AL) after renal transplantation with or without stem cell transplantation. Nephrol Dial Transplant 2011;26:2032–6.
59. Angel-Korman A, Stern L, Sarosiek S, et al. Long-term outcome of kidney trans-plantation in AL amyloidosis. Kidney Int 2019;95:405–11.

Liver and Gastrointestinal Involvement

Michael Rosenzweig, MD[a], Raymond L. Comenzo, MD[b],*

KEYWORDS

- Amyloidosis • Gastrointestinal • Hepatic liver

KEY POINTS

- Liver involvement with AL amyloid can cause abnormalities of coagulation that create a high risk of bleeding.
- Gastrointestinal involvement with AL amyloid can be a major cause of weight loss and anemia.
- Effective control and elimination of the pathologic immunoglobulin light chain can lead in time to restoration of normal liver, coagulation, splenic and GI function.

CASE 1

A 46-year-old woman slammed her hand in a closing car door and had continuous bleeding for 5 days. In the emergency room she was found to have a liver span of 18 cm in the midclavicular line on examination, a normal bilirubin but an elevated alkaline phosphatase of 654 mg/dL, Howell-Jolly bodies on the peripheral blood smear, a prolonged prothrombin time, and acquired factor X deficiency with a factor X level of 6%. Bone marrow and fat pad studies were obtained with aggressive plasma support. Fat pad showed amyloidosis and marrow showed 15% lambda-restricted plasma cells with trisomy 9. An immunoglobulin G (IgG) lambda measuring 0.7 g/dL on serum protein electrophoresis and lambda free light chains of 110 mg/L were identified. Echocardiogram and electrocardiogram were unremarkable. Bortezomib-based therapy was initiated and after 2 months a very good partial response (VGPR) was achieved but factor X level was 9%. She was vaccinated and underwent successful splenectomy with recombinant factor VIIa support with postoperative factor X level of 27%. Marrow showed 4% lambda-restricted plasma cells. Peripheral blood stem cells were mobilized with granulocyte colony-stimulating factor and plerixafor and she underwent an uncomplicated stem cell transplant with melphalan 200 mg/m^2 conditioning. At 3 months posttransplant, M-protein was 0.2 g/dL in the blood and FLC were normal. Alkaline phosphatase was normal and factor X level was 42%. At

---

[a] City of Hope Helford Clinical Research Hospital, City of Hope, 1500 East Duarte Road, Duarte, CA 91010, USA; [b] John C Davis Myeloma and Amyloid Program, Tufts University School of Medicine, Tufts Medical Center, Box 826, 800 Washington Street, Boston, MA 02111, USA
* Corresponding author.
E-mail address: rcomenzo@tuftsmedicalcenter.org

Hematol Oncol Clin N Am 34 (2020) 1081–1090
https://doi.org/10.1016/j.hoc.2020.09.001
0889-8588/20/© 2020 Elsevier Inc. All rights reserved.

12 months after stem cell transplantation, serum and urine immunofixation studies and free light chains were normal, hepatomegaly resolved, and the peripheral blood smear had no Howell-Jolly bodies.

LIVER INVOLVEMENT

The definition of liver involvement in systemic AL amyloidosis has not changed for almost 30 years.[1–3] Currently we continue to define it as the presence of interstitial amyloid on liver biopsy and/or as hepatomegaly with total liver span greater than 15 cm in the absence of heart failure with, in either case, an alkaline phosphatase level greater than 1.5 times the institutional upper limit of normal. On examination, the liver can feel hard and irregular in contour when percussed, a distinctly different examination finding from hepatomegaly due to passive congestion from heart failure. In a series of 816 patients with AL from 6 countries 16% had hepatic involvement.[4]

Symptoms of liver involvement include right upper quadrant discomfort, particularly with bending forward, early satiety, weight loss, and easy bruising. Complications of liver involvement include spontaneous hepatic rupture, hyperbilirubinemia due to severe intrahepatic cholestasis, ascites, and coagulation abnormalities.[5–8] In the case we present, there was an associated factor X deficiency, a critical signal that the patient likely had AL.[9] The mechanism of factor X and other coagulation factor deficiencies (factors IX and II) is thought to be related to the adsorption of factor X to amyloid fibrils and may be amplified by the accessibility of deposits to the circulation in patients with massive hepatosplenic amyloid.[10]

Of 368 patients seen in the 1990s at the Boston University Amyloidosis Center, 8.7% had factor X levels less than 50% of normal and more than half of them had bleeding events. Bleeding was more frequent and severe in the 12 patients with factor X levels less than 25% of normal; 2 of these patients had fatal bleeding events. In the case of our 46 year-old patient, we used recombinant factor VIIa to enable her and 2 others to undergo splenectomy before being treated on a phase II trial using stem cell transplant; all survived for more than a decade.[11] Importantly, such an approach may not be necessary today, given the effectiveness of daratumumab- and bortezomib-containing regimens.[12] The achievement of deep hematologic responses can be associated with the resorption of amyloid deposits from the liver and spleen and correction of coagulation abnormalities.[13] Unlike cardiac and renal involvement that have specific validated criteria of organ response, the improvements seen with therapy in hepatic and hepatosplenic amyloid have not been codified in the same fashion, although attempts have been made to use imaging techniques and elastography in the setting of clinical trials.[14]

CASE 2

A 42-year-old man began to experience weight loss, a bad taste in his mouth, and nausea. On evaluation by his primary care physician he was noted to have lost 25 pounds in less than a year. Endoscopy was performed and areas of friable mucosa were seen in the gastric antrum and biopsied. He was placed on proton pump inhibitor but his symptoms persisted. The biopsies revealed amyloidosis and a hematologic evaluation showed an IgA lambda paraprotein measuring 1.2 g/dL on serum protein electrophoresis and lambda free light chains of 456 mg/L. Marrow showed 20% lambda-restricted plasma cells. There was no evidence of cardiac involvement but gastric emptying scan showed delayed passage. He was treated with a bortezomib-based regimen, had a VGPR in 3 months, and was maintained on total parenteral nutrition (TPN). He underwent a peripheral blood stem cell transplant with conditioning with melphalan 200 mg/m^2 and was able to come off of TPN 6 months after transplant. He achieved a complete hematologic response and had resolution of all symptoms.

GASTROINTESTINAL INVOLVEMENT

AL can result in amyloid deposition virtually anywhere in the body apart from the brain.[15] The most commonly affected organs include the kidney and heart followed by the peripheral nervous system, liver, gastrointestinal (GI) tract, and soft tissues.[15] Clinicians should be aware of clinical manifestations of GI and liver involvement caused by AL as well as guidelines for management. Because the symptoms of GI amyloidosis often mimic those of other GI disorders, having a keen awareness of the need to evaluate for AL is critical in avoiding delay in diagnosis and intervention. As with all AL-related organ diseases, early treatment can prevent progression of tissue damage and improve outcomes.

GI involvement in AL is defined as the presence of GI symptoms with direct biopsy verification.[2] Although renal and cardiac involvement are the predominant organs involved with AL, involvement of the GI tract is less frequent and reported in 8% of cases.[16,17] A recent case series of more than 2000 patients noted dominant GI amyloidosis in just 3% of cases.[18] AL involvement of the GI tract can occur as a result of a localized plasma cell dyscrasia or systemic disease. Those with localized disease have isolated GI involvement with no other organs involved and no evidence of a plasma cell dyscrasia in the bone marrow. Elevated serologic markers including an abnormal free light chain ratio, however, is common with localized disease. Patients with localized disease should be managed without the use of systemic chemotherapy, so making the correct distinction is paramount to management. In the same aforementioned case series of patients with dominant GI amyloidosis, 21% were noted to have had localized rather than systemic disease.[18]

Symptoms of GI amyloidosis are nonspecific and include dysphagia, weight loss, nausea, vomiting, and abdominal pain, and symptoms of malabsorption include diarrhea, steatorrhea, and anorexia.[17,19,20] In addition, patients can present with varying degrees of bleeding including hematemesis, mild hematochezia as well as massive and sometimes fatal hemorrhage.[21,22] GI symptoms are estimated to occur in up to 60% of patients with AL[23] and may or may not be directly related to amyloid deposition in the GI tract itself. It is important to recognize that symptoms including diarrhea, constipation, weight loss, and early satiety may be due to autonomic neuropathy rather than GI tract deposition. The nature of symptoms experienced by patients is often related to the section of the GI tract involved with amyloid deposition. Weight loss and malnutrition are common features of systemic amyloidosis and are associated with poor survival.[24] Gastrointestinal symptoms almost certainly have a role in weight loss but extraintestinal features including cardiac cachexia and liver infiltration can also contribute.[25]

The GI system starts with the oral cavity; macroglossia, a key feature of amyloid, is found in 10% to 20% of patients with AL.[20] Macroglossia is generally thought to be pathognomonic for AL rather than other types of amyloid; however, at least one case of macroglossia with TTR has been reported.[26] Macroglossia can result in oral dysphagia as well as difficulty chewing, malocclusion of the teeth, and dental indentations of the tongue.[27,28] Abnormalities of the tongue are not the only manifestations of oral amyloidosis. There may be swelling of the mouth floor or hardening of soft tissues in the perioral region that can result in difficulty opening the mouth.[29] In addition, submandibular salivary gland involvement can result in xerostomia and a Sjogren-like picture.[30]

Esophageal involvement occurs in 13% to 22% of cases. Symptoms include dysphagia, chest pain, reflux symptoms, and hematemesis.[20] Abnormalities of the lower esophageal sphincter such as diminished amplitude of contractions or pressure can result in heartburn symptoms.[31] Radiographically, the most common feature is a dilated, atonic esophagus with decreased peristalsis. Sometimes there is distal narrowing and proximal dilation associated with tracheobronchial aspiration.[20] Ulceration of the esophagus has also been reported.[32,33]

Patients with gastric involvement such as our 42-year-old man often have symptoms of nausea, vomiting, hematemesis, and epigastric pain. Rarely patients develop pyloric edema, submucosal tumors, or polyps resulting in gastric outlet obstruction.[34,35] Gastroparesis may be confirmed radiographically; symptoms of gastroparesis are not uncommon.[36] Clinical presentations from small intestinal amyloid deposition are variable and result from either mechanical effect of direct amyloid infiltration of the mucosal tissue or dysmotility. Diarrhea is the most common symptom of GI amyloidosis and can be caused by either mechanism. Malabsorption due to amyloid infiltration of the small bowel mucosa may present as diarrhea, steatorrhea, or abdominal pain in the presence of specific laboratory abnormalities and evidence of a protein losing enteropathy possibly including a coagulopathy due to vitamin K deficiency.[24] Malabsorption is found in fewer than 5% of patients with AL and generally occurs in patients with small bowel amyloid infiltration.[24] It may also be caused by autonomic neuropathy leading to dysmotility, pancreatic insufficiency, bacterial overgrowth, or bowel wall ischemia.[20,37] In addition to typical symptoms of diarrhea and abdominal pain, patients with malabsorption may present with dizziness, orthostasis, anorexia, and weight loss. One case series of patients with malabsorption reported a median weight loss of 30 pounds.[24] Death due to inanition is not uncommon and perhaps second only to amyloid cardiomyopathy.

In addition to malabsorption, multiple other mechanisms may explain diarrhea in patients with AL. Amyloid infiltration of the Auerbach and Meissner plexi and autonomic ganglia can cause autonomic dysfunction and rapid GI transit time. One study demonstrated a 10-fold faster recovery of polyethylene glycol in patients with amyloidosis compared with healthy individuals when diarrhea was induced.[38] Delayed transit time in contrast may result in bacterial overgrowth, which can induce or exacerbate diarrhea; treatment with antibiotics may be helpful.[39] Treatment of diarrhea can be challenging and often the symptoms are intractable. Pharmacologic agents including loperamide, lomotil, octreotide, and particularly tincture of opium can be helpful.

Pseudo-obstruction due to amyloidosis can involve the small bowel, the colon, or both. Clinical manifestations of pseudo-obstruction include hematemesis, nausea, vomiting, and melena.[40] Patients typically present with mechanical obstruction with a paralytic ileus on imaging.[41] Characteristic computed tomography findings include diffuse bowel wall thickening, intestinal dilation, and fluid accumulation throughout the GI tract. In patients presenting with chronic intestinal pseudo-obstruction of unknown cause, a rectal or duodenal biopsy may diagnose amyloidosis as the cause. In a case series of patients with small bowel amyloidosis, only patients with AL or AH (heavy chain amyloid) presented with mechanical obstruction or chronic pseudointestinal obstruction.[42] Treatment of pseudo-obstruction due to amyloidosis remains a challenge. Medications including metoclopramide, erythromycin, and laxatives can be tried but are often ineffective.[43] Surgical management remains challenging and should be considered with extreme caution.[44]

Bleeding is a frequent and sometimes catastrophic consequence of amyloid deposition. GI bleeding has been reported in 36% of patients with dominant GI amyloidosis, a finding distinct from neuropathic involvement.[18] Bleeding from the GI tract occurs due to deposition of nonsoluble amyloid fibrils leading to diffuse erythema and friability of the gastric and duodenal mucosa as seen in our case. Reduced motility and increased rigidity of the musculature due to amyloid infiltration can lead to tearing of the muscularis mucosa and massive hemorrhage.[21] GI hemorrhage has also been reported in the setting of multiple GI polyps.[22] Bleeding may also be further complicated by coagulopathy due to hepatic involvement, factor X deficiency, or decreased vitamin K as a result of malabsorption. In addition, thrombocytopenia and/or platelet dysfunction from uremia can increase risk of bleeding.[45]

The risk of hemorrhage can be reduced with close surveillance that includes monitoring of prothrombin time with repletion of vitamin K, maintaining platelet counts greater than 50,000, and hemoglobin greater than 10 g/dL. Proton pump inhibitors can be prescribed, and aspirin products, antiplatelet agents, and nonsteroidal antiinflammatory medications other than acetaminophen should be avoided. Interventions including antifibrinolytic agents and splenectomy to reduce bleeding diatheses due to factor deficiencies have been used successfully.[46] Acute bleeding may be difficult to control due to diffuse involvement of the GI tract. Management includes intravenous administration of vitamin K, histamine H2 receptor antagonist, transfusion of platelets, packed red blood cells, fresh frozen plasma, or cryoprecipitate. Surgery of the GI tract is generally contraindicated even in cases of acute bleeding due to the often diffuse involvement of GI tract and impaired wound healing.[24,25] Interventions including embolization with placement of micro-coils has been used with limited success.[21]

Direct tissue biopsy is required for a definitive diagnosis of GI amyloidosis; however, a positive fat pad aspirate and bone marrow biopsy is diagnostic of systemic AL in 85% of cases.[47] For those with symptoms consistent with gastrointestinal amyloidosis, a presumptive diagnosis of GI involvement can be reasonably made without direct biopsy or tissue from the GI tract. The prevalence of radiographic abnormalities is highest in the small intestine, followed by the stomach, colorectum, and esophagus.[48] In those requiring endoscopy, a tissue biopsy confirming GI involvement should be obtained. Any site can be affected but amyloid most commonly involves the small bowel. A rectal biopsy is reasonable for screening in the event of a negative fat pad biopsy because of ease of access and a sensitivity of 75% to 94%.[20]

Endoscopic biopsy specimen reveals amyloidosis deposition most commonly in the duodenum followed by the stomach, colorectum, and esophagus.[49] Within the GI

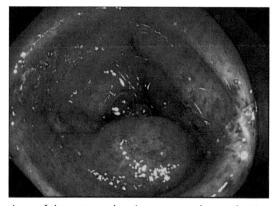

Fig. 1. Endoscopic views of the rectum, showing punctate hemorrhagic mucosa with absent vascularity and edema consistent with moderately severe hemorrhagic colitis in a patient with AL.

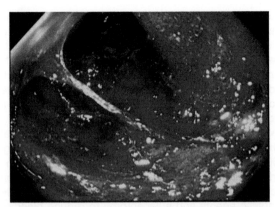

Fig. 2. Endoscopic views of the proximal colon, showing diffuse spontaneous mucosal bleeding consistent with severe, hemorrhagic colitis in a patient with AL.

tract, amyloid deposition occurs most commonly in the muscularis mucosa adjacent to nerves, nerve plexi, and vasculature, leading to vessel fragility, decreased compliance of the gut wall, and interference with peristalsis.[50,51] Endoscopic findings of the GI tract are nonspecific and can include erythema, erosions/ulcerations, granular or plaque-like lesions, friable mucosa, prepyloric ulcers, polypoid protrusions, and elevated lesions such as submucosal tumors.[52] In an undiagnosed patient, an endoscopist should consider systemic amyloidosis on visualization of nonspecific lesions, which are especially prominent in the upper GI tract.[53]

With the duodenum and small intestine most frequently involved with amyloid deposition, endoscopic abnormalities may be most marked in the duodenum.[49] Small bowel endoscopy revealing plaque lesions, thickened folds, and polypoid protrusions as well as ulceration are useful in deciding where to biopsy and make a diagnosis.[54] Endoscopic findings are also seen in the large intestine and are associated with an array of mucosal abnormalities including hemorrhagic bullous colitis caused by amyloid infiltration leading to cleavage between the submucosa and muscularis mucosa.[55,56] In addition, petechial mucosal ecchymosis can occur due to vascular infiltration by amyloid fibrils.[57] In patients with active bleeding, hemorrhagic colitis with diffuse edema can involve the GI tract diffusely and is often quite remarkable (**Figs. 1** and **2**).

Endoscopic findings vary by the type of amyloid involvement. In a series of 30 patients with amyloidosis of the small intestine, a fine granular appearance was found in significantly more AA cases compared with AL, beta-2 microglobulin, or transthyretin cases. Multiple polypoid protrusions and thickening of the small bowel folds were observed only in cases of AL. Histologically, wide granular deposits in the propria mucosa were seen significantly more often in AA, whereas massive amyloid deposits in the muscularis mucosa, submucosa, and muscularis propria were the more dominant findings in AL.[42]

SUMMARY

Early diagnosis of AL and appreciation of the nutritional and coagulation abnormalities associated with liver and GI involvement are critically important in treatment and management. In cases of severe malabsorption TPN can be extremely helpful as a bridge to organ improvement. Rarely the use of antifibrinolytic agents such as oral aminocaproic acid with transfusion support may control severe bleeding in patients with coagulation abnormalities. Anticipated toxicities of agents such as bortezomib in patients with elevated bilirubin or neuropathic symptoms should be kept in mind and the doses reduced and increased appropriately. Steroids also can be problematic in patients with GI involvement due to increased risk of bleeding; ensuring that they are taken with food or in some cases given intravenously may be particularly helpful for patients. It is important to keep in mind that organ improvement should follow in lag phase after the reduction in the pathologic free light chain with treatment. Closely following light chain levels may permit brief holidays from treatment and enable periods of recovery before resuming therapy in patients with prompt early and deep hematologic responses. Decisions regarding the role of stem cell transplant, as reflected in our 2 cases, involve weighing both the hematologic status and the organ-related picture of each patient on a case-by-case basis.

CLINICS CARE POINTS

- Splenic involvement can cause Howell-Jolly bodies on the blood smear and also thrombocytosis.
- Total parenteral nutrition can be used during therapy, even during stem cell transplant, to provide necessary nutritional support in patients with severe GI involvement.
- Surrogate site biopsies (abdominal fat, gingiva, rectum) are preferable to liver biopsy for diagnostic purposes because of the risk of bleeding with liver biopsy.

DISCLOSURE

The authors have nothing to disclose.

REFERENCES

1. Falk RH, Comenzo RL, Skinner M. The systemic amyloidoses. N Engl J Med 1997; 337(13):898–909.

2. Gertz MA, Comenzo R, Falk RH, et al. Definition of organ involvement and treatment response in immunoglobulin light chain amyloidosis (AL): a consensus opinion from the 10th International Symposium on Amyloid and Amyloidosis, Tours, France, 18-22 April 2004. Am J Hematol 2005;79(4):319-28.

3. Comenzo RL, Reece D, Palladini G, et al. Consensus guidelines for the conduct and reporting of clinical trials in systemic light-chain amyloidosis. Leukemia 2012; 26(11):2317–25.

4. Palladini G, Dispenzieri A, Gertz MA, et al. New criteria for response to treatment in immunoglobulin light chain amyloidosis based on free light chain measurement and cardiac biomarkers: impact on survival outcomes. J Clin Oncol 2012;30(36): 4541–9.

5. Naito KS, Ichiyama T, Kawakami S, et al. AL amyloidosis with spontaneous hepatic rupture: successful treatment by transcatheter hepatic artery embolization. Amyloid 2008;15(2):137–9.

6. Varela M, De Las Heras D, Miquel R. Hepatic failure due to primary AL amyloidosis. J Hepatol 2003;39(2):290.

7. Kitamura Y, Yokomori H. Hepatic amyloidosis manifesting severe intrahepatic cholestasis. Intern Med 2005;44(6):675–6.

8. Ferreira S, Baldaia C, Fatela N, et al. Severe intrahepatic cholestasis, erythrocytosis and hypoglycemia: Unusual presenting features of systemic AL amyloidosis. Scand J Gastroenterol 2007;43(3):375–9.
9. Uprichard J, Perry DJ. Factor X deficiency. Blood Rev 2002;16(2):97–110.
10. Furie B, Voo L, McAdam KP, et al. Mechanism of factor X deficiency in systemic amyloidosis. N Engl J Med 1981;304(14):827–30.
11. Cohen AD, Zhou P, Chou J, et al. Risk-adapted autologous stem cell transplantation with adjuvant dexamethasone +/- thalidomide for systemic light-chain amyloidosis: results of a phase II trial. Br J Haematol 2007;139(2):224–33.
12. Palladini G, Kastritis E, Maurer MS, et al. Daratumumab plus cybord for patients with newly diagnosed al amyloidosis: safety run-in results of ANDROMEDA. Blood 2020;136(1):71–80.
13. Landau HJ, Gertz MA, Comenzo RL. Autologous hematopoietic cell transplantation for systemic light chain (AL-) amyloidosis. Thomas' hematopoietic cell transplantation. Hoboken: John Wiley & Sons, Ltd; 2016. p. 724–41.
14. Richards DB, Cookson LM, Berges AC, et al. Therapeutic clearance of amyloid by antibodies to serum amyloid p component. N Engl J Med 2015;373(12):1106–14.
15. Merlini G, Dispenzieri A, Sanchorawala V, et al. Systemic immunoglobulin light chain amyloidosis. Nat Rev Dis Primers 2018;4(1):38.
16. Merlini G, Bellotti V. Molecular mechanisms of amyloidosis. N Engl J Med 2003;349(6):583–96.
17. Menke DM, Kyle RA, Fleming CR, et al. Symptomatic gastric amyloidosis in patients with primary systemic amyloidosis. Mayo Clin Proc 1993;68(8):763–7.
18. Cowan AJ, Skinner M, Seldin DC, et al. Amyloidosis of the gastrointestinal tract: a 13-year, single-center, referral experience. Haematologica 2013;98(1):141–6.
19. Hayman SR, Bailey RJ, Jalal SM, et al. Translocations involving the immunoglobulin heavy-chain locus are possible early genetic events in patients with primary systemic amyloidosis. Blood 2001;98(7):2266–8.
20. Ebert EC, Nagar M. Gastrointestinal manifestations of amyloidosis. Am J Gastroenterol 2008;103(3):776–87.
21. Kim SH, Kang EJ, Park JW, et al. Gastrointestinal amyloidosis presenting with multiple episodes of gastrointestinal bleeding. Cardiovasc Intervent Radiol 2009;32(3):577–80.
22. Suchartlikitwong S, Tantrachoti P, Mingbunjerdsuk T, et al. Gastrointestinal polyps and hemorrhage as a presentation of primary systemic light chain amyloidosis. ACG Case Rep J 2018;5:e44.
23. James DG, Zuckerman GR, Sayuk GS, et al. Clinical recognition of Al type amyloidosis of the luminal gastrointestinal tract. Clin Gastroenterol Hepatol 2007;5(5):582–8.
24. Hayman SR, Lacy MQ, Kyle RA, et al. Primary systemic amyloidosis: a cause of malabsorption syndrome. Am J Med 2001;111(7):535–40.
25. Sattianayagam P, Gibbs S, Hawkins P, et al. Systemic AL (light-chain) amyloidosis and the gastrointestinal tract. Scand J Gastroenterol 2009;44(11):1384–5.
26. Cowan AJ, Skinner M, Berk JL, et al. Macroglossia - not always AL amyloidosis. Amyloid 2011;18(2):83–6.
27. Jacobs P, Sellars S, King HS. Massive macroglossia, amyloidosis and myeloma. Postgrad Med J 1988;64(755):696–8.
28. Al-Hashimi I, Drinnan AJ, Uthman AA, et al. Oral amyloidosis: two unusual case presentations. Oral Surg Oral Med Oral Pathol 1987;63(5):586–91.

29. Pereira CM, Gasparetto PF, Correa ME, et al. Primary oral and perioral amyloidosis associated with multiple myeloma. Gen Dent 2005;53(5):340–1.

30. Gogel HK, Searles RP, Volpicelli NA, et al. Primary amyloidosis presenting as Sjogren's syndrome. Arch Intern Med 1983;143(12):2325–6.

31. Rubinow A, Burakoff R, Cohen AS, et al. Esophageal manometry in systemic amyloidosis. A study of 30 patients. Am J Med 1983;75(6):951–6.

32. Gonzalez J, Wahab A, Kesari K. Dysphagia unveiling systemic immunoglobulin light-chain amyloidosis with multiple myeloma. BMJ Case Rep 2018;2018.

33. Heitzman EJ, Heitzman GC, Elliott CF. Primary esophageal amyloidosis. Report of a case with bleeding, perforation, and survival following resection. Arch Intern Med 1962;109:595–600.

34. Cohen JA, An J, Brown AW, et al. Gastric outlet obstruction due to gastrointestinal amyloidosis. J Gastrointest Surg 2017;21(3):600–1.

35. Jensen K, Raynor S, Rose SG, et al. Amyloid tumors of the gastrointestinal tract: a report of two cases and review of the literature. Am J Gastroenterol 1985;80(10): 784–6.

36. Hoscheit M, Kamal A, Cline M. Gastroparesis in a patient with gastric AL amyloidosis. Case Rep Gastroenterol 2018;12(2):317–21.

37. Ectors N, Geboes K, Kerremans R, et al. Small bowel amyloidosis, pathology and diagnosis. Acta Gastroenterol Belg 1992;55(2):228–38.

38. Guirl MJ, Hogenauer C, Santa Ana CA, et al. Rapid intestinal transit as a primary cause of severe chronic diarrhea in patients with amyloidosis. Am J Gastroenterol 2003;98(10):2219–25.

39. Matsumoto T, Iida M, Hirakawa M, et al. Breath hydrogen test using water-diluted lactulose in patients with gastrointestinal amyloidosis. Dig Dis Sci 1991;36(12): 1756–60.

40. Shiratori Y, Fukuda K, Ikeya T, et al. Primary gastrointestinal amyloidosis with gastrointestinal hemorrhage and intestinal pseudo-obstruction: a report of a rare case. Clin J Gastroenterol 2019;12(3):258–62.

41. Iida T, Hirayama D, Sudo G, et al. Chronic intestinal pseudo-obstruction due to al amyloidosis: a case report and literature review. Clin J Gastroenterol 2019;12(2): 176–81.

42. Tada S, Iida M, Yao T, et al. Endoscopic features in amyloidosis of the small intestine: clinical and morphologic differences between chemical types of amyloid protein. Gastrointest Endosc 1994;40(1):45–50.

43. Tada S, Iida M, Yao T, et al. Intestinal pseudo-obstruction in patients with amyloidosis: clinicopathologic differences between chemical types of amyloid protein. Gut 1993;34(10):1412–7.

44. Leong RY, Nio K, Plumley L, et al. Systemic amyloidosis causing intestinal hemorrhage and pseudo-obstruction. J Surg Case Rep 2014;2014(9):rju087.

45. Koop AH, Mousa OY, Wang MH. Clinical and endoscopic manifestations of gastrointestinal amyloidosis: a case series. Clujul Med 2018;91(4):469–73.

46. Greipp PR, Kyle RA, Bowie EJ. Factor X deficiency in primary amyloidosis: resolution after splenectomy. N Engl J Med 1979;301(19):1050–1.

47. Gertz MA. Immunoglobulin light chain amyloidosis: 2018 Update on diagnosis, prognosis, and treatment. Am J Hematol 2018;93(9):1169–80.

48. Tada S, Iida M, Yao T, et al. Gastrointestinal amyloidosis: radiologic features by chemical types. Radiology 1994;190(1):37–42.

49. Tada S, Iida M, Iwashita A, et al. Endoscopic and biopsy findings of the upper digestive tract in patients with amyloidosis. Gastrointest Endosc 1990;36(1):10–4.

50. Rowe K, Pankow J, Nehme F, et al. Gastrointestinal amyloidosis: review of the literature. Cureus 2017;9(5):e1228.
51. Kaiserling E, Krober S. Massive intestinal hemorrhage associated with intestinal amyloidosis. An investigation of underlying pathologic processes. Gen Diagn Pathol 1995;141(2):147–54.
52. Iida T, Yamano H, Nakase H. Systemic amyloidosis with gastrointestinal involvement: Diagnosis from endoscopic and histological views. J Gastroenterol Hepatol 2018;33(3):583–90.
53. Sattianayagam PT, Hawkins PN, Gillmore JD. Systemic amyloidosis and the gastrointestinal tract. Nat Rev Gastroenterol Hepatol 2009;6(10):608.
54. Mandelli G, Radaelli F, Amato A, et al. The spectrum of small-bowel lesions of AL-type amyloidosis at capsule endoscopy. Endoscopy 2009;41(S 02):E51–2.
55. Dray X, Treton X, Joly F, et al. Hemorrhagic bullous colitis as a primary manifestation of AL amyloidosis. Endoscopy 2006;38(Suppl 2):E15–6.
56. Cho SH, Kim SW, Kim WC, et al. Hemorrhagic bullous colitis in a patient with multiple myeloma. Endoscopy 2013;45(Suppl 2 UCTN):E157–8.
57. Schmidt H, Fruhmorgen P, Riemann JF, et al. Mucosal suggillation in the colon in secondary amyloidosis. Endoscopy 1981;13(4):181–3.

Peripheral Nervous System Involvement

Pariwat Thaisetthawatkul, MD[a], P. James B. Dyck, MD[b],*

KEYWORDS

- Light chain amyloid • Amyloid neuropathy • Amyloid myopathy • Primary systemic
- Amyloidosis • AL amyloidosis • Amyloid autonomic neuropathy

KEY POINTS

- Peripheral nervous system involvement can be seen in up to 35% of light chain amyloid amyloidosis and can be a presenting symptom.
- Amyloid neuropathy typically presents with progressive symmetric length-dependent small-fiber predominant axonal sensorimotor neuropathy, typically accompanied by autonomic neuropathy.
- Amyloid myopathy typically presents with proximal or proximal and distal weakness with dysphagia, fatigue, and macroglossia.
- Peripheral nervous system involvement often is accompanied by systemic symptoms suggesting involvement of the other organs, such as cardiac or renal failure, nephrotic syndrome, peripheral edema, weight loss, or diarrhea.
- It is important to recognize the diagnosis because earlier treatment with less organ involvement may improve the prognosis.

INTRODUCTION

Peripheral nervous system involvement in primary systemic amyloidosis can be seen in 2 settings: amyloid neuropathy and amyloid myopathy. Involvement of light chain amyloid (AL) in peripheral nerves has been reported in 17% to 35% in patients with AL amyloidosis[1,2] while the prevalence of muscle involvement is unclear but the frequency of positive muscle biopsy for amyloid deposits is reported to be 1.5% in a large series of patients with Al amyloidosis.[3] As AL amyloidosis is a multisystem disorder, symptoms related to the other organs, such as nephrotic syndrome, congestive heart failure, ecchymoses, weight loss, hepatomegaly, diarrhea, and fatigue can be seen in association with peripheral nervous system involvement and these coexisting problems may suggest the diagnosis.[4] When peripheral neuropathy is the presenting

[a] Department of Neurological Sciences, University of Nebraska Medical Center, 988435 Nebraska Medical Center, Omaha, NE 68198-8435, USA; [b] Department of Neurology, Mayo Clinic College of Medicine, 200 1st street SW, Rochester, MN 55905, USA
* Corresponding author.
E-mail address: Dyck.PJames@mayo.edu

Hematol Oncol Clin N Am 34 (2020) 1091–1098
https://doi.org/10.1016/j.hoc.2020.07.004
0889-8588/20/© 2020 Elsevier Inc. All rights reserved.

problem and precedes the other systemic manifestations, the diagnosis may be missed and delayed as the features of amyloid neuropathy or myopathy often mimic other forms of neuropathy or myopathy. The prognosis of AL amyloidosis has improved significantly with newer modes of treatment giving better survival.[5] It is therefore important to recognize the major clinical manifestations of AL amyloidosis presenting with peripheral neuropathy or myopathy and to make a prompt diagnosis so that a patient with AL amyloidosis gets appropriate treatment before the disease becomes advanced.

LIGHT CHAIN AMYLOID NEUROPATHY

Peripheral nerve involvement in AL amyloidosis results from deposits of amyloid protein consisting of light chain immunoglobulins in the peripheral nerves.[2] The mechanism of how amyloid deposition causes neuropathy is poorly understood. Misfolded monoclonal light chain is produced from a malignant plasma cell clone in the bone marrow. It does not conform to the normal alpha-helical configuration, becomes insoluble and deposits into tissues causing tissue damage.[6] Amyloid deposits in the nerve appear as an amorphous acellular substance seen in the epineurium, perineurium and endoneurium, often around the blood vessels.[7] It can be visualized in hematoxylin-eosin and methyl violet preparations in pink color and in salmon color with Congo red staining (**Fig. 1**A). Under polarized microscopy, amyloid appears as apple green and birefringent (**Fig. 1**B).[7] The mechanism of nerve injury in AL amyloidosis remains controversial and essentially unknown. Many mechanisms have been postulated such as ischemia due to amyloid surrounding blood vessels, amyloid nodules compressing nerve fibers causing distortion of the nerve architecture and degeneration of nerve cells when amyloid is found in the ganglia.[7] Detection of C5b-9 complement complex on amyloid deposits in in vivo sural nerve preparation suggests that complement activation may play a role in axonal degeneration seen in amyloid neuropathy.[8] Even though peripheral nerve involvement can be seen in 17% to 35%[1,2] of AL amyloidosis cases, peripheral neuropathy is the presenting symptoms in about 20%[9] of them. When peripheral neuropathy is the presenting symptom, time to make the diagnosis of AL amyloidosis may take an additional 12 to 48 months.[1,9,10] Time to make the diagnosis of AL amyloidosis is usually shorter when congestive heart failure (3 months[1]) or nephrotic syndrome or renal failure (3 months[1]) is the presenting symptom. This delay in diagnosis suggests that the symptoms of amyloid neuropathy are similar to the other types of neuropathy. Amyloid neuropathy has been misdiagnosed as chronic inflammatory demyelinating polyradiculoneuropathy (CIDP) and may have similar electrodiagnostic features but the patients with AL amyloid polyneuropathy do not respond to immunotherapy.[11,12] This misdiagnosis as CIDP has also been seen in familial amyloid polyneuropathy (hATTR).[4] AL amyloid neuropathy is seen more commonly in men,[5,9,13] mostly older than 50 years.[13] As amyloid affects unmyelinated or small myelinated nerve fibers first,[3] small-fiber sensory symptoms often initially predominate.[13] This is usually prominent and experienced as numbness and neuropathic pain, often described as burning, stabbing or shooting pain, starting distally and symmetrically in the lower extremities and ascending to the upper extremities over time. When large nerve fibers are affected at later timepoints, patients can develop increased sensory loss, numbness, motor weakness and muscle atrophy. Weakness is usually present at the time of diagnosis.[13] Autonomic function, subserved by unmyelinated and small myelinated nerves, is also commonly affected and can be seen from 18% to 74% of the time.[5,13] The most common autonomic symptoms are orthostatic hypotension and syncope.[13] The other autonomic symptoms, such as loss of

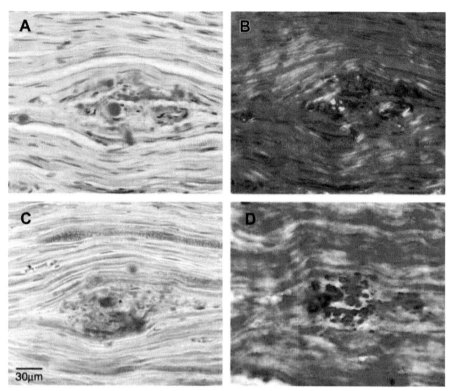

Fig. 1. A sural nerve biopsy from a patient with AL amyloid neuropathy. (*A*) Congophilic deposits surrounding endoneurial microvessels (Congo red stain). (*B*) Apple green birefringence under polarized light. (*C*) Amyloid stained in violet color (methyl violet). (*D*) Positive lambda reactivity. (*Adapted from* Bosch EP, Reeder CB, Dyck PJB: Predominant peripheral nerve involvement in AL amyloidosis. In Companion to Peripheral Neuropathy, Illustrated Cases and New Developments, PJ Dyck, PJB Dyck, JK Engelstad, PA Low, KK Amrami, RJ Spinner, CJ Klein, Editors, Saunders Elsevier, Section 2, Chapter 55:237-239, 2010.)

libido, erectile dysfunction, diarrhea (about 35%) and bladder dysfunction (approximately 29%), can also be seen.[13] Typically, amyloid neuropathy has a feature of progressive, symmetric, length-dependent, lower-limb predominant, small-fiber predominant, sensorimotor neuropathy associated with prominent autonomic symptoms. Carpal tunnel syndrome is a common entrapment neuropathy seen in AL amyloidosis and can be the presenting symptom in approximately 21% to 23%.[1,13] It can be unilateral or bilateral. Carpal tunnel syndrome typically causes paresthesia and pain in the hands and fingers supplied by the median nerve, that is, the first 3 fingers, the lateral half of the fourth finger and the palmar surface of the thenar area. The presence of carpal tunnel syndrome and polyneuropathy with symptoms in the feet accompanied by systemic symptoms should raise suspicion of amyloidosis (either AL or ATTR). Atypical presentations such as upper limb multiple asymmetrical mononeuropathies,[14] asymmetrical lower limb and cranial neuropathies,[15] isolated radial mononeuropathy,[16] lumbosacral radiculoplexus neuropathy,[17] and multiple cranial neuropathy[18,19] have also been reported. Amyloid neuropathy could be accompanied by systemic symptoms indicating involvement of the other organs such as weight loss, fatigue, nephrotic syndrome, renal failure, congestive heart failure, diarrhea, hepatomegaly, enlarged and vascular tongue, periorbital purpura, leg edema, hoarse voice, vocal cord paralysis, and lymphadenopathy.[1] These systemic symptoms can be clues to the diagnosis. Cardiac amyloidosis is important to recognize as it does not only make an evaluator suspicious of the diagnosis but also is underrecognized and its presence gives a poor prognosis for AL amyloidosis[20] and is briefly discussed here.

Amyloid cardiomyopathy, similar to amyloid neuropathy, results from extracellular deposition of light chain immunoglobulin in the cardiac tissue. It can be seen in approximately 70% of patients with systemic AL amyloidosis.[20] Heart failure initially affects diastolic function while preserving left ventricular ejection fraction but eventually systolic function declines.[20] An echocardiogram may detect sparkling myocardium with granular texture[20] but most commonly it shows increased ventricular wall thickness and impaired relaxation.[21]

Electrophysiologic studies and autonomic screening tests are very important in characterizing physiologic abnormalities in patients with amyloid neuropathy. The abnormalities in nerve conduction studies are typically those of axonal length-dependent sensorimotor neuropathy with mildly reduced conduction velocities, reduced amplitudes and mildly prolonged distal latencies.[5,13] Sensory nerve conduction studies usually yield absent response in sensory studies. There are findings to suggest carpal tunnel syndrome with prolonged median motor and sensory distal latencies.[5,13] Needle electromyography typically reveals distal and symmetric abnormalities with fibrillation potentials and neurogenic motor unit potentials involving the lower extremities more than the upper extremities.[5,13] Autonomic screening typically shows a pattern of generalized autonomic failure including widespread loss or decrease of sweat, cardio-vagal and adrenergic failure associated with orthostatic hypotension and impaired baroreflex.[22] The key laboratory test in AL amyloidosis is the demonstration of the presence of monoclonal protein, either an immunoglobulin or light chain.[23] A monoclonal light chain can be detected from immunofixation of the serum and the urine in about 90% of cases[23] and are an appropriate screening tool for a patient with a clinical syndrome compatible with AL amyloidosis.[24] A free light chain assay adds to the sensitivity if immunofixation in both serum and urine are negative.[24] If all 3 tests are negative, AL amyloidosis is unlikely and other causes of the symptoms, such as hereditary amyloidosis, should be explored.[24] In AL amyloidosis, lambda light chain proteinemia is predominantly seen and is a hallmark of this disease entity.[24] In immunoglobulin (Ig)M amyloid neuropathy, antibody against myelin-associated glycoprotein (anti-MAG) can be seen in approximately 33% of cases but does not appear to affect the neuropathy or require treatment directed to the antibody.[25] The presence of anti-MAG in IgM-associated neuropathy therefore does not exclude IgM amyloid neuropathy.[25] Amyloid-like IgM deposits have been reported in rare patients with IgM-associated neuropathy.[26] These patients had IgM intranerve deposits that have similar morphology to amyloid but do not stain with Congo red or have amyloid associated proteins such as amyloid-P component or apolipoprotein E.[26] These deposits are made up of both the heavy and light chain and are not Congophilic. The clinical pictures of this clinical entity are progressive asymmetric distal sensory neuropathy with rare autonomic and no cardiac or renal involvement.[26]

Once a patient with suspicious symptoms of AL amyloidosis has a positive monoclonal light chain, a tissue biopsy showing amyloid is required to make a definite diagnosis. It is reasonable to biopsy from the organ that is most affected but a less invasive biopsy carries less risk and discomfort.[23] Biopsy of iliac crest bone marrow combined with abdominal subcutaneous fat aspiration have been reported to yield 85% sensitivity.[24] If the bone marrow biopsy and fat aspiration are negative for amyloid, a biopsy of the affected organ is the next step.[24] A sural nerve biopsy (or other sensory cutaneous nerve biopsy) may yield positive results between 86%[27] and 100%[13] in patients presenting with peripheral neuropathy. The other organs that may yield high positive results are salivary gland, rectum, small intestine, liver, kidney, muscle and cardiac endo-myocardium.[13,24] Bone marrow biopsy may not only show amyloid deposit but also show proliferation of clonal plasma cells or, in some cases, multiple myeloma, which can be seen with AL amyloidosis.[28] Approximately 15% of patients with multiple myeloma have AL amyloidosis.[29] When tissue biopsy shows amyloid, further typing of amyloid protein in the tissue by either immunohistochemistry,[30] mass spectrometric-based proteomic analysis[31] or immunoelectron microscopy[1] is required.

Monoclonal gammopathy of uncertain significance (MGUS) has been reported in 20% to 40% of patients with hereditary transthyretin amyloidosis[29,32] and 2 types of amyloidosis (light chain immunoglobulin and wild-type transthyretin) presenting in a single patient is extremely rare but has been reported.[33] High-resolution magnetic resonance neurography (MRN) has a role in visualizing and quantifying peripheral neuropathy in AL amyloidosis in vivo with high sensitivity; imaging biomarkers can reliably detect early AL amyloid neuropathy.[34] MRN detects predominant involvement of the proximal nerve segment in AL amyloid neuropathy and there is a strong correlation between MRN pattern and clinical severity of AL amyloid neuropathy.[34] A nerve biopsy in AL amyloid neuropathy typically shows axonal degeneration, involving small myelinated and unmyelinated fibers more than large myelinated nerve fibers, and fiber loss.[7] Amyloid deposits, either in multifocal or diffuse forms, are seen in the connective tissue of the epineurium, the perineurium or the endoneurium or thicken the epineurium or endoneurium blood vessels compromising the lumens of the blood vessels (**Fig.** 1C, D).[7] Amyloid deposits are also seen on dorsal root and autonomic ganglia.[7]

LIGHT CHAIN AMYLOID MYOPATHY

Muscle involvement in AL amyloidosis is rare and the prevalence of amyloid myopathy is unknown. In a large series of 3434 patients with AL amyloidosis, only 1.5% had muscle biopsy positive for amyloid deposits.[3] Amyloid deposits in the muscle can be seen in the intramuscular vessel walls, perimysium or endomysium and encasing the muscle fibers.[35] Similar to AL amyloid neuropathy, all cases of AL amyloid myopathy are in patients older than 40 years and most are men.[3] The most common symptoms are muscle weakness, predominantly proximal weakness but combined distal and proximal weakness is not uncommon.[3] The other symptoms include atrophy, pseudohypertrophy, tenderness, dysphagia, generalized fatigue, shortness of breath, and macroglossia.[3] More rare clinical manifestations of AL amyloid myopathy are dropped head syndrome,[36,37] external ophthalmoplegia,[38] and muscle amyloidoma.[39] When myopathy is the presenting symptom the time to diagnosis is about 24 months.[3] AL amyloid myopathy is often underdiagnosed and the diagnosis is often delayed.[40] Many patients were misdiagnosed as inflammatory myopathy and received immunotherapy before the correct diagnosis was revealed.[3,41] Similar to AL amyloid neuropathy, involvement of other organs is usually present.[3] Electrophysiologic studies typically show myopathic changes (small, rapidly recruiting motor unit potentials) and fibrillation potentials in approximately 90% of cases and accompanying evidence of axonal neuropathy can be seen in approximately 50%[3] of cases. Elevated creatine kinase can be seen in only 34% of cases while elevated cardiac troponin T can be seen in 70% of cases even when there is no known cardiac involvement.[3] Similar to AL amyloid neuropathy, demonstration of monoclonal light chain in serum or urine immunofixation and free light chain abnormalities are the key to the diagnosis. A muscle biopsy is required to make a definite diagnosis which is confirmed by positive Congo red staining (apple green birefringence) or by electron microscopic findings of fibrillary amyloid material.[42] The presence of amyloid in the muscle could also suggest isolated amyloid myopathy such as those from anoctaminopathy-5 or dysferlinopathy.[35] However, isolated amyloid myopathy typically has a much higher level of creatine kinase, more severe calf atrophy, unaccompanied by peripheral neuropathy and present more with asymptomatic hyperCKemia.[35]

TREATMENT AND PROGNOSIS

The treatment of peripheral nervous system involvement with AL amyloidosis is similar to the treatment of AL amyloidosis in general and is discussed in depth elsewhere in this volume. Briefly, an autologous stem cells transplantation, when done in properly selected patients, can achieve hematological and organ responsiveness as long-term survival.[6] Autologous stem cell transplantation may halt progression and improve survival in AL amyloid polyneuropathy. In patients who decline or are not eligible for autologous stem cell transplantation, chemotherapy with regimens including proteasome inhibitors, melphalan, corticosteroids, and monoclonal antibodies are available.[6] The major determinant of prognosis in AL amyloid is the presence of cardiac involvement.[29] The presence of severe cardiac involvement can exclude a patient from autologous stem cell transplantation.[6,29] It is therefore important to make a diagnosis earlier in AL amyloid patients who present with peripheral nervous system involvement to enable them to have a better prognosis.

In conclusion, peripheral neuropathy in AL amyloidosis presents initially with small-fiber symptoms or pain and autonomic dysfunction but progresses to a generalized sensorimotor peripheral neuropathy with numbness and weakness. It is often associated with other systemic symptoms of weight loss, and heart or kidney failure. Tissue confirmation of amyloidosis in association with a monoclonal protein is necessary for diagnosis. It is a progressive disorder but responds reasonably well to treatment, especially autologous stem cell transplant.

CLINICS CARE POINTS

- All patients with progressive symmetric length-dependent small-fiber predominant axonal sensorimotor neuropathy with profound autonomic involvement should have screening tests for AL amyloidosis with serum and urine immunofixation and the free light chain assay.
- AL amyloidosis requires tissue biopsy to make a definite diagnosis. When amyloid is identified in a nerve or muscle biopsy, further typing of amyloid mass by immunohistochemistry, immunoelectron microscopy or mass spectrometry is indicated. The presence of monoclonal protein does not always mean AL amyloidosis because monoclonal gammopathy is prevalent in older patients and can be seen in association with hereditary or wild-type transthyretin amyloidosis (ATTR).
- It is important to recognize the syndrome of AL amyloidosis as earlier diagnosis without extensive organ involvement may lead to treatment that can improve prognosis.

DISCLOSURE

P. Thaisetthawatkul and P.J.B. Dyck have nothing to disclose.

REFERENCES

1. Kyle RA, Gertz MA. Primary systemic amyloidosis: clinical and laboratory feature in 474 cases. Semin Hematol 1995;32:45–59.
2. Matsuda M, Gono T, Morita H, et al. Peripheral nerve involvement in primary systemic AL amyloidosis: a clinical and electrophysiological study. Eur J Neurol 2011;18:604–10.
3. Muchtar E, Derudas D, Mauermann M, et al. Systemic immunoglobulin light chain amyloidosis-associated myopathy: presentation, diagnostic pitfalls, and outcome. Mayo Clin Proc 2016;91:1354–61.
4. Kaku M, Berk JL. Neuropathy associated with systemic amyloidosis. Semin Neurol 2019;39:578–88.
5. Vaxman I, Dispenzieri A, Muchtar E, et al. New developments in diagnosis, risk assessment and management in systemic amyloidosis. Blood Rev 2019;100636. https://doi.org/10.1016/j.blre.2019.100636.
6. Vaxman I, Gertz M. Recent advances in the diagnosis, risk stratification, and management of systemic light-chain amyloidosis. Acta Haematol 2019;141: 93–106.
7. Dyck PJ, Dyck PJB, Engelstad J. Pathologic alterations of nerves. In: Dyck PJ, Thomas PK, editors. Peripheral neuropathy. 4th edition. Philadelphia: Elsevier Saunders; 2005. p. 733–829.
8. Hafer-Macko CE, Dyck PJ, Koski CL. Complement activation in acquired and hereditary amyloid neuropathy. J Peripher Nerv Syst 2000;5:131–9.
9. Duston MA, Skinner M, Anderson J, et al. Peripheral neuropathy as an early marker of AL amyloidosis. Arch Intern Med 1989;149:358–60.
10. Adams D, Lozeron P, Theaudin M, et al. Varied patterns of inaugural light-chain (AL) amyloid polyneuropathy: a monocentric study of 24 patients. Amyloid 2011;18(Suppl 1):98–100.
11. Mathis S, Magy L, Diallo L, et al. Amyloid neuropathy mimicking chronic inflammatory demyelinating polyneuropathy. Muscle Nerve 2012;45:26–31.
12. Luigetti M, Papacci M, Bartoletti S, et al. AL amyloid neuropathy mimicking a chronic inflammatory demyelinating polyneuropathy. Amyloid 2012;19:53–5.
13. Kelly JJ Jr, Kyle RA, O'Brien PC, et al. The natural history of peripheral neuropathy in primary systemic amyloidosis. Ann Neurol 1979;6:1–7.
14. Tracy JA1, Dyck PJ, Dyck PJB. Primary amyloidosis presenting as upper limb multiple mononeuropathies. Muscle Nerve 2010;41:710–5.
15. Sadek I, Mauermann MI, Hayman SR, et al. Primary systemic amyloidosis presenting with asymmetric multiple mononeuropathies. J Clin Oncol 2010;28: e429–32.
16. Cheng RR, Eskandari R, Welsh CT, et al. A case of isolated amyloid light-chain amyloidosis of the radial nerve. J Neurosurg 2016;125:598–602.
17. Ladha SS, Dyck PJ, Spinner RJ, et al. Isolated amyloidosis presenting with lumbosacral radiculoplexopathy: description of two cases and pathogenic review. J Peripher Nerv Syst 2006;11:346–52.
18. Traynor AE, Gertz MA, Kyle RA. Cranial neuropathy associated with primary amyloidosis. Ann Neurol 1991;29:451–4.
19. Massey EW, Massey JM. Facial diplegia due to amyloidosis. South Med J 1986; 79:1458–9.
20. Manolis AS, Manolis AA, Manolis TA, et al. Cardiac amyloidosis: An underdiagnosed/underappreciated disease. Eur J Intern Med 2019;67:1–13.

21. Kyriakou P, Mouselimis D, Tsarouchas A, et al. Diagnosis of cardiac amyloidosis: a systematic review on the role of imaging and biomarkers. BMC Cardiovasc Disord 2018;18:221.

22. Low PA, Tomalia VA, Park KJ. Autonomic function tests: some clinical applications. J Clin Neurol 2013;9:1–8.

23. Gertz MA, Lacy MQ, Dispenzieri A. Amyloidosis: recognition, confirmation, prognosis, and therapy. Mayo Clin Proc 1999;74:490–4.

24. Gertz MA. Immunoglobulin light chain amyloidosis: 2018 Update on diagnosis, prognosis, and treatment. Am J Hematol 2018;93:1169–80.

25. Garces-Sanchez M, Dyck PJ, Kyle RA, et al. Antibodies to myelin-associated glycoprotein (anti-Mag) in IgM amyloidosis may influence expression of neuropathy in rare patients. Muscle Nerve 2008;37:490–5.

26. Figueroa JJ, Bosch EP, Dyck PJB, et al. Amyloid-like IgM deposition neuropathy: a distinct clinico-pathologic and proteomic profiled disorder. J Peripher Nerv Syst 2012;17:182–90.

27. Kapoor M, Rossor AM, Jaunmuktane Z, et al. Diagnosis of amyloid neuropathy. Pract Neurol 2019;19:250–8.

28. Kelly JJ Jr, Kyle RA, Miles JM, et al. The spectrum of peripheral neuropathy in myeloma. Neurology 1981;31:24–31.

29. Gertz MA. Immunoglobulin light chain amyloidosis diagnosis and treatment algorithm 2018. Blood Cancer J 2018;8:44.

30. Li K, Kyle RA, Dyck PJ. Immunohistochemical characterization of amyloid proteins in sural nerves and clinical associations in amyloid neuropathy. Am J Pathol 1992;141:217–26.

31. Klein CJ, Vrana JA, Theis JD, et al. Mass spectrometric-based proteomic analysis of amyloid neuropathy type in nerve tissue. Arch Neurol 2011;68:195–9.

32. Phull P, Sanchorawala V, Connors LH, et al. Monoclonal gammopathy of undetermined significance in systemic transthyretin amyloidosis (ATTR). Amyloid 2018; 25:62–7.

33. Sidiqi MH, McPhail ED, Theis JD, et al. Two types of amyloidosis presenting in a single patient: a case series. Blood Cancer J 2019;9:30.

34. Kollmer J, Weiler M, Purrucker J, et al. MR neurography biomarkers to characterize peripheral neuropathy in AL amyloidosis. Neurology 2018;91:e625–34.

35. Liewluck T, Milone M. Characterization of isolated amyloid myopathy. Eur J Neurol 2017;24:1437–45.

36. Chuquilin M, Al-Lozi M. Primary amyloidosis presenting as "dropped head syndrome. Muscle Nerve 2011;43:905–9.

37. Laurent C, Aouizerate J, Hourdille A, et al. Dropped head syndrome with proximal myopathy revealing AL amyloidosis. Joint Bone Spine 2018;85:779–81.

38. Hoshi A, Ebitani M, Tanaka G, et al. Amyloid myopathy with external ophthalmoparesis. J Neurol 2009;256:676–8.

39. Ikezawa Y, Oka K, Nagayama R, et al. Bence-Jones protein-type myeloma with amyloid myopathy presenting as amyloidomas and extensive amyloid deposits in the muscularis propria: a rapidly fatal autopsy case. Int J Surg Pathol 2012; 20:83–8.

40. Spuler S, Emslie-Smith A, Engel AG. Amyloid myopathy: an underdiagnosed entity. Ann Neurol 1998;43:719–28.

41. Moore S, Symmons DP, DuPlessis D, et al. Amyloid myopathy masquerading as polymyositis. Clin Exp Rheumatol 2015;33:590–1.

42. Prayson RA. Amyloid myopathy: clinicopathologic study of 16 cases. Hum Pathol 1998;29:463–8.

Systemic Amyloidosis Caused by Monoclonal Immunoglobulins

Soft Tissue and Vascular Involvement

James E. Hoffman, MD[a], Naomi G. Dempsey, MD[a],
Vaishali Sanchorawala, MD[b,*]

KEYWORDS

- Macroglossia • Shoulder-pad sign • Raccoon eyes • Periorbital ecchymosis
- Carpal tunnel syndrome • Amyloid arthropathy • Amyloid myopathy

KEY POINTS

- Macroglossia, periorbital ecchymosis, and the shoulder-pad sign of deltoid pseudohypertrophy are considered pathognomonic for amyloid light-chain (AL) amyloidosis.
- In any patient with a rheumatologic diagnosis of seronegative arthritis that does not adequately fit with the clinical presentation and laboratory findings, amyloid arthropathy should be considered in the differential diagnosis.
- Carpal tunnel syndrome (CTS) commonly presents earlier in the course of AL amyloidosis than cardiomyopathy, so bilateral CTS or a history of carpal tunnel release surgery may be an early warning sign of underlying amyloidosis.
- The increased capillary pressure caused by rubbing eyes, vomiting, coughing, forced respiration, Valsalva maneuver, or Trendelenburg position can be the inciting factor for periorbital ecchymosis in patients with AL amyloidosis.

INTRODUCTION

Amyloid light-chain (AL) amyloidosis can affect any tissue outside of the brain, and there are many soft tissue manifestations that are classic for AL amyloidosis. Clinical features of soft tissue AL amyloidosis include macroglossia, arthropathy, muscle pseudohypertrophy, skin plaques, carpal tunnel syndrome (CTS), and lymphadenopathy, with varying frequency. Vascular manifestations of AL amyloidosis include periorbital ecchymosis, jaw or limb claudication, and even myocardial infarction caused by occlusion of small vessel coronary arteries.[1–3]

---

[a] Department of Medicine, Division of Hematology, University of Miami/Sylvester Comprehensive Cancer Center, 1475 Northwest 12th Avenue, Miami, FL 33136, USA; [b] Boston University School of Medicine and Boston Medical Center, 72 East Concord Street, K-503, Boston, MA 02118, USA
* Corresponding author.
E-mail address: vaishali.sanchorawala@bmc.org

Hematol Oncol Clin N Am 34 (2020) 1099–1113
https://doi.org/10.1016/j.hoc.2020.08.004
0889-8588/20/© 2020 Elsevier Inc. All rights reserved.

Some of these features, such as macroglossia, periorbital ecchymosis, and the so-called shoulder-pad sign of deltoid pseudohypertrophy, are considered pathognomonic for AL amyloidosis and can also help to distinguish AL amyloidosis from Transthyretin amyloidosis (ATTR amyloidosis).[4,5] Although pathognomonic for AL amyloidosis, it can sometimes (although rarely) be seen in ATTR amyloidosis as well.[6] In some cases, these findings are the initial presenting features of the disease, and their recognition is very important for the diagnosis and early intervention on the underlying plasma cell disease. This article discusses the soft tissue and vascular manifestations of AL amyloidosis.

DISCUSSION
Macroglossia

Tongue enlargement occurs along a spectrum of severity in AL amyloidosis and it can be life threatening if the tongue obstructs the airway. The tongue is the most common intraoral location of amyloid deposition. When amyloid deposition in the tongue is extensive, causing functional or esthetic problems, it is termed macroglossia.[4,7] An early retrospective study of 236 patients with amyloidosis performed by Kyle and colleagues[8] showed that up to 26% of patients with systemic amyloidosis had clinically apparent macroglossia. Other series report an incidence of 20% to 40%.[2,4,5,8] In 1 study of 30 patients with multiple myeloma, random biopsies of the tongue were performed. Seven biopsy specimens were found to be positive for amyloid, even though only 3 of those patients had symptomatic macroglossia, suggesting that progressive accumulation of amyloid is required before macroglossia can be appreciated on physical examination.[9]

Patients with macroglossia may complain of progressive difficulty with speaking, chewing, or swallowing. Voice changes, including a raspy or hoarse voice, as well as changes in taste sensation have been reported. On physical examination, the earliest findings are scalloping of the edges of the tongue where indentations of the teeth are noted, which may range from subtle (**Fig. 1**) to pronounced (**Fig. 2**). The tongue can enlarge in all directions, feels rubbery, firm, and dry on palpation, and may show loss of papillae[10] (**Fig. 3**). The patient may not be able to touch the tip of the tongue to the tip of the nose or to the chin. There may be ulcerations, papules, plaques (**Fig. 4**), nodular masses (**Fig. 5**), and indurated areas on the tongue as well, which may be painful. The tongue may appear pale or, less commonly, red.[11] Concomitant involvement of the submandibular salivary glands and lips is common (**Fig. 6**). When macroglossia becomes advanced, the tongue may prevent mouth closure and lead to constant drooling and xerostomia (**Fig. 7**). This stage of tongue involvement understandably causes significant psychological impacts and social impairment. Some patients are only able to eat liquids or soft foods because of tongue immobility. Once the tongue causes pharyngeal blockage, sleep apnea and even dyspnea while awake can ensue.[12]

Pathologic examination of amyloid deposits in the tongue typically show acellular, amorphous, eosinophilic material in the lamina propria and submucosa. The epithelium is spared from amyloid deposition but is atrophic. Inflammation is sparse or absent. The walls of small blood vessels may be involved, characterized by dilatation and thin walls with macrophages and giant cells present. These deposits stain with Congo red, showing apple-green birefringence. Immunohistochemistry may show κ or λ monoclonality, but plasma cells are absent.[7,9,10] In more severe cases, skeletal muscle fibers are almost completely replaced with amyloid.[13]

Treatment of macroglossia in AL amyloidosis is multidisciplinary and depends on the extent of disability caused by the macroglossia. Initial treatment is directed at

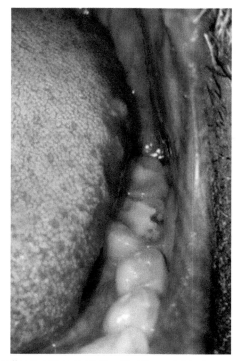

Fig. 1. Mild tongue scalloping in a patient with AL amyloidosis.

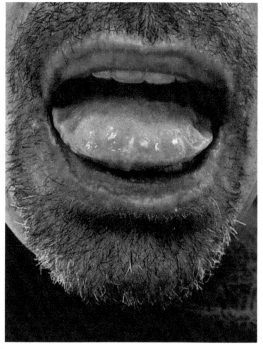

Fig. 2. Pronounced tongue indentations.

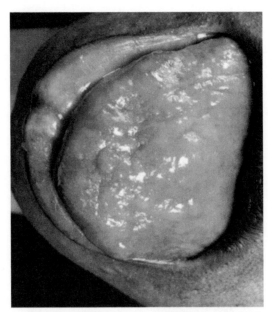

Fig. 3. Macroglossia with smooth tongue and loss of papillae. Amyloid tongue and lip nodules also present.

decreasing plasma cell burden but, even when hematologic response is noted, macroglossia may be irreversible. Radiation therapy with 20-Gy external beam radiotherapy has been attempted without success at 14-month follow-up in 1 case report by Thibault and Vallieres.[12]

Glossectomy is controversial and is generally viewed as a palliative approach because macroglossia often persists or recurs after surgery. This type of surgery is also risky because the blood vessels are fragile because of amyloid deposition and because perioperative bleeding may be difficult to control. Postoperative aspiration caused by uncontrolled bleeding, airway obstruction caused by tongue edema, poor healing, loss of taste, tongue anesthesia, and decrease of tongue mobility

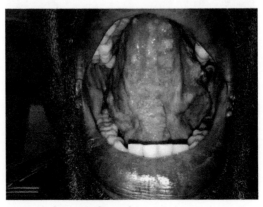

Fig. 4. Amyloid plaque on inferior surface of tongue.

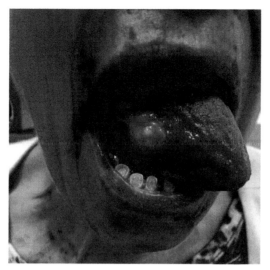

Fig. 5. Nodular amyloid mass on the lateral surface of the tongue. Perioral cutaneous hemorrhage is present.

caused by scarring have been reported.[14] For these reasons, partial glossectomy is usually reserved for severe cases where a patient's vital functions are compromised or there are concerns about airway obstruction.[11] Some studies report an improvement in quality of life after partial glossectomy restored some degree of speech or swallowing. Other investigators advocate for tracheostomy and gastrostomy as a lower-risk, more predictable option in patients at risk for airway compromise or nutritional deficits because of macroglossia.[4]

Submandibular Gland Enlargement

Enlarged submandibular glands are common in the setting of macroglossia. AL amyloidosis sometimes infiltrates salivary and lacrimal glands, causing localized

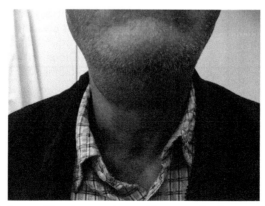

Fig. 6. Submandibular swelling in a patient with macroglossia caused by salivary gland involvement.

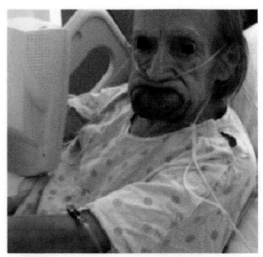

Fig. 7. Severe macroglossia caused by AL amyloidosis with tongue protrusion. This patient also has mild periorbital hemorrhage.

swelling and xerostomia/xerophthalmia.[15] In a group of 191 patients with AL amyloidosis, submandibular gland enlargement was the most common type of soft tissue involvement and was noted in 31.9%. Of those who had any other type of soft tissue involvement, submandibular gland enlargement occurred in 74.4%.[2] The physical examination shows firm, nontender submandibular swelling, often with associated macroglossia. The patient may report sicca symptoms, which, along with the submandibular swelling, can mimic Sjögren syndrome.

Ultrasonography is currently used as part of the criteria for Sjögren syndrome to increase diagnostic accuracy. Certain salivary gland ultrasonography features are thought in the rheumatology community to be specific for Sjögren syndrome. For this reason, a study was done to evaluate whether ultrasonography can distinguish the submandibular swelling noted in AL amyloidosis and sarcoidosis from Sjögren syndrome, and all of these patients were compared with controls. Twenty-seven percent of patients with AL amyloidosis had ultrasonography features that would have met the ultrasonography portion of the criteria for Sjögren syndrome. Given these results and that Sjögren syndrome is diagnosed clinically, signs and symptoms of Sjögren syndrome seen in conjunction with other inconsistent manifestations should raise suspicion for AL amyloidosis.[16] Biopsy of the enlarged gland can ultimately be used to distinguish amyloidosis from other causes of submandibular gland swelling.

Arthropathy

Amyloidosis rarely affects the joints, but, when amyloid arthropathy is noted, the subtype is almost exclusively AL or AB2M (beta 2-microglobulin) amyloidosis. As a result, this feature can clinically distinguish this condition from ATTR when present.[17] In studies of patients diagnosed with AL amyloidosis or multiple myeloma, amyloid arthropathy is reported in about 3% to 7% of patients.[2,17–19] Although amyloid arthropathy is not life threatening, it can affect quality of life as negatively as any other feature of multiple myeloma.

Arthropathy caused by AL amyloidosis can present along a spectrum from indolent arthritis to rapidly destructive inflammatory arthritis. Amyloid can affect any joint in the body and can mimic several rheumatologic diseases, such as rheumatoid arthritis (RA), mixed connective tissue disease, and polymyalgia rheumatica. As a consequence, in any patient with a rheumatologic diagnosis of seronegative arthritis that does not adequately fit with the clinical presentation and laboratory findings, amyloid arthropathy should be considered in the differential diagnosis. The first involved joint is often a larger joint, such as shoulder, knee, or hip, and may be bilateral. Shoulders are the most commonly affected joints. The presentation is most commonly polyarthritis that precedes the diagnosis of plasma cell disease, but it may also be monoarthritis or oligoarthritis and may follow the discovery of a monoclonal gammopathy.[2,17,18,20]

Patients with shoulder involvement complain of difficulty raising arms above head, shaving or brushing hair, or lifting heavy objects. Patients with hip involvement complain of pain with walking and reduced ability to walk for a prolonged period and also crossing legs. When wrists are affected, patients complain of concomitant CTS in nearly every case. A RA-like polyarthritis affecting bilateral hands causes pain and prolonged morning stiffness that can mimic RA.[18]

On physical examination, affected joints are often swollen with diminished range of motion, but signs of acute inflammation such as erythema, tenderness, and warmth are classically absent. Palpation of joint swelling imparts a sense of firmness and induration and may ultimately progress to contractures.[17,21] Subcutaneous nodules may be palpated on the extensor surface of the olecranon, similar to rheumatoid nodules. However, the subcutaneous nodules of RA are almost always seen in the presence of positive rheumatoid factor, and in amyloid arthropathy rheumatoid factor is negative.[17,20,21]

Amyloid deposition occurs in the synovial membrane, synovial fluid, or articular cartilage, and can be shown on biopsy of these tissues or synovial fluid analysis. The bone marrow of a large joint such as a hip may be replaced with a tumefaction of amyloid, which results in fractures.[21] Synovial fluid analysis can show a noninflammatory, mildly inflammatory (degenerative) or, less commonly, a highly inflammatory pattern. Synovial tissue biopsy shows a bland synovitis with amyloid deposition and no plasma cells. Immunohistochemistry showing κ or λ monoclonality can confirm AL amyloidosis as the amyloid subtype.[18]

Joint imaging frequently shows osteopenia or osteoporosis, and cysts at the site of synovium insertion. Osteolytic lesions and fractures caused by myeloma may be apparent on plain film if that is the underlying plasma cell disorder, but amyloid can also cause bone lesions independent of multiple myeloma. Erosive joint changes are rare, but they can occur in about 5% of patients with amyloid arthropathy.[17] Joint space widening likely reflects underlying amyloid accumulation causing synovium hypertrophy. Bone scintigraphy shows uptake in affected joints, but MRI is the most informative imaging modality.[20]

Treatment is directed at the underlying plasma cell disease, and generally when hematologic response is noted joint pain improves. However, the joint swelling and stiffness often remain even with adequate control of plasma cell burden. One study showed that, in patients with intense synovitis on MRI, glucocorticoid injections were effective for managing symptoms in patients with monoarticular or oligoarticular arthritis.[18] When amyloid arthropathy is misdiagnosed as a rheumatologic condition, such as RA, steroids are often the first line of treatment. Because plasma cell disease responds to steroids, initial responses are common and consequently the true diagnosis is not revealed until other organs are affected.

Carpal Tunnel Syndrome

The most common rheumatologic manifestation of AL amyloidosis is CTS. Although CTS is more common in ATTR amyloidosis, it is seen in about 13% to 38% of patients with AL amyloidosis and often precedes the diagnosis of plasma cell disease by a year or more.[2,8,18,19] One study retrospectively evaluated more than 500 patients from a large database of patients with amyloidosis. Frequency of CTS was evaluated based on a history of carpal tunnel release surgery. That study reported no increase in CTS between patients with AL amyloidosis and the general population, but this may be because there was no reporting of CTS symptoms, only the history of a surgical intervention.[22]

CTS commonly presents earlier in the course of AL amyloidosis than cardiomyopathy, so bilateral CTS or a history of carpal tunnel release surgery may be an early warning sign of an underlying systemic disease. Amyloid deposits in the flexor tenosynovium and transverse carpal ligament cause impingement on the median nerve, resulting in classic CTS symptoms.[23] This process is important, because a small amount of amyloid deposition causes CTS symptoms, but further amyloid deposition is required before symptomatic cardiomyopathy develops. Cardiomyopathy is the limiting prognostic factor in patients with AL amyloidosis, so early detection based on a diagnosis of CTS can positively influence the course of the disease. As a result, hand surgeons and hematologists alike advocate for routine screening biopsy during carpal tunnel release surgery.[24]

Myopathy

Amyloid infiltrates muscles and causes concomitant hypertrophy and weakness. The most commonly affected muscles include quadriceps, hamstring, triceps, deltoids, biceps, gluteus maximus, and gastrocnemius. By the time muscles become affected by AL amyloidosis, other organ systems are generally affected as well. The initial presenting symptom is usually proximal muscle weakness, which may mimic polymyalgia rheumatica or inflammatory myopathy with difficulty rising from a chair or brushing hair. When the neck flexors are severely affected, the patients may have to support their heads when sitting up from the supine position to prevent hyperextension.

Distal weakness, myalgia, and dysphagia may be associated and atrophy may be noted on physical examination. Pseudohypertrophy develops later in the disease course and, when present, makes identification of amyloidosis as the underlying cause more obvious.[25] When deltoid muscles develop pseudohypertrophy, the classic shoulder-pad sign may be noted on physical examination and is pathognomonic for AL amyloidosis[17,26] (**Fig. 8**). In 1 study, 1.6% of patients with AL amyloidosis had findings of muscle pseudohypertrophy.[2] Infiltration of intraocular muscles can cause proptosis and ophthalmoplegia.[19] Involvement of the diaphragm has been reported to cause respiratory failure requiring mechanical ventilation. In these patients, respiratory failure will be the cause of death.[25,27]

Electromyograms show myopathic changes but do not generally yield a diagnosis. Creatine kinase level may be normal or increased and can fluctuate, so it is not a good screening marker for amyloid myopathy. Imaging is nonspecific and biopsy is often required to identify the cause if other end-organ damage has not already suggested amyloidosis as the diagnosis. Tissue specimens show denervation atrophy and regenerating and necrotic fibers, consistent with myopathy. Amyloid deposition in vessel walls is universal and is also likely to be present in perimysium/endomysium or encasing muscle fibers. This deposition interferes with normal propagation of action potentials along the sarcolemma.[19] Even after biopsy, patients are often misdiagnosed, so

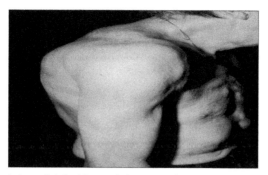

Fig. 8. Shoulder-pad sign of deltoid pseudohypertrophy.

monoclonal gammopathy work-up should be standard in the evaluation of myopathy.[28]

Cutaneous Manifestations

Skin findings in AL amyloidosis are varied and occur in 30% to 40% of cases. The most common manifestation is purpura caused by vascular infiltration with amyloid, which is discussed later. Otherwise, characteristic skin lesions are smooth, shiny, waxy, nontender, nonpruritic papules, nodules, or plaques, which may be skin colored, amber, brown, or yellow. The lesions sometimes also have a hemorrhagic appearance or they may resemble vesicles. The eyelids are a common location for these lesions and they may only become apparent when the eyes are closed (**Fig. 9**). Other common locations include flexural areas, retroauricular, neck, axillae, umbilicus, inguinal, or anogenital regions[29] (**Fig. 10**).

Nodules often resemble condyloma lata in the anogenital area and xanthomas in other areas. Plaques can be isolated or can coalesce and form a large tumefactive lesion, which can exclude the external auditory meatus. The presentation can mimic scleroderma with thickening of face, hands, and feet. Keratosis of the fingers can lead to contractures and loss of mobility. It can also resemble myxedema with rigid expression, drooping eyelids, and enlarged ears. Scalp involvement can cause alopecia and nails may appear dystrophic with striations, brittleness, and crumbling

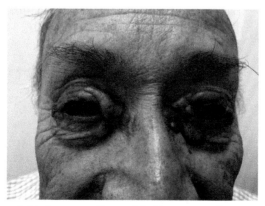

Fig. 9. Cutaneous amyloid plaques on the eyelids. Plaques are also present in the nasolabial fold.

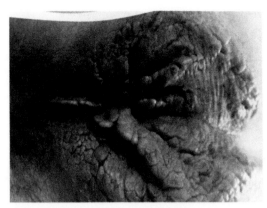

Fig. 10. Anal amyloid lesions that resemble condyloma.

(**Fig. 11**). Bullous lesions form when there is shearing of the dermal amyloid deposits in skin or mucosal areas. When occurring on the hands, these bullae can simulate porphyria cutanea tarda.[29] Penile ulcers have also been reported as a manifestation of AL amyloidosis.[30]

AL amyloidosis of the skin without systemic involvement is possible and is histologically indistinguishable from amyloidosis related to systemic disease. Localized cutaneous AL amyloidosis of the nodular subtype progresses to systemic disease in up to 50% of cases. Skin biopsy of any type of cutaneous amyloid shows deposition of amorphous, eosinophilic, fissured material in the papillary dermis with thinning or obliteration of the rete ridges that stains with Congo red and shows apple-green birefringence under polarized light.[31] The amyloid deposits generally do not have associated inflammatory infiltrate. Local blood vessel walls, pilosebaceous units, arrector pili muscles, lamina propria of sweat glands and ducts, and individual fat cells are surrounded by amyloid, which appears as amyloid rings.[29] Biopsy of clinically normal skin in patients with systemic amyloidosis is positive in about 50% to 55% of cases.[19,29]

Periorbital Ecchymosis

Vascular amyloid deposition can manifest as a structural abnormality, such as an increase in vessel wall thickness, or as functional abnormality, such as endothelial

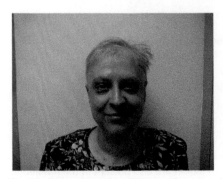
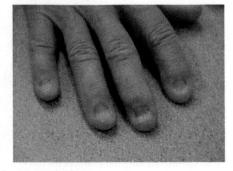

Fig. 11. Alopecia and nail dystrophy caused by AL amyloidosis.

dysfunction. Common findings caused by vascular infiltration include the classic raccoon-eye sign of periorbital hemorrhage, jaw and limb claudication, and angina in the absence of coronary artery disease. Vascular involvement of tissues throughout the body is extremely common in patients with AL amyloidosis, seen on biopsies in up to 88% to 90% of patients in various studies, which is in stark contrast with the low incidence of vascular involvement by ATTR amyloidosis.[32,33]

Although vessels throughout the body are affected, purpura tends to manifest in areas with thin skin where the vessels are most fragile. For this reason, the periorbital areas are preferentially affected and can be triggered by minor trauma (**Fig. 12**). The increased pressure caused by vomiting, coughing, forced respiration, Valsalva maneuver, or Trendelenburg position can be the inciting factor for periorbital hemorrhage. Postproctoscopy after prolonged Trendelenburg position is a classic situation in which raccoon eyes develop because of venous congestion. Even gentle eye scratching, rubbing, or pinching can cause cutaneous hemorrhage or skin shedding.[19] Eye taping and removal during general anesthesia of a patient with AL amyloid should be done with care to avoid causing periorbital hemorrhage.

Petechiae and purpura can occur in other areas as well, especially areas with skin folds such as nasolabial fold, neck, axillae, umbilicus, and anogenital regions. Overall, cutaneous hemorrhage is noted in about 15% of patients with AL amyloidosis.[8] These purpuric areas may become hyperpigmented. Removal of electrocardiogram leads or tape can also trigger hemorrhage. Because AL amyloidosis can cause factor X deficiency along with vascular fragility, these patients are at increased risk for hemorrhage.[34]

Claudications

Jaw claudication is classically considered a symptom of giant cell arteritis (GCA) in which vasculitis causes jaw fatigue with mastication. This situation leads to a biopsy of the temporal artery, in which a finding of amyloidosis is often a surprise. Amyloid infiltrates the media of arteries and arterioles, including the temporal artery, and renders them fixed and nonexpansile, which leads to ischemia.[19,35] Amyloid can also

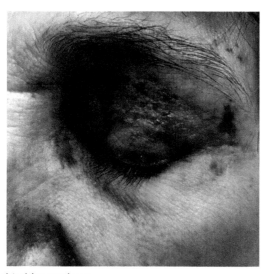

Fig. 12. Mild periorbital hemorrhage.

infiltrate the muscles of mastication. This involvement leads to symptoms that mimic GCA, such as jaw claudication, temporal headaches, and blurred vision.[36,37]

About 10% of patients with AL amyloidosis report symptoms of jaw claudication. Arm and leg claudication are less common vascular manifestations of AL amyloidosis. Arm or leg claudication in combination with the other symptoms provides a clue that symptoms mimicking GCA are related to a systemic issue and are not solely limited to the temporal artery. Another clue that GCA is not the true diagnosis is a lack of response to corticosteroids.[37] The erythrocyte sedimentation rate is not specific, and it may or may not be increased in amyloidosis. When the temporal artery is biopsied, the classic inflammation of GCA is absent, but amyloid would be identified if Congo red staining is done. Because AL amyloidosis affects vessels much more commonly and extensively than other types of amyloid, this type of presentation mimicking GCA is more common in AL amyloidosis than in ATTR amyloidosis. For this reason, if a temporal artery biopsy does not show inflammation, Congo red staining is necessary.[36] If amyloid is discovered, immunohistochemistry can be done for subtyping. Claudication may improve with systemic therapy, but usually does not resolve completely.[1]

Myocardial Ischemia

Amyloid can also deposit in small intramyocardial arteries. This deposition can occur independently of the interstitial cardiac amyloid deposition that leads to restrictive cardiomyopathy. Vascular deposition starts in the media of the vessel and, once severe, the deposition can extend transmurally. Extensive myocardial vascular involvement can cause stenosis or luminal obliteration of the vessel, which leads to focal subendocardial ischemic injury, myocardial necrosis, focal scarring, and ischemic cardiomyopathy. In a series of 108 patients with cardiac amyloidosis of all subtypes who were evaluated at autopsy, 5 patients (4.6%) had severe intramyocardial vascular amyloid deposition associated with local areas of myocardial ischemia. Four of these 5 patients had AL amyloidosis, although most of the patients in the study had ATTR amyloidosis. Epicardial coronary arteries, which are normally affected by coronary artery disease in cases of ischemic heart disease, were relatively free of atherosclerotic changes on pathologic evaluation.[38] This finding suggests that ischemic cardiomyopathy caused by microvascular involvement may have a significant impact on the cardiac morbidity of amyloidosis in patients with the AL subtype given the vascular predilection.

Patients with significant cardiac ischemia caused by amyloidosis present with either typical exertional angina, atypical chest pain, or acute myocardial infarction. Microvascular disease causes decreased coronary flow reserve, but coronary arteries appear relatively normal on cardiac catheterization. In another study of 153 patients with chest pain and normal coronaries on angiography, 5 were later found to have AL amyloidosis. Four presented with angina and 1 with myocardial infarction. Echocardiography at presentation showed no signs of cardiac amyloidosis in any of the 5 patients. Exercise stress test reproduced their angina and showed ST segment depression, and exercise stress imaging showed reversible perfusion defects similar to those commonly seen in myocardial ischemia caused by coronary artery disease. Typical cardiac medications such as angiotensin-converting enzyme inhibitors, nitrates, and calcium channel blockers did not result in improvement, and some patients worsened. Right ventricular biopsy was ultimately performed in 2 of the patients and showed amyloid deposition within the media of the walls of the intramyocardial vessels without luminal obstruction. AL amyloidosis was diagnosed 9 to 48 months after initial presentation when more common signs of amyloidosis, such as renal insufficiency and cardiomyopathy, manifested. All patients eventually developed congestive heart failure; 4 of the 5 died of cardiac causes.[39]

SUMMARY

The soft tissue and vascular manifestations of AL amyloidosis comprise a wide spectrum of clinical presentations that may not be immediately apparent as belonging to a single systemic illness. Many of the signs and symptoms lead to misdiagnosis of various rheumatologic diseases, such as RA, polymyalgia rheumatica, scleroderma, or GCA. Although these manifestations are usually not life threatening, if they are iden tified accurately as part of the AL amyloidosis syndrome, the underlying plasma cell disorder can be treated. With early treatment, the life-threatening organ dysfunction of amyloidosis, such as heart failure and renal failure, can be averted or delayed. As such, all clinicians should have a low threshold to screen for monoclonal gammopathy when key clinical findings do not fit a given diagnosis.

CLINICS CARE POINTS

- Macroglossia, periorbital ecchymosis, and the shoulder-pad sign of deltoid pseudohypertrophy are considered pathognomonic for AL amyloidosis.
- In any patient with a rheumatologic diagnosis that does not adequately fit with the clinical presentation and laboratory findings, amyloid arthropathy should be considered in the differential diagnosis.
- CTS commonly presents earlier in the course of AL amyloidosis than cardiomyopathy, so bilateral CTS or a history of carpal tunnel release surgery may be an early warning sign of underlying amyloidosis.
- The increased capillary pressure caused by vomiting, coughing, forced respiration, Valsalva maneuver, or Trendelenburg position can be the inciting factor for periorbital ecchymosis in a patient with AL amyloidosis.

DISCLOSURE

The authors have nothing to disclose.

REFERENCES

1. Gertz M, Comenzo R, Falk RH, et al. Definition of Organ Involvement and Treatment Response in Immunoglobulin Light Chain Amyloidosis (AL): A Consensus Opinion From the 10th International Symposium on Amyloid in Amyloidosis. Am J Hematol 2005;79(3 19):319–28.
2. Prokaeva T, Spencer B. Soft Tissue, Joint, and Bone Manifestations of AL Amyloidosis. Arthritis Rheum 2007;56(11):3858–68.
3. Tsai SB, Seldin DC, O'Hara C, et al. Myocardial infarction with 'clean coronaries' caused by light-chain AL amyloidosis: a case report and literature review. Amyloid 2011;18:160–4.
4. Guijarro-Martinez R, Alba LM, Puchades RV, et al. Rational Management of Macroglossia Due to Acquired Systemic Amyloidosis: Does Surgery Play a Role? J Oral Maxillofac Surg 2009;67:2013–7.
5. Cuddy S, Falk RH. Amyloidosis as a Systemic Disease in Context. Can J Cardiol 2020;36:396–407.
6. Cowan AJ, Skinner M, Berk JL, et al. Macroglossia - not always AL amyloidosis. Amyloid 2011;18:83–6.

7. Angiero F, Seramondi R, Magistro S, et al. Amyloid Deposition in the Tongue: Clinical and Histopathological Profile. Anticancer Res 2010;30:3009–14.
8. Kyle RA, Bayrd ED. Amyloidosis: Review of 236 Cases. Medicine 1975;51(4):271–99.
9. Raubenheimer EJ, Dauth J, Pretorius FJ. Multiple myeloma and amyloidosis of the tongue. J Oral Pathol 1988;17:554–9.
10. Penner CR, Muller S. Head and neck amyloidosis: A clinicopathologic study of 15 cases. Oral Oncol 2006;42:421–9.
11. Reinish EI, Raviv M, Srolovitz H, et al. Tongue, primary amyloidosis, and multiple myeloma. Oral Surg Oral Med Oral Pathol 1994;77:121–5.
12. Thibault I, Vallieres I. Macroglossia due to Systemic Amyloidosis: Is There a Role for Radiotherapy. Case Rep Oncol 2011;4:392–9.
13. Cobb AR, Boyapati R, Walker DM, et al. The surgical management of severe macroglossia in systemic AL amyloidosis. Br J Oral Maxillofac Surg 2013;51:e72–374.
14. Topouzelis N, Iliopoulos C, Kolokitha OE. Macroglossia. Int Dent J 2011;61:63–9.
15. Yoon SH, Cho JH, Jung HY, et al. Exceptional mucocutaneous manifestations with amyloid nephropathy: a case report. J Med Case Rep 2018;12:1760–6.
16. Law ST, Jafarzadeh SR, Govender P, et al. Comparison of Ultrasound Features of Major Salivary Glands in Sarcoidosis, Amyloidosis, and Sjögren's syndrome. Arthritis Care Res 2019. https://doi.org/10.1002/acr.24029.
17. Lakhanpal S, Li CY, Gertz MA, et al. Synovial Fluid Analysis for Diagnosis of Amyloid Arthropathy. Arthritis Rheum 1987;30(4):419–23.
18. Fautrel B, Fermand JP, Nochy D, et al. Amyloid Arthropathy in the Course of Multiple Myeloma. J Rheumatol 2002;29:1473–81.
19. Kyle A, Griepp PR. Amyloidosis (AL): Clinical and Laboratory Features in 229 cases. Mayo Clin Proc 1983;58:665–83.
20. Elsaman AM, Radwan AR, Akmatov MK, et al. Amyloid arthropathy associated with multiple myeloma: A systematic analysis of 101 reported cases. Semin Arthritis Rheum 2013;43:405–12.
21. Wiernik P. Amyloid Joint Disease. Medicine 1972;51(6):465–79.
22. Milandri A, Farioli A, Gagliardi C, et al. Carpal tunnel syndrome in cardiac amyloidosis: implications for early diagnosis and prognostic role across the spectrum of aetiologies. Eur Soc Cardiol 2019. https://doi.org/10.1002/ejhf.1742.
23. Sperry BW, Reyes BA, Ikram A, et al. Tenosynovial and Cardiac Amyloidosis in Patients Undergoing Carpal Tunnel Release. J Am Coll Cardiol 2018;72(17):2040–50.
24. Donnelly JP, Hanna M, Sperry BW, et al. Carpal Tunnel Syndrome: A Potential Early, Red-Flag Sign of Amyloidosis. J Hand Surg Am 2019;44(10):868–76.
25. Gertz M, Kyle RA. Myopathy in primary systemic amyloidosis. J Neurol Neurosurg Psychiatry 1996;60:655–60.
26. Liepnieks JJ, Burt C, Benson MD. Shoulder-Pad Sign of Amyloidosis: Structure of an Ig Kappa III Protein. Scand J Immunol 2001;54:404–8.
27. Berk JL, Wiesman JF, Skinner M, et al. Diaphragm paralysis in primary systemic amyloidosis. Amyloid 2005;12:193–6.
28. Muchtar E, Derudas D, Mauermann M, et al. Systemic Immunoglobulin Light Chain Amyloidosis-Associated Myopathy: Presentation, Diagnostic Pitfalls, and Outcome. Mayo Clin Proc 2016;91(10):1354–61.
29. Breathnach SM. Amyloid and Amyloidosis. J Am Acad Dermatol 1988;18(1):1–16.

30. Arun M, Shelton A, Sanchorawala V. Penile ulcers complicating systemic AL amyloidosis: a case report. Amyloid 2016;23:203–4.
31. Terushkin V, Boyd KP, Patel RR, et al. Primary localized cutaneous amyloidosis. Dermatol Online J 2013;19(12):1–3.
32. Modesto M, Dispenzieri A, Gertz M, et al. Vascular abnormalities in primary amyloidosis. Eur Heart J 2007;28:1019–24.
33. Crotty TB, Chin-Yang L, Edwards D, et al. Amyloidosis and Endomyocardial Biopsy: Correlation of Extent and Pattern of Deposition with Amyloid Immunophenotype in 100 Cases. Cardiovasc Pathol 1995;4(1):39–42.
34. Weingarten TN, Hall BA, Richardson BF, et al. Periorbital Ecchymoses During General Anesthesia in a Patient with Primary Amyloidosis: A Harbinger for Bleeding? Anesth Analg 2007;105(6):1561–3.
35. Subbarao K, Jacobson HG. Amyloidosis and Plasma Cell Dyscrasias of the Musculoskeletal System. Semin Roentgenol 1986;21(2):139–49.
36. Churchill CH, Abril A, Krishna M, et al. Jaw Claudication in Primary Amyloidosis: Unusual Presentation of a Rare Disease. J Rheumatol 2003;30:2283–6.
37. Salvarani C, Gabriel SE, Gertz M, et al. Primary Systemic Amyloidosis Presenting as Giant Cell Arteritis and Polymyalgia Rheumatica. Arthritis Rheum 1994;37(11):1621–6.
38. Smith RR, Hutchins GM. Ischemic Heart Disease Secondary to Amyloidosis of Intramyocardial Arteries. Am J Cardiol 1979;44:413–7.
39. Al Suwaidi J, Velianou JL, Gertz MA, et al. Systemic Amyloidosis Presenting with Angina Pectoris. Ann Intern Med 1999;131(11):838–41.

Options for Chemotherapy and Scoring Response and Relapse

Cindy Varga, MD[a],*, Chakra Chaulagain, MD[b]

KEYWORDS

- AL amyloidosis • Novel agents • Proteasome inhibitor • Immunomodulator
- Cardiac amyloidosis • Renal amyloidosis

KEY POINTS

- The treatment of amyloid light chain (AL) amyloidosis depends on stem cell transplant eligibility. For transplant-ineligible patients, a bortezomib-based regimen is used first line.
- Alkylating agents, such as cyclophosphamide/melphalan, often are combined with bortezomib as frontline therapy. Immunomodulators are reserved for relapse due to their high toxicity profile.
- Targeted therapy with venetoclax, a B-cell lymphoma 2 inhibitor, is proving to be a promising agent with a relatively mild toxicity profile.
- Prognosis of AL amyloidosis depends on the number and extent of organs affected at the time of diagnosis. Cardiac involvement carries the worst prognosis. Early diagnosis and prompt treatment are key for prolonged survival.
- There are well-validated response and progression criteria. Incorporating these criteria into clinical practice and into clinical trials is encouraged.

INTRODUCTION

The primary goal in amyloid light chain (AL) amyloidosis is the rapid achievement of a hematologic response and ultimately the reversal of organ dysfunction. Although anti–plasma cell agents can halt the production of pathologic light chains effectively, the precursor protein responsible for widespread organ damage, they do not target the circulating or deposited amyloid fibrils. Because there currently are no Food Drug and Administration (FDA)-approved drugs in AL amyloidosis, physicians rely on the same combination of medications currently approved in the treatment of multiple myeloma (MM). Due to differences in disease biology, there are major challenges

a The John Conant Davis Myeloma and Amyloid Program, Division of Hematology/Oncology, Tufts Medical Center, 800 Washington Street, Boston, MA 02111, USA; b Department of Hematology and Oncology, Maroone Cancer Center, Cleveland Clinic Florida, 2950 Cleveland Clinic Boulevard, Weston, FL 33331, USA
* Corresponding author.
E-mail address: cvarga1@tuftsmedicalcenter.org
Twitter: @ChaulagainMD (C.C.)

Hematol Oncol Clin N Am 34 (2020) 1115–1131
https://doi.org/10.1016/j.hoc.2020.07.005
0889-8588/20/© 2020 Elsevier Inc. All rights reserved.

when adapting myeloma drugs to fit the needs of patients with amyloidosis; dose adjustments are required to accommodate for organ dysfunction and to address the lower toxicity threshold encountered in this patient population. For example, the use of high-dose melphalan (HDM) and stem cell transplantation (SCT), a cornerstone in the treatment of MM, has a more limited role in AL amyloidosis due to advanced heart failure, poor performance status, and multiorgan involvement. Conservative treatment with alkylating agents and novel anti–plasma cell therapies, such as proteasome inhibitors (PIs) and immunomodulators (IMiDs), have led to a paradigm shift in this disease, resulting in improved outcomes over the past 2 decades. This article comprehensively reviews the treatment options for AL amyloid patients who are ineligible for SCT.

ALKYLATING AGENTS

Alkylating agents are an important class of antineoplastic drugs that prevent cell division by cross-linking DNA strands, thus preventing DNA synthesis and halting tumor growth. They have no cellular specificity but the high chance of interacting with dividing cells forms the basis for their antitumor effects.[1]

Melphalan

Melphalan is one of the oldest agents used in AL amyloidosis and at one point was the standard-first line therapy in this disease. Melphalan can be administered in both oral and intravenous forms. Intravenous melphalan in high doses is the modality of choice for conditioning prior to an SCT, whereas lower-dose oral melphalan tends to be used in the outpatient setting. A multicenter randomized trial, comparing HDM/SCT with oral melphalan and dexamethasone (MDex), demonstrated inferior median overall survival (OS) in the transplant arm compared with the nontransplant arm (22.2 months vs 56.9 months, respectively) after a median follow-up of 3 years.[1] The main critique of this trial was the 24% treatment-related mortality in the SCT arm, indicating that many of the patients were not fit to undergo SCT. With the use of stricter eligibility criteria and careful patient selection, HDM/SCT has become an extremely effective treatment modality in amyloidosis, with complete response (CR) rates that range from 40% to 60%.[2,3] The indication and efficacy of HDM/SCT are discussed in detail in Morie A. Gertz and Stefan Schonland's article, "Stem Cell Mobilization and Autologous Transplant for Immunoglobulin Light-Chain Amyloidosis" in this issue.

In a large, randomized, single-center study conducted in the final decades of the twentieth century, 220 patients with AL amyloidosis were assigned to receive melphalan and prednisone, melphalan-prednisone-colchicine, or colchicine alone.[4] Therapy that included melphalan and prednisone resulted in higher objective response rates and led to improved OS compared with the colchicine-alone arm (median OS of 18 months vs 8.5 months, respectively; $P<.001$).

In another study, the pairing of MDex also was examined among transplant-ineligible patients. MDex led to impressive outcomes, with an overall hematologic response (OHR) of 67% and a CR rate of 33%. CRs were durable and maintained in 70% of patients for at least 3 years.[5]

Although oral melphalan no longer is the drug of choice for first line therapy in North America, it still is used by many amyloid specialists in Europe today.

Bendamustine

Bendamustine is a bifunctional alkylating agent that has been used effectively in various indolent lymphoproliferative disorders, such as chronic lymphocytic leukemia, follicular lymphoma, and Waldenström macroglobulinemia.[6–8] In addition to crosslinking DNA strands, it also acts through other unclear mechanisms, which may explain its efficacy in patients who are refractory to other chemotherapeutic agents.[9]

A phase 2, multicenter trial was conducted to evaluate the efficacy and safety of bendamustine and dexamethasone in 31 patients with relapsed or refractory AL amyloidosis (RRAL); 57% of patients achieved a partial response (PR) or better (11% CR and 18% very good PR [VGPR]). The overall organ response was 29% (46% renal and 13% cardiac) whereas 42% experienced organ progression. The median OS was 18.2 months but it was significantly longer in patients who had achieved a hematologic response after 2 cycles (median OS not reached). Median progression-free survival (PFS) was 11.3 months; 65% of patients had treatment-related grade 3 or grade 4 adverse events (AEs), the most common leukopenia (26%), fatigue (19%), renal dysfunction (13%), rash (6%), and mood symptoms (6%).[10]

Overall, Bendamustine is a feasible option in patients with RRAL who have progressed on multiple lines of therapy, even if treated with a prior alkylator.

Cyclophosphamide

Cyclophosphamide is one of the most commonly used alkylating agents in the treatment of AL amyloidosis. It often is combined with bortezomib and dexamethasone to form a popular triplet therapy utilized as frontline therapy. This regimen is discussed in further detail.

PROTEASOME INHIBITORS

The proteasome and its multicatalytic enzymatic activity play a key role in the ubiquitin-proteasome system. Proteasomes regulate protein homeostasis within the cell by rapidly degrading ubiquitinated target proteins directly involved in cell cycle regulation, transcription, DNA repair, and apoptosis.[11] PIs may be especially effective against malignant plasma cells, given the high rate of protein synthesis in the form of light and heavy chains making up the immunoglobulin structure. In AL amyloidosis, bortezomib, carfilzomib (CFZ), and ixazomib (Ixa) all have been evaluated.

Bortezomib

Several retrospective studies demonstrated the efficacy of intravenous bortezomib in both RRAL and newly diagnosed AL amyloidosis patients. Although bortezomib led to impressive organ responses at a rate of 30% to 40%, this was at the expense of a high discontinuation rate due to the development of peripheral neuropathy (PN).[12,13]

In a first prospective phase 1/2 study, intravenous bortezomib was evaluated as a once-weekly (1.6-mg/m^2) or twice-weekly (1.3-mg/m^2) regimen in patients with RRAL.[14,15] The overall CR rates were 37.5% and 24.2%, respectively, and the median time to first response was 2.1 and 0.7 months, respectively. In both cohorts, a majority of responses were maintained beyond 1 year. One-year hematologic PFS rates were 72.2% and 74.6%, respectively, and 1-year OS rates were 93.8% and 84.0%, respectively. As expected, rates of grade greater than or equal to 3 AEs were significantly greater in the twice-weekly dosing cohort (79% vs 50%, respectively) although no grade 3 PN was reported in either group. Once-a-week dosing of bortezomib has been the preferred frequency among amyloid physicians globally.

Triple-therapy combinations involving bortezomib, steroid, and an alkylator, such as cyclophosphamide or melphalan, have been adopted as popular first lines of therapy in AL amyloidosis patients who are not eligible for HDM/SCT. In 2014, a large international, multicenter, retrospective study evaluated 60 patients with Mayo Clinic stage III cardiac amyloidosis (**Tables 1** and **2** lists staging criteria) who received

Table 1
The cardiac staging system in amyloid light chain amyloidosis

Staging System	Markers	Cutoffs	Cardiac Stage	N	Key References
Standard Mayo	NT-proBNP, cTnT	>332 ng/L >0.035 ng/mL	I = both markers below cutoff II = 1 marker elevated III = both markers elevated	Non-ASCT = 242 ASCT = 98	Dispenzieri et al,[66] 2004; Dispenzieri et al,[67] 2004
Revised Mayo	NT-proBNP, cTnT dFLC	>1800 ng/L >0.025 ng/mL >180 mg/L	I = all markers below cutoff II = 1 marker elevated III = 2 markers elevated IV = all markers elevated	808	Kumar et al,[68] 2012
BU	TnI BNP	>0.1 ng/mL >81pg/mL	I = both markers below cutoff II = 1 marker above cutoff III = both markers above cutoff	Derivation cohort = 249 Complementary cohort = 592	Lilleness et al,[69] 2019

Abbreviations: ASCT, Autologous stem cell transplantation; BU, Boston university; JCO, *Journal of Clinical Oncology.*
Data from Refs.[66–69]

Table 2
The renal staging system in amyloid light chain amyloidosis

Markers	Cutoffs	Renal Stage	N	Key Reference
24-h proteinuria	>5 g	I = both markers below cutoff	732	Palladini et al,[70] 2014
eGFR	<50 mL/min/1.73 m^2	II = 1 marker elevated		
		III = both markers elevated		

Data from Palladini G, Hegenbart U, Milani P, Kimmich C, Foli A, Ho AD, et al. A staging system for renal outcome and early markers of renal response to chemotherapy in AL amyloidosis. Blood. 2014;124(15):2325-32.

cyclophosphamide-bortezomib-dexamethasone (CVD). The overall response rate was 68% but, among the patients who survived longer than 3 months, the OHR was an impressive 86%. A cardiac response (**Tables 3** and **4** lists response and progression criteria) was reported in one-third of patients. The estimated 1-year OS for the entire cohort was 57%, with 40% of patients ultimately succumbing to their disease. Neuropathy was reported in only 18% of patients.[16]

The largest study to examine the efficacy of the CVD regimen was a European retrospective series of 230 newly diagnosed AL amyloidosis patients. In this study, the OHR was 60% (VGPR 43%). Renal and cardiac responses were 25% and 17%, respectively. The cardiac cohort had a survival benefit with the achievement of a hematologic response though patients with advanced disease (N-terminal pro-BNP [NT-proBNP] >8500 ng/L) had an inferior median OS of only 7 months.[17]

The combination of melphalan-bortezomib-dexamethasone (BMDex) was studied in a matched case-control study and demonstrated a higher OHR over MDex alone (42% vs 19%, respectively), although this did not translate into superior OS.[18] In a phase 3 multicenter study, MDex was compared with BMDex in newly diagnosed AL

Table 3
Hematologic response and progression criteria in amyloid light chain amyloidosis

Hematologic Response	Response Criteria	Key References
CR	Normalization of FLC levels and ratio, negative serum and urine immunofixation	Comenzo et al,[73] 2012 Palladini et al,[74] 2012
VGPR	Decline in the dFLC to <40 mg/L	
PR	>50% reduction in the dFLC	
NR	Less than a PR	
Progression	From CR: any reappearance of monoclonal protein or abnormal FLC ratio (light chain must double) From PR: a 50% increase in serum M protein to >0.5 g/dL or 50% increase in urine M protein to >200 mg/d or an FLC increase of 50% to >100 mg/L	

Abbreviations: M protein, monoclonal protein; NR, no response.
Data from Comenzo RL, Reece D, Palladini G, Seldin D, Sanchorawala V, Landau H, et al. Consensus guidelines for the conduct and reporting of clinical trials in systemic light-chain amyloidosis. Leukemia. 2012;26(11):2317-25; and Palladini G, Dispenzieri A, Gertz MA, Kumar S, Wechalekar A, Hawkins PN, et al. New criteria for response to treatment in immunoglobulin light chain amyloidosis based on free light chain measurement and cardiac biomarkers: impact on survival outcomes. J Clin Oncol. 2012;30(36):4541-9.

Table 4
Organ response and progression criteria for amyloid light chain amyloidosis

Organ	Response Criteria	Progression Criteria	Key References
Heart	NT-proBNP response (>30% and >300 ng/L decrease in patients with baseline NT-proBNP ≥650 ng/L) or NYHA class response (≥2 class decrease in subjects with baseline NYHA class 3 or 4)	NT-proBNP progression (>30% and >300 ng/L increase) or cTn progression (≥33% increase) or ejection fraction progression (≥10% decrease)	Comenzo et al,[73] 2012 Palladini et al,[74] 2012
Kidney	50% decrease (at least 0.5 g/d) of 24-h urine protein (urine protein must be >0.5 g/d pretreatment). Creatinine and creatinine clearance must not worsen by 25% over baseline	50% increase (at least 1 g/d) of 24-h urine protein to >1 g/d or 25% worsening of serum creatinine or creatinine clearance	
Liver	50% decrease in abnormal ALP value. Decrease in liver size radiographically at least 2 cm.	50% increase of ALP above the lowest value	

Data from Comenzo RL, Reece D, Palladini G, Seldin D, Sanchorawala V, Landau H, et al. Consensus guidelines for the conduct and reporting of clinical trials in systemic light-chain amyloidosis. Leukemia. 2012;26(11):2317-25; and Palladini G, Dispenzieri A, Gertz MA, Kumar S, Wechalekar A, Hawkins PN, et al. New criteria for response to treatment in immunoglobulin light chain amyloidosis based on free light chain measurement and cardiac biomarkers: impact on survival outcomes. J Clin Oncol. 2012;30(36):4541-9.

amyloidosis patients. The OHR and CR/VGPR rates were significantly higher in the BMDex arms. Cardiac response was 24% in the MDex arm and 38% in the BMDex arm.

Generally, although bortezomib is a very effective agent in AL amyloidosis, it bears limitations, particularly its high rate of PN. Approximately one-fifth of AL amyloidosis patients initially present with disease-related PN; thus, bortezomib may require dose reduction or may be contraindicated in some cases.[19] In an attempt to reduce neurotoxicity, subcutaneous delivery now is the modality of choice and has been shown to result in similar high rates of hematologic responses equivalent to historic controls.[20]

Cytogenetic information also is an important factor when considering bortezomib for first-line therapy; there is some evidence demonstrating that patients harboring a translocation[11,14] have inferior outcomes with bortezomib and instead should be considered for alkylator-based treatments.[21] Larger studies still are required to confirm these results.

Carfilzomib

CFZ is a highly selective, irreversible second-generation PI with well-documented efficacy both in patients with newly diagnosed MM and those with relapsed refractory MM (RRMM).[22,23] CFZ has a marked selectivity for the active site of the proteasome[24]; thus, it results in fewer off-target effects.[25,26] In the myeloma literature, CFZ has demonstrated a significantly lower incidence of PN[27-30] and is an attractive option for patients with disease-related PN at baseline.

CFZ was administered to 28 patients with RRAL in a phase 1/2 study at increasing doses (27 mg/m^2, 36 mg/m^2, and 45 mg/m^2). The 36-mg/m^2 dose was the maximum tolerated dose (MTD) in this cohort. Fatigue (36%) was the most common drug-related AE reported, followed by an increase in creatinine (29%), nausea (25%), dyspnea (18%), anemia (18%), diarrhea (14%), and hypertension (11%). There was a high rate of grade greater than or equal to 3 AEs (71%), which included a decrease in ejection fraction and ventricular tachycardia in 1 patient. The OHR was impressive at 63% (CR 12%), with a fifth of responding patients achieving an organ response. Although CFZ proved effective in this study, the cardiac toxicity raises concern in this particular patient population. Eleven patients (39%) had NT-proBNP increases of grade greater than or equal to 30%, half of whom were clinically symptomatic.[31]

Due to cardiac toxicity concerns, CFZ has not been widely adopted in AL amyloidosis. Nevertheless, the potential of this drug cannot be denied, and, with cardiac surveillance, CFZ may be cautiously considered in patients with peripheral and/or autonomic neuropathy in whom bortezomib would be contraindicated and without severe cardiac or renal involvement.

Ixazomib

Ixa is the first orally available second-generation PI. Ixa was first FDA approved in 2015 for use in combination with lenalidomide and dexamethasone in RRMM. Similar to CFZ, Ixa has demonstrated a low incidence of PN.[32,33]

In a phase 1/2 trial, patients with RRAL were given Ixa on days 1, 8, and 15 of a 28-day cycle for up to 12 cycles. The MTD was 4 mg. AEs were mild and included nausea, skin disorders, diarrhea, and fatigue. The OHR was 52%, with organ responses reported in 56% of patients. Median PFS was 14.8 months. This PI was particularly effective in patients who were not previously exposed to bortezomib. The 1-year OS was 85%.[34]

A phase 3 study of dexamethasone and Ixa (Ixa-Dex) versus physician's choice in relapsed disease (NCT01659658) was discontinued in June 2019 due to its failure to demonstrate a significant improvement in OHR: 53% versus 51%, respectively, although CR rates were 26% and 18%. The second primary endpoint of 2-year vital organ deterioration or death was not mature at the time of the analysis. Expanded results were presented at the American Society of Hematology in December 2019.[35] Median duration of hematologic response was more than double in the Ixa-Dex arm (46.5 vs 20.2 months, respectively). Vital organ PFS was also longer in the Ixa-Dex cohort, 18.0 months versus 11.0 months, respectively. Time to treatment failure and time to subsequent therapy both favored the Ixa-Dex cohort. Drug-related AEs were similar in both groups. Unfortunately, due to the premature closure of this trial, the true potential of Ixa in relapsed could not be explored fully.

Currently, Ixa is being investigated as a maintenance drug (NCT03618537) after initial line of therapy. Tolerability has been encouraging in a phase 1/2 study (NCT03236792) of ixazomib-cyclophosphamide-dexamethasone in newly diagnosed AL amyloidosis.[36] Ixa also is being investigated in combination with daratumumab-dexamethasone (NCT03283917).

IMMUNOMODULATORS

IMiDs can exert their effects on the immune system by various mechanisms: the costimulation of both CD4$^+$ and CD8$^+$ T cells, the suppression of regulatory T cells, and the enhancement of antibody-dependent cellular cytotoxicity. IMiDs also can inhibit vascular endothelial growth factor, resulting in antiangiogenesis while influencing other mediators, such as interleukin and receptor activator of nuclear factor kappa-B ligand.[37]

Thalidomide

Thalidomide is a first-in class IMiD with documented activity in patients with MM.[38] Its initial use in AL amyloidosis at high doses was not well tolerated in a phase 2 trial. Progressive edema, cognitive difficulties, and constipation occurred in approximately 75% of patients. Five of 12 patients developed progressive renal insufficiency. Half of the 12 subjects withdrew from the study due to the side-effect profile.[39] In another phase 2 trial, lower doses of thalidomide and dexamethasone led to an OHR of 48% (CR 19%). Organ responses also were seen in 26% of patients. Despite lower doses, treatment-related toxicities were reported in two-thirds of patients.[40]

In 1 trial, thalidomide combined with cyclophosphamide and dexamethasone (CTD) in transplant ineligible patients led to an OHR of 74% and a CR of 21%.[41] Thalidomide also was investigated for use as consolidation post-HDM/SCT in patients who did not achieve a CR as a risk-adapted approach; 42% of patients saw an improvement in hematologic response at 12 months post-SCT.[42]

When thalidomide was administered to patients with advanced cardiac amyloid (New York Heart Association [NYHA] class IV), the OHR was 36%, but approximately a third of patients died during treatment.[43]

A retrospective matched comparison of CVD versus risk-adapted CTD resulted in response rates of 71.0% versus 79.7%, respectively ($P = .32$). The CR rate was double in the CVD arm (40.5% vs 24.6%, respectively) although 1-year OS was the same. The median PFSs were 28.0 months and 14.0 months, respectively, for CVD and CTD, respectively ($P = .039$). The takeaway from this study was that CVD correlated with deeper responses and a prolonged PFS over CTD in the upfront setting.[44]

Overall, thalidomide has an expansive toxicity profile, making tolerance a major issue in this fragile population. Grade 3 or higher AEs were reported in more than 50% of participants in published studies. Fluid retention, symptomatic bradycardia, PN, and progression of renal failure are the most common events.[40,45]

Lenalidomide

Lenalidomide is a second-generation IMiD that commonly is used in first-line or second-line therapy in MM.[46,47] Several phase 2 studies have evaluated lenalidomide with or without dexamethasone in newly diagnosed and RRAL. In 1 trial, standard lenalidomide dosing (25 mg for 21 days of a 28-day cycle) was not well tolerated and the first 8 recruited participants required dose reductions to 15 mg and the protocol subsequently amended. The most common toxicities were myelosuppression and fatigue, with grade 3/4 neutropenia developing in a small percentage of patients. Other side effects included skin rash (59%) and venous thromboembolism (9%). Of the evaluable patients, the OHR was 67% (CR 29%) with an impressive renal response of 41%.[48] An unexpected observation in this study was the sudden deterioration of renal function among a large proportion of patients (20 of 34 enrolled). The median time from start of therapy to worsening organ function was only 44 days. Risk factors included renal amyloid involvement at baseline, older age, and greater proteinuria at start of therapy. There was no association between baseline estimated glomerular filtration rate (eGFR) and the development of renal failure. Some patients had renal recovery after the discontinuation of lenalidomide whereas patients who had to initiate dialysis had no recovery.[49] Brain natriuretic peptide (BNP) increases of greater than 30% also were noted among patients on trial, although this rise was not necessarily associated with heart failure symptoms; thus, the phenomenon was termed, *paradoxic*.

In a second trial, the activity of single-agent lenalidomide was limited, with only 1 patient achieving a hematologic response. The addition of dexamethasone did improve responses (OHR 41%). Similar to the prospective study discussed previously, there was a very high rate of grade greater than or equal to 3 AEs (86%) which included neutropenia, rash, and infection.[50]

Lenalidomide also has been evaluated in combination with different alkylating agents.[51–54] When combined with MDex in newly diagnosed AL amyloidosis patients, lenalidomide required dose reductions in nearly all subjects, many of whom had stage III cardiac involvement. Worsening cardiac failure and atrial fibrillation were the most common nonhematologic AEs observed. Renal function remained stable in most patients. At 6 months, the CR/VGPR rate was 50%. The overall organ response was 48%, some of whom had continued organ improvement 24 months after start of therapy.[51] In a lenalidomide-melphalan-dexamethasone phase 2 trial, the CR rate was 42%, with estimated 2-year OS and event-free survival rates of 80.8% and 53.8%, respectively. The MTD was determined to be 15 mg.[52]

The combination of lenalidomide with dexamethasone and oral cyclophosphamide, a well-tolerated alkylator, has resulted in OHR of approximately 60%.[53,54]

Pomalidomide

Pomalidomide is a well-tolerated second generation IMiD that was FDA approved in 2008 for the treatment of RRMM. In AL amyloidosis, pomalidomide has been investigated in combination with dexamethasone in phase 1/2 studies in.[55–57] All the studies resulted in impressive OHRs, ranging from 50% to 70%. Again, cytopenias and fatigue were the most common treatment-related AEs. Common grade greater than or equal to 3 AEs included fluid retention (25%), infection (25%), atrial fibrillation (7%), and deep venous thrombosis (7%). In 1 study, the median time to response was rapid, at 1 month, and even demonstrated a survival advantage in those who achieved a hematologic response.[57] Similar to lenalidomide, all the studies did report a paradoxic increase in cardiac biomarkers among a majority of participants, even in those who achieved hematologic responses. The mechanism behind this rise in biomarkers is unclear and may or may not represent true cadiotoxicity.[58]

In general, although lenalidomide and pomalidomide do have a role in the treatment of AL amyloidosis, they have been reserved mostly for use in the relapsed setting due to cardiac and renal toxicity concerns. Bortezomib-based regimens remain in the forefront, especially in transplant-ineligible patients.

SMALL MOLECULE: VENETOCLAX

The overexpression of antiapoptotic proteins, such as B-cell lymphoma 2 (BCL-2), BCL-XL, and MCL-1, plays a role in the survival of myeloma cells and possibly contributes to chemotherapy resistance.[59] Venetoclax is a selective, orally bioavailable inhibitor of BCL-2 that induces programmed cell death. Venetoclax currently is an approved drug for the treatment of chronic lymphocytic leukemia, small lymphocytic lymphoma, and acute myeloid leukemia.[60]

When venetoclax was evaluated in a phase 1 study in RRMM, the overall response rate was 21%; however, 86% of responders harbored the t(11;14). In this group, overall response rate was 40%, with 27% of patients achieving greater than or equal to VGPR.[61] Venetoclax is an extremely attractive drug for patients with AL amyloidosis, given its good tolerability and the high prevalence (50%–60%) of the t(11;14) mutation in this disease.[21] There are several case reports describing venetoclax's ability to induce a rapid complete hematologic and organ response among some AL amyloidosis patients with the t(11;14) mutation.[62–65] Unfortunately, a phase 1 trial (NCT03000660) of venetoclax and dexamethasone in RRAL was halted when the Bellini trial (NCT02755597), a phase 3 study of venetoclax-bortezomib-dexamethasone versus bortezomib- dexamethasone in RRMM, reported an increased mortality rate in the venetoclax arm versus placebo arm (21.1% vs 11.3%, respectively). Causes of death in the venetoclax arm were attributed to infection, sepsis, pneumonia, and cardiac arrest.

Venetoclax has great potential in AL amyloidosis in light of its rapid response and usually mild toxicity profile. For the moment, venetoclax should be reserved for a subgroup of AL amyloidosis patients who have been refractory to several lines of therapy and who harbor the t(11;14).

MONOCLONAL ANTIBODIES

Immunotherapy with monoclonal antibodies that target CD38 on plasma cells have been successfully incorporated into the treatment algorithm of MM. Daratumumab has been studied as monotherapy and in combination with other novel agents in AL amyloidosis with encouraging results. Isatuximab is another anti-CD38 monoclonal antibody approved for RRMM and currently is being evaluated in AL amyloidosis in a phase 2 Southwest Oncology Group study (NCT03499808). The role, mechanism of action, and tolerability of daratumumab and other monoclonal antibodies are discussed in further detail in Amandeep Godara and Giovanni Palladini's article, "Monoclonal Antibody Therapies in Systemic Light-Chain Amyloidosis" in this issue

PROGNOSTIC MODELS, STAGING, RESPONSE, AND PROGRESSION
Prognostic Models in Systemic Amyloid Light Chain Amyloidosis

Over the years, various prognostic classifications have been proposed for staging or for risk-stratifying patients with AL amyloidosis. Because cardiac involvement in AL amyloidosis dictates prognosis, the levels of cardiac biomarkers at the time of diagnosis have been used to develop the prognostic staging system. The staging systems (summarized in **Tables 1** and **2**) use baseline biomarkers that correlate well with prognosis. The staging systems are widely used, well validated, and not only provide prognostic information but also allow a risk-adapted therapeutic approach in patients with AL amyloidosis.

Standard Mayo staging system
This was the first staging system published by investigators at Mayo Clinic in 2004 based on the analysis of 242 newly diagnosed transplant-ineligible AL amyloidosis patients from a single center by using serum levels of 2 different cardiac biomarkers: cardiac troponin T (cTnT) and NT-proBNP.[66] Cutoff values of NT-proBNP less than 332 ng/L and cTnT less than 0.035 ng/mL were utilized. Stages I, II, and III patients had none, 1, or 2 markers above the cutoffs, respectively. Stage III accounted for 37% of the patients analyzed and was associated with extremely poor prognosis (median survival of 3.5 months); 33% of the patients were stage I and had the best prognosis (median survival of 26.4 months) and 30% were stage II with a median survival of 10.5 months. This staging system also was reproduced in another analysis of 98 patients with AL amyloidosis undergoing peripheral SCT.[67] This stratification added a new dimension in the care and monitoring of patients with AL amyloidosis. Baseline levels of cardiac biomarkers and their monitoring throughout therapy has become

the standard of care for both transplant-eligible and transplant-ineligible patients. Cardiac troponin (both troponin T and troponin I) elevation indicates cardiac myocyte injury due to underlying amyloid deposition and is a strong predictor of OS, with troponin-negative patients having the best prognosis. NT-proBNP elevation indicates cardiac strain and can provide valuable prognostic information as well.

Revised Mayo staging system

An improvised revision for the standard Mayo staging system was published in 2012 also from Mayo Clinic.[68] In a large cohort of patients (N = 808), in addition to the cardiac biomarkers, the serum free light chain (FLC) measurements were incorporated to account for the impact of underlying clonal plasma cell burden. The cutoff value for the NT-proBNP, cTnT, and the difference between involved and uninvolved FLCs (dFLC) used in this model can be found in **Table 1**. Based on the cutoff values of these biomarkers, the proportions of patients with stages I, II, III, and IV disease were 25%, 27%, 25%, and 23%, respectively, and their corresponding median OSs from diagnosis were 94.1 months, 40.3 months, 14 months, and 5.8 months, respectively. This classification system was validated in 2 different data sets made up of 303 patients and 103 patients. This staging system is novel in the sense that it incorporates the measurement of underlying clonal burden and the proliferative capacity/toxicity of serum FLCs for response assessment and progression of organ damage. The application of this system is useful particularly when the clonal light chain burden is very high but challenging when the dFLC is less than 50 mg/L, as seen in 15% to 20% patients with AL amyloidosis.

Boston University staging system

The Boston University scoring system is the newest biomarker staging system from the group at Boston University published in 2019.[69] This system uses brain-type natriuretic peptide (BNP), which is widely available compared with NT-proBNP, a marker with limited availability. This system has allowed centers without access to NT-proBNP to stage and prognosticate AL amyloidosis patients at diagnosis and assess for progression. Two cohorts of patients were used to validate this scoring system, a derivation cohort (N = 249) and a complementary cohort (N = 592). The biomarker cutoff values of BNP and TnI were greater than 81 pg/mL and greater than 0.1 ng/mL, respectively, which strongly correlated with Mayo Clinic staging systems in terms of predicting OS in patients with AL amyloidosis (see **Table 1**).

Renal staging system

In 2014, Palladini and colleagues[70] pioneered, validated, and published the renal staging system (see **Table 2**). All patients (N = 732) included the testing cohort (n = 461) and the validation cohort (n = 271) and had histologically confirmed renal involvement with proteinuria (>0.5 g/24 hours). A cutoff urinary protein level of greater than 5 g/24 hours and an eGFR of less than 50 mL/min/1.73 m^2 at the time of diagnosis were the best predictors of progression to dialysis over time. Proteinuria below and eGFR above the cutoffs indicated low risk for progression to end-stage renal disease and dialysis. Attainment of both a hematologic VGPR and a complete remission (CR) with therapy was associated with improved renal outcome and survival. Although cardiac involvement is the principal determinant of death, kidney involvement can increase morbidity significantly and can limit therapeutic options, including participation in clinical trials. Renal response criteria can help facilitate risk-adapted therapeutic interventions in this patient population.

Scoring Response and Progression in Amyloid Light Chain Amyloidosis

Hematologic response and progression

The goal of therapy in AL amyloidosis is to induce rapid hematologic response by employing therapeutic interventions targeting the underlying clonal plasma cell population (see **Table 3**). A deeper hematologic response is associated with improved organ response that translates into an OS benefit. After initial staging, patients should be monitored to determine disease response to the chosen therapy via regular clinic visits and laboratory studies. After each cycle of therapy (at least monthly), serum protein electrophoresis and serum FLC assay should be measured. A change in therapy should be considered if there is less than optimal hematologic response or evidence of hematologic or organ progression (see **Table 3**) despite an adequate trial of chemotherapy. Alternative therapy also is recommended if there is less than a 50% decline in dFLC after 2 cycles of therapy or if dFLC is greater than or equal to 40 mg/L after 6 cycles of chemotherapy or at 3 months post-SCT. In approximately 15% to 20% of patients, the dFLC is less than 50 mg/L at initial presentation. Because response assessment using hematologic criteria is not applicable in this subgroup of patients, they are excluded from participating in clinical trials. This particular cohort of patients tends to present with more renal involvement, which portends a better prognosis. Response to therapy generally has been better in this cohort; a reduction in dFLC after therapy to less than 10 mg/L has been associated with better OS and renal outcomes.[71,72]

Organ response and progression in amyloid light chain amyloidosis

For cardiac response, the authors recommend checking cTnT and NT-proBNP regularly (see **Table 4**). Electrocardiography and echocardiography also may be pursued, depending on clinical signs and symptoms. For renal response, serum creatinine, a 24-hour urine protein electrophoresis, and 24-hour quantification of proteinuria are indicated. Because NT-proBNP is cleared renally, it can be elevated in patients with progressively worsening renal function. In such a setting, NT-proBNP may not be a reliable marker for cardiac progression. A liver panel to assess for alkaline phosphatase (ALP) and imaging to obtain liver dimensions are indicated in a patient with hepatic involvement. A 2-cm decrease in liver size from baseline and at least a 50% decrease in the level of ALP indicate response whereas increases in liver dimensions and ALP are consistent with progression. The frequency of the testing should be individualized to each patient based on recommendations from a multidisciplinary team that may include hematology, cardiology, nephrology, and neurology. A minimum of monthly biomarker testing may be indicated in symptomatic patients undergoing chemotherapy, but less frequent testing can be considered in those who are minimally symptomatic and are being monitored after having achieved a deep clinical response. Evaluation of organ responses can be confounded by drug-related effects on biomarker readings; clinical judgment is required in that circumstance. A progressive rise in the pathologic FLC may indicate early hematologic progression and rising cardiac biomarkers in the absence of an alternative etiology may indicate organ progression. Renal progression is suspected when there is worsening eGFR or proteinuria. In cardiac amyloidosis, a rise in biomarker usually is accompanied by symptoms (dyspnea on exertion and fluid overload) and requires reinitiating of anti–plasma cell chemotherapy along with supportive care to optimize cardiac function and fluid balance.

SUMMARY

AL amyloidosis is a challenging disease, with a large majority of patients presenting with extensive involvement of multiple organ systems. Improved long-term outcomes have coincided with the incorporation of novel agents, such as PIs in frontline therapy and IMiDs and/or second-generation PIs at time of relapse. Eligible patients should be encouraged to participate in clinical trials when feasible. Methods for assessing hematologic and organ disease have expanded as well with the use of the FLC assay along with cardiac and renal biomarkers for accurate staging and monitoring responses to therapy. The future of this disease remains hopeful as the amyloid-specific landscape is broadened with emerging immunotherapeutic agents and other targeted therapies.

DISCLOSURE

The authors have nothing to disclose.

REFERENCES

1. Hall AG, Tilby MJ. Mechanisms of action of, and modes of resistance to, alkylating agents used in the treatment of haematological malignancies. Blood Rev 1992;6(3):163–73.
2. Comenzo RL, Vosburgh E, Falk RH, et al. Dose-intensive melphalan with blood stem-cell support for the treatment of AL (amyloid light-chain) amyloidosis: survival and responses in 25 patients. Blood 1998;91(10):3662–70.
3. Cibeira MT, Sanchorawala V, Seldin DC, et al. Outcome of AL amyloidosis after high-dose melphalan and autologous stem cell transplantation: long-term results in a series of 421 patients. Blood 2011;118(16):4346–52.
4. Kyle RA, Gertz MA, Greipp PR, et al. A trial of three regimens for primary amyloidosis: colchicine alone, melphalan and prednisone, and melphalan, prednisone, and colchicine. N Engl J Med 1997;336(17):1202–7.
5. Palladini G, Russo P, Nuvolone M, et al. Treatment with oral melphalan plus dexamethasone produces long-term remissions in AL amyloidosis. Blood 2007;110(2):787–8.
6. Knauf WU, Lissichkov T, Aldaoud A, et al. Phase III randomized study of bendamustine compared with chlorambucil in previously untreated patients with chronic lymphocytic leukemia. J Clin Oncol 2009;27(26):4378–84.
7. Rummel MJ, Niederle N, Maschmeyer G, et al. Bendamustine plus rituximab versus CHOP plus rituximab as first-line treatment for patients with indolent and mantle-cell lymphomas: an open-label, multicentre, randomised, phase 3 non-inferiority trial. Lancet 2013;381(9873):1203–10.
8. Rummel MJ, Al-Batran SE, Kim SZ, et al. Bendamustine plus rituximab is effective and has a favorable toxicity profile in the treatment of mantle cell and low-grade non-Hodgkin's lymphoma. J Clin Oncol 2005;23(15):3383–9.
9. Cheson BD, Rummel MJ. Bendamustine: rebirth of an old drug. J Clin Oncol 2009;27(9):1492–501.
10. Lentzsch S, Lagos GG, Comenzo RL, et al. Bendamustine with dexamethasone in relapsed/refractory systemic light-chain amyloidosis: results of a phase II study. J Clin Oncol 2020;38(13):1455–62.
11. Konstantinova IM, Tsimokha AS, Mittenberg AG. Role of proteasomes in cellular regulation. Int Rev Cell Mol Biol 2008;267:59–124.
12. Kastritis E, Wechalekar AD, Dimopoulos MA, et al. Bortezomib with or without dexamethasone in primary systemic (light chain) amyloidosis. J Clin Oncol 2010;28(6):1031–7.
13. Wechalekar AD, Lachmann HJ, Offer M, et al. Efficacy of bortezomib in systemic AL amyloidosis with relapsed/refractory clonal disease. Haematologica 2008;93(2):295–8.

14. Reece DE, Sanchorawala V, Hegenbart U, et al. Weekly and twice-weekly borte-zomib in patients with systemic AL amyloidosis: results of a phase 1 dose-escalation study. Blood 2009;114(8):1489–97.

15. Reece DE, Hegenbart U, Sanchorawala V, et al. Efficacy and safety of once-weekly and twice-weekly bortezomib in patients with relapsed systemic AL amyloidosis: results of a phase 1/2 study. Blood 2011;118(4):865–73.

16. Jaccard A, Comenzo RL, Hari P, et al. Efficacy of bortezomib, cyclophosphamide and dexamethasone in treatment-naive patients with high-risk cardiac AL amyloidosis (Mayo Clinic stage III). Haematologica 2014;99(9):1479–85.

17. Palladini G, Sachchithanantham S, Milani P, et al. A European collaborative study of cyclophosphamide, bortezomib, and dexamethasone in upfront treatment of systemic AL amyloidosis. Blood 2015;126(5):612–5.

18. Palladini G, Milani P, Foli A, et al. Melphalan and dexamethasone with or without bortezomib in newly diagnosed AL amyloidosis: a matched case-control study on 174 patients. Leukemia 2014;28(12):2311–6.

19. Duston MA, Skinner M, Anderson J, et al. Peripheral neuropathy as an early marker of AL amyloidosis. Arch Intern Med 1989;149(2):358–60.

20. Abbas H, Rybicki LA, Reu FJ, et al. Once weekly subcutaneous bortezomib, cyclophosphamide, and dexamethasone as induction therapy for all AL amyloid-osis. Blood 2016;128(22):5813.

21. Bochtler T, Hegenbart U, Kunz C, et al. Translocation t(11;14) is associated with adverse outcome in patients with newly diagnosed AL amyloidosis when treated with bortezomib-based regimens. J Clin Oncol 2015;33(12):1371–8.

22. Stewart AK, Rajkumar SV, Dimopoulos MA, et al. Carfilzomib, lenalidomide, and dexamethasone for relapsed multiple myeloma. N Engl J Med 2015;372(2):142–52.

23. Sheng Z, Li G, Li B, et al. Carfilzomib-containing combinations as frontline ther-apy for multiple myeloma: a meta-analysis of 13 trials. Eur J Haematol 2017;98(6):601–7.

24. Parlati F, Lee SJ, Aujay M, et al. Carfilzomib can induce tumor cell death through selective inhibition of the chymotrypsin-like activity of the proteasome. Blood 2009;114(16):3439–47.

25. Arastu-Kapur S, Anderl JL, Kraus M, et al. Nonproteasomal targets of the protea-some inhibitors bortezomib and carfilzomib: a link to clinical adverse events. Clin Cancer Res 2011;17(9):2734–43.

26. Kirk R, Laman H, Knowles PP, et al. Structure of a conserved dimerization domain within the F-box protein Fbxo7 and the PI31 proteasome inhibitor. J Biol Chem 2008;283(32):22325–35.

27. Bringhen S, Petrucci MT, Larocca A, et al. Carfilzomib, cyclophosphamide, and dexamethasone in patients with newly diagnosed multiple myeloma: a multi-center, phase 2 study. Blood 2014;124(1):63–9.

28. Dytfeld D, Jasielec J, Griffith KA, et al. Carfilzomib, lenalidomide, and low-dose dexamethasone in elderly patients with newly diagnosed multiple myeloma. Hae-matologica 2014;99(9):e162–4.

29. Lendvai N, Hilden P, Devlin S, et al. A phase 2 single-center study of carfilzomib 56 mg/m2 with or without low-dose dexamethasone in relapsed multiple myeloma. Blood 2014;124(6):899–906.

30. Mikhael JR, Reeder CB, Libby EN, et al. Phase Ib/II trial of CYKLONE (cyclophos-phamide, carfilzomib, thalidomide and dexamethasone) for newly diagnosed myeloma. Br J Haematol 2015;169(2):219–27.

31. Cohen AD, Landau H, Scott EC, et al. Safety and efficacy of carfilzomib (CFZ) in previously-treated systemic light-chain (AL) amyloidosis. Blood 2016; 128(22):645.

32. Dou QP, Zonder JA. Overview of proteasome inhibitor-based anti-cancer therapies: perspective on bortezomib and second generation proteasome inhibitors versus future generation inhibitors of ubiquitin-proteasome system. Curr Cancer Drug Targets 2014;14(6):517–36.

33. Moreau P, Masszi T, Grzasko N, et al. Oral ixazomib, lenalidomide, and dexamethasone for multiple myeloma. N Engl J Med 2016;374(17):1621–34.

34. Sanchorawala V, Palladini G, Kukreti V, et al. A phase 1/2 study of the oral proteasome inhibitor ixazomib in relapsed or refractory AL amyloidosis. Blood 2017; 130(5):597–605.

35. Dispenzieri A, Kastritis E, Wechalekar AD, et al. Primary results from the phase 3 tourmaline-AL1 trial of ixazomib-dexamethasone versus physician's choice of therapy in patients (Pts) with relapsed/refractory primary systemic AL amyloidosis (RRAL). Blood 2019;134(Supplement_1):139.

36. Sanchez L, Landau HJ, Rosenbaum CA, et al. A phase 1/2 study to assess safety and dose of ixazomib in combination with cyclophosphamide and dexamethasone in newly diagnosed patients with light chain (AL) amyloidosis. Blood 2019;134(Supplement_1):3128.

37. Quach H, Ritchie D, Stewart AK, et al. Mechanism of action of immunomodulatory drugs (IMiDS) in multiple myeloma. Leukemia 2010;24(1):22–32.

38. Weber D, Rankin K, Gavino M, et al. Thalidomide alone or with dexamethasone for previously untreated multiple myeloma. J Clin Oncol 2003;21(1):16–9.

39. Dispenzieri A, Lacy MQ, Rajkumar SV, et al. Poor tolerance to high doses of thalidomide in patients with primary systemic amyloidosis. Amyloid 2003;10(4): 257–61.

40. Palladini G, Perfetti V, Perlini S, et al. The combination of thalidomide and intermediate-dose dexamethasone is an effective but toxic treatment for patients with primary amyloidosis (AL). Blood 2005;105(7):2949–51.

41. Wechalekar AD, Goodman HJ, Lachmann HJ, et al. Safety and efficacy of risk-adapted cyclophosphamide, thalidomide, and dexamethasone in systemic AL amyloidosis. Blood 2007;109(2):457–64.

42. Cohen AD, Zhou P, Chou J, et al. Risk-adapted autologous stem cell transplantation with adjuvant dexamethasone +/- thalidomide for systemic light-chain amyloidosis: results of a phase II trial. Br J Haematol 2007;139(2):224–33.

43. Palladini G, Russo P, Lavatelli F, et al. Treatment of patients with advanced cardiac AL amyloidosis with oral melphalan, dexamethasone, and thalidomide. Ann Hematol 2009;88(4):347–50.

44. Venner CP, Gillmore JD, Sachchithanantham S, et al. A matched comparison of cyclophosphamide, bortezomib and dexamethasone (CVD) versus risk-adapted cyclophosphamide, thalidomide and dexamethasone (CTD) in AL amyloidosis. Leukemia 2014;28(12):2304–10.

45. Seldin DC, Choufani EB, Dember LM, et al. Tolerability and efficacy of thalidomide for the treatment of patients with light chain-associated (AL) amyloidosis. Clin Lymphoma 2003;3(4):241–6.

46. Richardson PG, Schlossman RL, Weller E, et al. Immunomodulatory drug CC-5013 overcomes drug resistance and is well tolerated in patients with relapsed multiple myeloma. Blood 2002;100(9):3063–7.

47. Rajkumar SV, Hayman SR, Lacy MQ, et al. Combination therapy with lenalidomide plus dexamethasone (Rev/Dex) for newly diagnosed myeloma. Blood 2005; 106(13):4050–3.

48. Sanchorawala V, Wright DG, Rosenzweig M, et al. Lenalidomide and dexamethasone in the treatment of AL amyloidosis: results of a phase 2 trial. Blood 2007; 109(2):492–6.

49. Specter R, Sanchorawala V, Seldin DC, et al. Kidney dysfunction during lenalidomide treatment for AL amyloidosis. Nephrol Dial Transplant 2011;26(3):881–6.

50. Dispenzieri A, Lacy MQ, Zeldenrust SR, et al. The activity of lenalidomide with or without dexamethasone in patients with primary systemic amyloidosis. Blood 2007;109(2):465–70.

51. Hegenbart U, Bochtler T, Benner A, et al. Lenalidomide/melphalan/dexamethasone in newly diagnosed patients with immunoglobulin light chain amyloidosis: results of a prospective phase 2 study with long-term follow up. Haematologica 2017;102(8):1424–31.

52. Moreau P, Jaccard A, Benboubker L, et al. Lenalidomide in combination with melphalan and dexamethasone in patients with newly diagnosed AL amyloidosis: a multicenter phase 1/2 dose-escalation study. Blood 2010;116(23):4777–82.

53. Kastritis E, Terpos E, Roussou M, et al. A phase 1/2 study of lenalidomide with low-dose oral cyclophosphamide and low-dose dexamethasone (RdC) in AL amyloidosis. Blood 2012;119(23):5384–90.

54. Kumar SK, Hayman SR, Buadi FK, et al. Lenalidomide, cyclophosphamide, and dexamethasone (CRd) for light-chain amyloidosis: long-term results from a phase 2 trial. Blood 2012;119(21):4860–7.

55. Dispenzieri A, Buadi F, Laumann K, et al. Activity of pomalidomide in patients with immunoglobulin light-chain amyloidosis. Blood 2012;119(23):5397–404.

56. Sanchorawala V, Shelton AC, Lo S, et al. Pomalidomide and dexamethasone in the treatment of AL amyloidosis: results of a phase 1 and 2 trial. Blood 2016; 128(8):1059–62.

57. Palladini G, Milani P, Foli A, et al. A phase 2 trial of pomalidomide and dexamethasone rescue treatment in patients with AL amyloidosis. Blood 2017;129(15): 2120–3.

58. Dispenzieri A, Dingli D, Kumar SK, et al. Discordance between serum cardiac biomarker and immunoglobulin-free light-chain response in patients with immunoglobulin light-chain amyloidosis treated with immune modulatory drugs. Am J Hematol 2010;85(10):757–9.

59. Touzeau C, Maciag P, Amiot M, et al. Targeting Bcl-2 for the treatment of multiple myeloma. Leukemia 2018;32(9):1899–907.

60. Mihalyova J, Jelinek T, Growkova K, et al. Venetoclax: a new wave in hematooncology. Exp Hematol 2018;61:10–25.

61. Kumar S, Kaufman JL, Gasparetto C, et al. Efficacy of venetoclax as targeted therapy for relapsed/refractory t(11;14) multiple myeloma. Blood 2017;130(22): 2401–9.

62. Leung N, Thome SD, Dispenzieri A. Venetoclax induced a complete response in a patient with immunoglobulin light chain amyloidosis plateaued on cyclophosphamide, bortezomib and dexamethasone. Haematologica 2018;103(3):e135–7.

63. Yip PL, Lau JSM, Lam CP. Venetoclax monotherapy induced rapid and sustained response in a frail patient with refractory AL amyloidosis: less is more? Int J Hematol 2020;112(2):234–7.

64. Ghilardi G, Stussi G, Mazzucchelli L, et al. Venetoclax plus daratumumab induce hematological CR and organ response in an AL amyloidosis patient with t(11;14). Amyloid 2019;26(3):173–4.
65. Gran C, Borg Bruchfeld J, Ellin F, et al. Rapid complete response to single-agent Bcl-2 inhibitor venetoclax in a heart-transplanted patient with triple refractory immunoglobulin light-chain amyloidosis. Acta Haematol 2020;1–4.
66. Dispenzieri A, Gertz MA, Kyle RA, et al. Serum cardiac troponins and N-terminal pro-brain natriuretic peptide: a staging system for primary systemic amyloidosis. J Clin Oncol 2004;22(18):3751–7.
67. Dispenzieri A, Gertz MA, Kyle RA, et al. Prognostication of survival using cardiac troponins and N-terminal pro-brain natriuretic peptide in patients with primary systemic amyloidosis undergoing peripheral blood stem cell transplantation. Blood 2004;104(6):1881–7.
68. Kumar S, Dispenzieri A, Lacy MQ, et al. Revised prognostic staging system for light chain amyloidosis incorporating cardiac biomarkers and serum free light chain measurements. J Clin Oncol 2012;30(9):989–95.
69. Lilleness B, Ruberg FL, Mussinelli R, et al. Development and validation of a survival staging system incorporating BNP in patients with light chain amyloidosis. Blood 2019;133(3):215–23.
70. Palladini G, Hegenbart U, Milani P, et al. A staging system for renal outcome and early markers of renal response to chemotherapy in AL amyloidosis. Blood 2014; 124(15):2325–32.
71. Milani P, Basset M, Russo F, et al. Patients with light-chain amyloidosis and low free light-chain burden have distinct clinical features and outcome. Blood 2017;130(5):625–31.
72. Dittrich T, Bochtler T, Kimmich C, et al. AL amyloidosis patients with low amyloidogenic free light chain levels at first diagnosis have an excellent prognosis. Blood 2017;130(5):632–42.
73. Comenzo RL, Reece D, Palladini G, et al. Consensus guidelines for the conduct and reporting of clinical trials in systemic light-chain amyloidosis. Leukemia 2012; 26(11):2317–25.
74. Palladini G, Dispenzieri A, Gertz MA, et al. New criteria for response to treatment in immunoglobulin light chain amyloidosis based on free light chain measurement and cardiac biomarkers: impact on survival outcomes. J Clin Oncol 2012;30(36): 4541–9.

Stem Cell Mobilization and Autologous Transplant for Immunoglobulin Light-Chain Amyloidosis

Morie A. Gertz, MD, MACP[a],*, Stefan Schonland, MD[b]

KEYWORDS

- Transplantation • High-dose chemotherapy • Mobilization • Melphalan

KEY POINTS

- Stem cell transplantation results in high hematologic and organ response rates in amyloidosis.
- Virtually all eligible patients can undergo safe stem cell transplantation.
- With proper patient selection, therapy-related mortality is now less than 3%.

BACKGROUND

Stem cell transplantation has been an established modality for the treatment of multiple myeloma for more than 30 years. This technique is applied globally and is considered a standard of care. Patients who achieve a complete response following stem cell transplantation with amyloidosis have a longer progression-free survival than patients who achieve a complete response following autologous stem cell transplant for multiple myeloma. This is understandable given the fact that patients with amyloidosis have a low tumor mass at diagnosis (average 10% plasma cells), have far less frequent unfavorable genetics (5% vs 25%), and have a nonproliferative clone of plasma cells unlike multiple myeloma. Conceptually, transplanting amyloidosis is as transplanting monoclonal gammopathy of unknown significance, and one would expect more durable responses and longer times to next treatment.

The differences between transplanting multiple myeloma and transplanting amyloidosis are significant, however. In multiple myeloma, the bone marrow is compromised, but organ function, particularly the heart, the liver, and the kidney,

[a] Division of Hematology, Mayo Clinic, 200 Southwest First Street, W10, Rochester, MN 55905, USA; [b] Department of Internal Medicine V, Division of Hematology/Oncology, Amyloidosis Center, Heidelberg University Hospital, Im Neuenheimer Feld 450, Heidelberg 69120, Germany
* Corresponding author.
E-mail address: gertz.morie@mayo.edu
Twitter: @moriegertz (M.A.G.)

Hematol Oncol Clin N Am 34 (2020) 1133–1144
https://doi.org/10.1016/j.hoc.2020.07.007
0889-8588/20/© 2020 Elsevier Inc. All rights reserved.

are functioning well. The converse is the case in light-chain amyloidosis. The bone marrow is minimally involved, there is a very low tumor mass, but these patients typically have advanced cardiac or renal or hepatic dysfunction. Organ compromise leads to significant complications with the application of myeloablative chemotherapy. These issues of organ dysfunction and late diagnosis of amyloidosis translate into a proportion of patients with light-chain amyloid eligible for stem cell transplant at no more than 20% to 25%.

Treatment-Related Mortality and Eligibility Criteria

The primary consideration for proceeding with stem cell transplantation for amyloidosis is safety. Currently, treatment-related mortality from all causes by day 100 in myeloma is less than 1%. Given the availability of many new drugs for amyloidosis, mortality rates in excess of 3% should be considered unacceptable. In the early days of transplantation, there were few alternatives for therapy and included melphalan-dexamethasone and vincristine-doxorubicin-dexamethasone. With those regimens, deep responses were uncommon, and patients often had little alternative but to undergo stem cell transplantation. With the availability of new agents, including proteasome inhibitors, immunomodulatory drugs (IMIDs), and monoclonal antibodies, subjecting a patient to a stem cell transplant if the expected morbidity and mortality is high is considered unacceptable.[1] However, with careful patient selection, autologous stem cell transplantation is an effective therapy for light-chain amyloidosis. In publications over the last 5 years where patient selection has been refined, complete hematological and organ responses can be seen in 50% to 60% of the patients.[2] Patients who had brain natriuretic peptide levels less than 300 pg/mL and troponin I levels less than or equal to 0.07 ng/mL had better outcomes.[3] Because of refinements in patient selection and the availability of alternative, highly effective chemotherapies for patients with amyloidosis, the early mortality over time has fallen substantially.[4] When the Mayo program began, therapy-related mortality was as high as 14.5%. It is currently 2.4%. We believe that safety of transplantation is the paramount consideration for eligibility.[4]

Stem Cell Transplant in Patients with Renal Failure

Although refined patient selection is required for good outcomes, it is not to say that excellent outcomes cannot be achieved in subsets of patients historically deemed unsuitable for stem cell transplantation. Accounts of patients on steady-state dialysis with successful stem cell transplantation for light-chain amyloidosis have been reported,[5] with a complete hematologic response in 70% of evaluable patients 1 year after stem cell transplant and a median overall survival of 5.8 years. This has a positive impact on the survival of patients with amyloid light-chain (AL) amyloidosis. In one trial, significant differences in overall survival were seen, depending on when acute renal failure occurs. Patients transplanted on steady-state dialysis can do remarkably well. Patients who develop acute renal insufficiency and require dialysis within 30 days of autologous stem cell transplant have unacceptably high rates of treatment-related mortality. If it is expected that the patient will sustain acute renal insufficiency, either associated with very low serum albumin levels or markedly elevated urinary protein levels, the patient should not be considered for transplantation.[6] The Mayo group has transplanted a cohort of patients with an estimated glomerular filtration rate of less than 45 mL/min. Dialysis was required in 6.7% within 100 days of autologous stem cell transplant, and dialysis was required in 22% in patients with renal stage 3 disease. In this cohort, 100-day mortality was 14%. Impaired renal function does predict for a higher rate of hospitalization, progression to dialysis, and early mortality.[7] A powerful predictor of acute renal injury during stem cell transplant for renal amyloidosis is severe hypoalbuminemia, serum albumin less than 2 g/dL. Evidence of acute renal failure requiring hemodialysis was 25% when the albumin was this low. Extreme caution should be used in conditioning patients for transplant who have a serum albumin less than 2 g/dL, and melphalan dose modification should be strongly considered.[8] With careful patient selection, the overall response rate was 75%, the complete response rate was 25%, and the progression-free survival was 40 months.

Stem Cell Transplant in Elderly Patients

In patients older than 70 years the treatment-related mortality was 3%, and transplant can be performed safely. The authors have transplanted patients with 3 or more organs involved. They found that this can be done safely as long as the severity of cardiac involvement is mild to moderate. An NT-proBNP level greater than 2000 was a powerful predictor of overall survival and was far more important than the number of organs involved. Number of organs should not be considered a contraindication to safe transplantation if cardiac function is preserved.[9]

Patients who have lung, liver, gastrointestinal, neurologic, and soft tissue involvement have also been safely transplanted.[10] In one trial, 46 patients received induction therapy before transplant. The 100-day treatment-related mortality was 3.8%. Median progression-free and overall survivals were 36 and 73 months, respectively. Stem cell transplantation in selected patients with AL with gastrointestinal, hepatic, pulmonary, and soft tissue involvement can be considered safe for transplantation. Mayo has also transplanted patients with factor X deficiency and a bleeding diathesis. After stem cell transplant, factor X levels increased in all patients evaluated, but the degree of improvement in factor X levels were correlated with an improvement in markers of renal involvement by amyloid. Patients with factor X deficiency with appropriate support can be safely transplanted.[11] However, splenic rupture has been reported in a patient with factor X deficiency undergoing autologous stem cell transplant, so caution is required.[12]

As in all patients receiving myeloablative chemotherapy, bacterial infections are common. They have been reported in 24% of patients. And when they occur, treatment-related mortality was 10%. Infections are Gram positive in 51%, anaerobic in 16%, Gram negative in 13%, and fungal in 9%. Serum creatinine greater than 2 mg/dL was a risk factor for infection.[13] Among 377 patients with AL acute kidney injury during leukocyte engraftment was very common and attributed to the engraftment syndrome. Patients who have a serum creatinine increase at the time of leukocyte engraftment should be considered to have engraftment syndrome and be considered for corticosteroid therapy.[14]

Induction Therapy

It is controversial whether patients with light-chain amyloidosis and a small plasma cell burden require induction chemotherapy before autologous stem cell transplantation. The HOVON reported extended follow-up with vincristine-doxorubicin-dexamethasone induction followed by high-dose melphalan in a phase 2 trial. Four-year overall survival rate was 62% and after transplantation, it was 78%. Median survival of all patients was 96 months. The investigators concluded that vincristine-doxorubicin-dexamethasone should not be applied as induction therapy for amyloidosis but did recommend a 2-step approach consisting of induction therapy followed by high-dose melphalan.[15] The most common induction regimen is the bortezomib-containing regimen. Induction therapy with bortezomib and dexamethasone was reported in 56 patients. The complete remission rate in the bortezomib high-dose melphalan arm was 68%. In this randomized study, those patients who did not have induction therapy but transplant only had a complete response rate of only 36% (*P* = .03); moreover, a survival advantage was reported for those transplanted patients who received bortezomib induction, suggesting that bortezomib-dexamethasone induction with transplant was superior to transplant alone.[16] In a nonrandomized trial where half of the patients received bortezomib pretransplant and the other half went directly to transplant, the overall response rate in the bortezomib-treated group was 92% versus 69% in the group that received no treatment. Time to best response was also shorter in the bortezomib-treated group (3 vs 14 months).[17] A nonrandomized trial of novel-agent induction was reported, consisting of a proteasome inhibitor in 13, an IMID in 16, a proteasome inhibitor and cyclophosphamide in 3, and an IMID and a proteasome inhibitor in 3. A progression-free survival advantage at 3 years in patients receiving novel-agent induction was 79% and was 53% for those who went directly to transplant without induction. This suggests that a novel-agent induction regimen before stem cell transplant could improve outcomes.[18] The Mayo group reported on 415 patients with AL who had induction before stem cell transplant. Hematologic complete and very good partial response rates were significantly higher in those patients who had less than 10% plasma cells in the bone marrow. Multivariate analysis risk factors for inferior survival included failure to give induction therapy, advanced amyloid stage, and bone marrow greater than 10% plasma cells. Induction therapy pretransplant may improve outcomes among patients with AL due to a rapid reduction of toxic light chains.[19] At MD Anderson, IMID or proteasome inhibitor–based induction was associated with a longer overall survival compared with patients who receive no induction before autologous stem cell transplant. They reported a 2-year overall survival of 87% with induction therapy compared with 73% without induction therapy. Response depth was also greater in the induction therapy cohort.[20] In the long-term follow-up from Boston University, the incorporation of bortezomib into induction yielded durable hematologic responses with corresponding organ responses and prolonged survival. The overall response rate was 100%, and the median overall and progression-free survival had not been reached with a median follow-up of 77 months.[21]

In the HOVON 104 trial, bortezomib-based induction followed by stem cell transplant was performed on 50 patients. Treatment-related mortality was 0%. Hematologic responses at 6 months after transplant were 86%, with 46% complete and 26% very good partial response, confirming the high efficacy of bortezomib as an induction regimen for patients with AL amyloidosis.

The preponderance of evidence suggests that induction therapy with bortezomib-based regimens should be strongly considered in all patients with transplant-eligible light-chain amyloidosis.

Mobilization

Stem cell mobilization (SCM) can be performed with different strategies that combine chemomobilization and plerixafor administration. Main studies reporting results on SCM in AL amyloidosis are reported in **Table 1**. SCM is associated with unusual morbidity in AL amyloidosis compared with multiple myeloma, even when performed without chemotherapy. In a large monocentric series, 11% of patients with SCM with granulocyte colony-stimulating factor (G-CSF) did not proceed to stem cell transplantation due to complications and 4% died during SCM. Hypoxia and hypotension are rare life-threatening events during SCM with G-CSF and may be the result of a capillary leak syndrome triggered by the growth factor. Capillary leak syndrome may also

Table 1
Studies on peripheral blood stem cell mobilization in patients with amyloid light-chain amyloidosis

Study	N° of Patients	Mobilization Approach	Observed AEs	Median Collected CD34+ Cells	Main Remarks
Skinner,[38] et al.[a]	312	G-CSF	4% mortality	>2.0 × 10^6/kg	11% of patients did not proceed to HSCT due to perimobilization morbidity/mortality
Perotti,[39] et al.	42	G-CSF alone G-CSF and CTX	4.7% grade ≥2 AEs	8.2 × 10^6/kg 8.9 × 10^6/kg	Mobilization effective in 95% of cases, with a median number of collections of 1.8
Gertz,[40] et al.[a]	434	G-CSF	10% marked fluid retention	7.16 × 10^6/kg	Patients who had perimobilization fluid retention required 1 mo of recovery before HSCT
Lee,[41] et al.	5	Plerixafor and G-CSF	No mobilization-related AEs	5.9 × 10^6/kg	Plerixafor is effective and well tolerated in cardiac AL amyloidosis
Kaul,[42] et al.	12	Plerixafor and G-CSF	25% grade 1 AEs	13.8 × 10^6/kg	Plerixafor allows collection of sufficient CD34+ cells for HSCT and cryopreservation
Dhakal,[43] et al.	49	G-CSF alone Plerixafor and G-CSF	28% hospitalization 37% hospitalization	6.3 × 10^6/kg 12.8 × 10^6/kg	Combination of plerixafor and G-CSF results in a more effective PBSC collection
Lisenko,[44] et al.	110	G-CSF alone CAD and G-CSF Ifosfamide and G-CSF	10% grade 3 AEs 26% grade 3 AEs 43% grade 3 AEs	4.9 × 10^6/kg 8.8 × 10^6/kg 19.1 × 10^6/kg	CAD mobilization is an effective approach, and tolerability may be implemented suspending doxorubicin. G-CSF alone is also effective and safe
Yeh,[45] et al.	101	G-CSF (and plerixafor if needed)	14% hospitalization 4% mortality	-	Low serum albumin, high NT-proBNP, and increased IVS thickness were associated with higher morbidity/mortality
Badar,[46] et al.	53	Plerixafor and G-CSF	2% grade 2 AEs	12.4 × 10^6/kg	Mobilization with plerixafor and G-CSF is effective and safe in AL amyloidosis

Abbreviations: AE, adverse event; CAD, cyclophosphamide, doxorubicin, and dexamethasone; CTX, cyclophosphamide; G-CSF, granulocyte colony-stimulating factor; HSCT, hematopoietic stem cell; PBSC, peripheral stem blood cell.

[a] These 2 papers reported a large series of patients with AL amyloidosis treated with HSCT by Boston and Mayo Clinic groups. Only information about mobilization are reported in the table. In Skinner's paper, a requirement for HSCT was the collection of at least 2.0 × 10^6 CD34+ cells/kg (median value not reported).

be responsible of worsening of fluid retention. This is particularly relevant in patients with cardiac and renal AL amyloidosis who present with heart failure and nephrotic syndrome. In another study, 10% had worsening of fluid retention during G-CSF SCM that resulted in a delay in stem cell transplantation. In chemomobilization, G-CSF dosage is half than in SCM with G-CSF alone. The Heidelberg group reported a series of patients in whom SCM was performed with G-CSF alone or with chemotherapy that was cyclophosphamide, doxorubicin, and dexamethasone (CAD) in most cases. CAD mobilization was highly effective, with a median of 8×10^6 CD34+/Kg body weight (range, 0–46) collected cells with a median of one leukapheresis procedure. Main adverse events during CAD mobilization were cardiovascular events, gastrointestinal toxicity, and infections. When compared with G-CSF-alone SCM, no differences in rates of grade III or IV adverse events were seen (20% vs 10% and 4% vs 0%). In order to improve chemomobilization tolerability, an SCM with only cyclophosphamide and dexamethasone was proposed. In poor mobilizers, as in patients previously exposed to melphalan, the addition of plerixafor is effective to reach the requisite number of CD34+ cells. This drug has been proved effective and safe in several series of patients with AL amyloidosis. Particularly, a study comparing SCM with G-CSF alone and G-CSF and plerixafor showed that adding plerixafor resulted in higher numbers of collected CD34+ cells with no obvious differences in toxicity.

Mobilization strategy, either with or without chemotherapy, should be aimed to obtain the requested CD34+ cell collection in the shortest time, in order to proceed rapidly to stem cell transplant. Mobilization-related toxicity may also result in a delay in high-dose treatment and should be carefully considered. Recently, a study reported that low serum albumin and high NT-proBNP are associated with higher perimobilization morbidity/mortality. Thus, patients' selection remains of utmost importance. Finally, SCM should provide an adequate number of CD34+ cells to have a long-term recovery of bone marrow hematopoietic function. The Heidelberg group showed that infusion of greater than 6.5×10^6 CD34+ cells/Kg resulted in shorter duration of leukocyte reconstitution and higher platelet count at 12 months from high-dose treatment. Reconstitution of good hematopoietic function after stem cell transplant might result in a better hematologic tolerability of a second-line treatment and be associated with a reduction of secondary hematologic neoplasia.

Conditioning

Proper dosing of melphalan, the standard conditioning agent for amyloidosis, is important to optimize outcomes. Southwest Oncology Group investigated 2 sequential cycles of modified high-dose melphalan at 100 mg/m^2 and reported a treatment-related mortality of 12% and grade 3 and higher nonhematologic adverse events in 81% of patients. Reported outcomes with this approach do not seem to be superior to single induction with melphalan 200 mg/m^2.[22] Risk adjustment of the melphalan dose is used at some centers. One center reported success by using melphalan 200 mg/m^2 in patients who had a performance status of zero or one, 2 or less organs involved, a creatinine of 1.5 mg/dL or less, an ejection fraction greater than 50%, and a BNP of 200 pg/mL or less. All other patients received 140 mg/m^2. In this schema, there was no treatment-related mortality.[23] In the Mayo Clinic experience, full-dose conditioning at melphalan 200 is associated with a higher rate of very good partial response or better, complete response and organ response compared with reduced-dose conditioning. We also found progression-free survival to be superior in the full-intensity group at 4 years, 55% versus 31% in the reduced-intensity group, as well as a higher overall survival rate at 4 years. Conditioning dose remained an independent factor for progression-free and overall survival. As a consequence at Mayo and Heidelberg, we generally will not transplant a patient if we believe they will not tolerate full-dose melphalan 200, as we have been unable to demonstrate that melphalan 140 is better than current novel agent–based chemotherapy.[24] Boston University does use a risk-adapted modified conditioning dose of melphalan for patients with poor baseline functional status, advanced age, renal compromise, and cardiac involvement. In this very large cohort median overall survival was 6.1 years. Median event-free survival was 4.3 years and was driven by hematologic complete response. The treatment-related mortality was 3%. This group continues to use modified doses of melphalan for conditioning.[25] The Boston group has also reported on a second course of high-dose melphalan for the treatment of relapsed disease. Eleven patients achieved a hematologic complete response at 1 year. Three patients died of progressive disease. Only one-third of patients who relapsed after a first stem cell transplant achieve hematologic complete response with a second stem cell transplant.[26]

Consolidation Treatment

We have explored the possibility of using consolidation chemotherapy following autologous stem cell transplant to deepen response and maintain the response. We identified 72 patients receiving consolidation. In patients who achieved a very good partial response or better at day 100, consolidation therapy postautologous transplant did not improve progression-free or overall survival. However, for patients who achieve less than a very good partial response at day +100, consolidation improves progression-free survival for patients and should be strongly considered for patients who, at day 100, have not achieved a very good partial response. In one trial patients with persistent clonal plasma cell disease 3 months post-SCT received 9 months of adjuvant thalidomide/dexamethasone. Forty-two percent achieved an improvement in hematological response. By intention-to-treat, overall hematological response rate was 71% (36% complete response), with 44% having organ responses.[27] In a risk-adapted trial of stem cell transplantation in 40 patients those patients with less than complete hematological response received bortezomib dexamethasone consolidation. Twenty-three patients received consolidation and in 86% response improved demonstrating the value of consolidation therapy in patients whose responses felt not to be sufficiently deep to result in an organ response.[28] This trial was subsequently updated to include 143 patients receiving risk adapted transplantation. The complete response rate was particularly high (62%) in patients offered bortezomib consolidation. Median event-free survival with risk-adapted stem cell transplantation was 4.04 years and median overall survival was 10.4 years.[29]

PROGNOSIS

Several attempts have been made to assess prognosis following autologous stem cell transplantation. In a case series of 82 patients undergoing stem cell transplantation, 2-dimensional global longitudinal strain echocardiography was highly predictive of survival in patients with AL amyloidosis. A global longitudinal strain of -17% was associated with improved survival.[30] Predictors of early treatment failure following initial therapy for AL amyloidosis has also been assessed. Patients with early treatment failure were older, had a higher prevalence of cardiac and multiorgan involvement, and had a higher proportion of patients with the t(11;14) genetic abnormality. In a multivariate analysis, the presence of t(11;14) and failure to proceed with autologous stem cell transplant were significant predictors of early treatment failure, suggesting that stem cell transplant is a very important component of management.[31]

The most important endpoint following stem cell transplant in amyloidosis is normalization of the serum-free light chain and, in fact, the achievement of minimal residue disease negativity. In amyloidosis, since the light chain is the precursor of the amyloid protein, virtual complete eradication of the amyloidogenic light chain is required for optimal response. In one Mayo Clinic study of 313 patients, higher values of the free light chain at diagnosis predicted overall response, and an early overall response predicted an improved overall survival.[32] A stringent complete response is the optimal endpoint after stem cell transplantation in immunoglobulin light-chain amyloidosis. We assessed a total of 540 patients, of whom 220 achieved a complete response. Progression-free survival was significantly shorter in patients failing to achieve a stringent complete response. A bone marrow examination posttransplant is important because it can identify patients who fail to achieve a stringent complete response and thereby predicts earlier progression.[33] The endpoint of treatment with stem cell transplantation should be stringent complete response with normalization of the light chain ratio.

OUTCOMES

Long-term outcomes have been well reported for autologous stem cell transplant. In a Mayo Clinic report of 10-year survival after stem cell transplant, 43% of patients were 10-year survivors.[30] We recently updated this to our 15-year overall survival rate.[31] A higher proportion of patients with 15-year survivorship received full-dose melphalan conditioning and achieved a complete response. The median overall survival among those patients who achieved a complete response was 19.3 years. Fifteen-year overall survival was observed in 30% of patients. A report from the Bone Marrow Transplant Registry has shown improved outcomes after autologous stem cell transplant for light-chain amyloidosis.[32] Posttransplantation survival in AL has improved with a dramatic reduction in early posttransplant mortality and excellent 5-year survival. From 2007 to 2012, therapy-related mortality at 100 days posttransplant was 5%. In addition, 5-year overall survival improved to 77%.[32] We have identified that a bone marrow plasma cell percentage of 20% or greater has an important impact on response and survival. These patients have a poor outcome independent of their cardiac risk factors and stem cell transplant eligibility.[33]

There are special subsets of patients with amyloidosis. One is IgM amyloidosis present in 7% of patients with light-chain amyloidosis. These patients have similar survival but very different presentations, with a higher incidence of neurologic and pulmonary involvement. When these patients undergo stem cell transplant, it is effective, and therapy is safe. The median progression-free survival is 93 months for patients achieving a response.[34]

The National Amyloidosis Center of Britain reported 264 patients transplanted. The median overall survival posttransplant was 87%, and a hematological response was achieved in 94.8%. The reported treatment-related mortality from 2013 to 2018 was 1.1%.[35] Stem cell transplantation was compared directly with melphalan plus dexamethasone in the treatment of light-chain amyloidosis. In a matched control series, patients undergoing stem cell transplant had a 3-year overall survival rate of 83.6% and was far superior to melphalan and dexamethasone, with an overall mortality hazard ratio of 2.56.[36] Another comparative trial of outcomes using stem cell transplant versus standard chemotherapy was reported.[37] Most of the patients in the chemotherapy cohort received bortezomib-based treatment. The median progression-free and overall survivals were superior in the transplant cohort not reached versus 9 months, and overall survival was 74 months versus 8 months. A multivariable analysis demonstrated an improved progression-free survival and overall survival were associated with stem cell transplant compared with chemotherapy. The first phase 3 study comparing chemotherapy with transplantation in 100 patients was inconclusive because of very high therapy-related mortality associated with stem cell transplant (9 deaths among 37patients) and that many patients assigned to stem cell transplant were never transplanted (26%).

SUMMARY

Autologous stem cell transplant is a highly effective technique for the treatment of amyloidosis. Patients can be selected to reduce therapy-related mortality less than 3%. The goal of therapy is normalization of the involved immunoglobulin-free light chain and its ratio.

CLINICS CARE POINTS

- Stem cell transplantation is an important and effective therapy for the management of amyloidosis.
- The procedure should only be undertaken if the estimated therapy-related mortality is less than 3%.
- SCM is successful in more than 95% of patients and can be done using cyclophosphamide with filgrastim or filgrastim and plerixafor

DISCLOSURE

S. Schonland research support from Janssen and Sanofi, serves on the advisory boards for Janssen and Prothena and has received honoraria from Janssen, Takeda, and Prothena; M.A. Gertz personal fees from Ionis/Akcea, personal fees from Alnylam, personal fees from Prothena, personal fees from Celgene, personal fees from Janssen, grants and personal fees from Spectrum, personal fees from Annexon, personal fees from Appellis, personal fees from Amgen, personal fees from Medscape, personal fees from Physicians Education Resource, personal fees for Data Safety Monitoring board from Abbvie, personal fees from Research to Practice, speaker fees from Teva, Speaker fees from Johnson and Johnson; Speaker fees from Medscape, Speaker fees DAVA oncology; Advisory Board for Pharmacyclics Advisory Board for Proclara outside the submitted work; Development of educational materials for i3Health.

REFERENCES

1. Dispenzieri A, Seenithamby K, Lacy MQ, et al. Patients with immunoglobulin light chain amyloidosis undergoing autologous stem cell transplantation have superior outcomes compared with patients with multiple myeloma: a retrospective review from a tertiary referral center. Bone Marrow Transplant 2013;48(10):1302–7.

2. Jimenez-Zepeda VH, Franke N, Reece DE, et al. Autologous stem cell transplant is an effective therapy for carefully selected patients with AL amyloidosis: experience of a single institution. Br J Haematol 2014;164(5):722–8.

3. Venner CP, Gillmore JD, Sachchithanantham S, et al. Stringent patient selection improves outcomes in systemic light-chain amyloidosis after autologous stem cell transplantation in the upfront and relapsed setting. Haematologica 2014; 99(12):e260–3.

4. Sidiqi MH, Aljama MA, Buadi FK, et al. Stem Cell transplantation for light chain amyloidosis: decreased early mortality over time. J Clin Oncol 2018;36(13): 1323–9.

5. Batalini F, Econimo L, Quillen K, et al. High-dose melphalan and stem cell transplantation in patients on dialysis due to immunoglobulin light-chain amyloidosis and monoclonal immunoglobulin deposition disease. Biol Blood Marrow Transplant 2018;24(1):127–32.

6. Leung N, Kumar SK, Glavey SV, et al. The impact of dialysis on the survival of patients with immunoglobulin light chain (AL) amyloidosis undergoing autologous stem cell transplantation. Nephrol Dial Transplant 2016;31(8):1284–9.

7. Sidiqi MH, Nadiminti K, Al Saleh AS, et al. Autologous stem cell transplantation in patients with AL amyloidosis with impaired renal function. Bone Marrow Transplant 2019;54(11):1775–9.

8. Lee SY, Meehan RS, Seldin DC, et al. Effect of severe hypoalbuminemia on toxicity of high-dose melphalan and autologous stem cell transplantation in patients with AL amyloidosis. Bone Marrow Transplant 2016;51(10):1318–22.

9. Al Saleh AS, Sidiqi MH, Muchtar E, et al. Outcomes of patients with light chain amyloidosis who had autologous stem cell transplantation with 3 or more organs involved. Biol Blood Marrow Transplant 2019;25(8):1520–5.

10. Afrough A, Saliba RM, Hamdi A, et al. Outcome of patients with immunoglobulin light-chain amyloidosis with lung, liver, gastrointestinal, neurologic, and soft tissue involvement after autologous hematopoietic stem cell transplantation. Biol Blood Marrow Transplant 2015;21(8):1413–7.

11. Cordes S, Gertz MA, Buadi FK, et al. Autologous stem cell transplantation in immunoglobulin light chain amyloidosis with factor X deficiency. Blood Coagul Fibrinolysis 2016;27(1):101–8.

12. Fernandez de Larrea C, Cibeira MT, Rovira M, et al. Spontaneous rupture of the spleen as immediate complication in autologous transplantation for primary systemic amyloidosis. Eur J Haematol 2008;80(2):182–4.

13. Taimur S, Nader C, Lloyd-Travaglini C, et al. Microbiologically documented infections in patients undergoing high-dose melphalan and autologous stem cell transplantation for the treatment of light chain amyloidosis. Transpl Infect Dis 2013;15(2):187–94.

14. Irazabal MV, Eirin A, Gertz MA, et al. Acute kidney injury during leukocyte engraftment after autologous stem cell transplantation in patients with light-chain amyloidosis. Am J Hematol 2012;87(1):51–4.

15. Hazenberg BP, Croockewit A, van der Holt B, et al. Extended follow up of high-dose melphalan and autologous stem cell transplantation after vincristine, doxorubicin, dexamethasone induction in amyloid light chain amyloidosis of the prospective phase II HOVON-41 study by the Dutch-Belgian Co-operative Trial Group for Hematology Oncology. Haematologica 2015;100(5):677–82.

16. Huang X, Wang Q, Chen W, et al. Induction therapy with bortezomib and dexamethasone followed by autologous stem cell transplantation versus autologous stem cell transplantation alone in the treatment of renal AL amyloidosis: a randomized controlled trial. BMC Med 2014;12:2.

17. Scott EC, Heitner SB, Dibb W, et al. Induction bortezomib in Al amyloidosis followed by high dose melphalan and autologous stem cell transplantation: a single institution retrospective study. Clin Lymphoma Myeloma Leuk 2014;14(5): 424–430 e1.

18. Cowan AJ, Klippel ZK, Stevenson PA, et al. Pre-transplantation novel agent induction predicts progression-free survival for patients with immunoglobulin

light-chain amyloidosis undergoing high-dose melphalan and autologous stem cell transplantation. Amyloid 2016;23(4):254–9.

19. Hwa YL, Kumar SK, Gertz MA, et al. Induction therapy pre-autologous stem cell transplantation in immunoglobulin light chain amyloidosis: a retrospective evaluation. Am J Hematol 2016;91(10):984–8.

20. Afrough A, Saliba RM, Hamdi A, et al. Impact of induction therapy on the outcome of immunoglobulin light chain amyloidosis after autologous hematopoietic stem cell transplantation. Biol Blood Marrow Transplant 2018;24(11):2197–203.

21. Gupta VK, Brauneis D, Shelton AC, et al. Induction therapy with bortezomib and dexamethasone and conditioning with high-dose melphalan and bortezomib followed by autologous stem cell transplantation for immunoglobulin light chain amyloidosis: long-term follow-up analysis. Biol Blood Marrow Transplant 2019; 25(5):e169–73.

22. Sanchorawala V, Hoering A, Seldin DC, et al. Modified high-dose melphalan and autologous SCT for AL amyloidosis or high-risk myeloma: analysis of SWOG trial S0115. Bone Marrow Transplant 2013;48(12):1537–42.

23. Hayashi T, Ikeda H, Igarashi T, et al. Autologous stem cell transplantation for AL amyloidosis: adjustment of melphalan dose by factors including BNP. Int J Hematol 2014;100(6):554–8.

24. Tandon N, Muchtar E, Sidana S, et al. Revisiting conditioning dose in newly diagnosed light chain amyloidosis undergoing frontline autologous stem cell transplant: impact on response and survival. Bone Marrow Transplant 2017;52(8): 1126–32.

25. Nguyen VP, Landau H, Quillen K, et al. Modified high-dose melphalan and autologous stem cell transplantation for immunoglobulin light chain amyloidosis. Biol Blood Marrow Transplant 2018;24(9):1823–7.

26. Quillen K, Seldin DC, Finn KT, et al. A second course of high-dose melphalan and auto-SCT for the treatment of relapsed AL amyloidosis. Bone Marrow Transplant 2011;46(7):976–80.

27. Cohen AD, Zhou P, Chou J, et al. Risk-adapted autologous stem cell transplantation with adjuvant dexamethasone +/- thalidomide for systemic light-chain amyloidosis: results of a phase II trial. Br J Haematol 2007;139(2):224–33.

28. Landau H, Hassoun H, Rosenzweig MA, et al. Bortezomib and dexamethasone consolidation following risk-adapted melphalan and stem cell transplantation for patients with newly diagnosed light-chain amyloidosis. Leukemia 2013; 27(4):823–8.

29. Landau H, Smith M, Landry C, et al. Long-term event-free and overall survival after risk-adapted melphalan and SCT for systemic light chain amyloidosis. Leukemia 2017;31(1):136–42.

30. Cordes S, Dispenzieri A, Lacy MQ, et al. Ten-year survival after autologous stem cell transplantation for immunoglobulin light chain amyloidosis. Cancer 2012; 118(24):6105–9.

31. Sidana S, Sidiqi MH, Dispenzieri A, et al. Fifteen year overall survival rates after autologous stem cell transplantation for AL amyloidosis. Am J Hematol 2019; 94(9):1020–6.

32. D'Souza A, Dispenzieri A, Wirk B, et al. Improved outcomes after autologous hematopoietic cell transplantation for light chain amyloidosis: a center for international blood and marrow transplant research study. J Clin Oncol 2015;33(32): 3741–9.

33. Muchtar E, Gertz MA, Kourelis TV, et al. Bone marrow plasma cells 20% or greater discriminate presentation, response, and survival in AL amyloidosis. Leukemia 2019;34(4):1135–43.
34. Sidiqi MH, Buadi FK, Dispenzieri A, et al. Autologous stem cell transplant for IgM-associated amyloid light-chain amyloidosis. Biol Blood Marrow Transplant 2019; 25(3):e108–11.
35. Sharpley FA, Petrie A, Mahmood S, et al. A 24-year experience of autologous stem cell transplantation for light chain amyloidosis patients in the United Kingdom. Br J Haematol 2019;187(5):642–52.
36. Gertz MA, Lacy MQ, Dispenzieri A, et al. Stem cell transplantation compared with melphalan plus dexamethasone in the treatment of immunoglobulin light-chain amyloidosis. Cancer 2016;122(14):2197–205.
37. Oke O, Sethi T, Goodman S, et al. Outcomes from autologous hematopoietic cell transplantation versus chemotherapy alone for the management of light chain amyloidosis. Biol Blood Marrow Transplant 2017;23(9):1473–7.
38. Skinner M, Sanchorawala V, Seldin DC, et al. High-dose melphalan and autologous stem-cell transplantation in patients with AL amyloidosis: an 8-year study. Ann Intern Med 2004;140(2):85–93.
39. Perotti C, Del Fante C, Viarengo G, et al. Peripheral blood progenitor cell mobilization and collection in 42 patients with primary systemic amyloidosis. Transfusion 2005;45(11):1729–34.
40. Gertz MA, Lacy MQ, Dispenzieri A, et al. Effect of hematologic response on outcome of patients undergoing transplantation for primary amyloidosis: importance of achieving a complete response. Haematologica 2007;92(10):1415–8.
41. Lee SY, Sanchorawala V, Seldin DC, et al. Plerixafor-augmented peripheral blood stem cell mobilization in AL amyloidosis with cardiac involvement: a case series. Amyloid 2014;21(3):149–53.
42. Kaul E, Shah G, Chaulagain C, et al. Plerixafor and G-CSF for autologous stem cell mobilization in AL amyloidosis. Bone Marrow Transplant 2014;49(9):1233.
43. Dhakal B, Strouse C, D'Souza A, et al. Plerixafor and abbreviated-course granulocyte colony-stimulating factor for mobilizing hematopoietic progenitor cells in light chain amyloidosis. Biol Blood Marrow Transplant 2014;20(12). 1926–193.
44. Lisenko K, Wuchter P, Hansberg M, et al. Comparison of Different Stem Cell Mobilization Regimens in AL Amyloidosis Patients. Biol Blood Marrow Transplant 2017; 23(11):1870–8.
45. Yeh JC, Shank BR, Milton DR, et al. Adverse prognostic factors for morbidity and mortality during peripheral blood stem cell mobilization in patients with light chain amyloidosis. Biol Blood Marrow Transplant 2018;24(4):815–9.
46. Badar T, Dhakal B, Szabo A, et al. An updated single center experience with plerixafor and granulocyte colony-stimulating factor for stem cell mobilization in light chain amyloidosis. J Clin Apher 2019;34(6):686–91.

Monoclonal Antibody Therapies in Systemic Light-Chain Amyloidosis

Amandeep Godara, MD[a], Giovanni Palladini, MD, PhD[b],*

KEYWORDS

- Light-Chain amyloidosis • Monoclonal antibodies • Multiple myeloma • Plasma cell
- Daratumumab • Elotuzumab • Rituximab • Anti-amyloid antibodies

KEY POINTS

- Monoclonal antibody targets in systemic light-chain amyloidosis include both clonal plasma (or B) cells and amyloid aggregates.
- Daratumumab is an anti-CD38 antibody, which is well-tolerated in patients with systemic light-chain amyloidosis and leads to high rates of hematologic and organ responses in upfront or relapsed/refractory setting.
- Clinical trials of anti-amyloid therapies have failed to exhibit an obvious clinical benefit and no drugs have received approval from the US Food and Drug Administration to date.

BACKGROUND

Systemic light-chain amyloidosis (AL) results from deposition of amyloid fibrils produced by unstable precursor light-chains secreted by a clonal cell (plasma cell or B cell).[1,2] The organ damage in AL amyloidosis is compounded by the direct toxicity of free light-chains and disruption of tissue architecture by the amyloid fibrils.[3,4] Despite the lower burden of plasma cells in the bone marrow niche in AL amyloidosis compared with multiple myeloma (MM), the manifestations of these proteotoxic light-chains on various organs are manifold and a significant fraction of newly diagnosed patients die within 6 months of diagnosis, usually from cardiac disease.[5,6] The mainstay of treatment is to target the disease clone and cease the production of precursor light-chains, thus eliminating the substrate for amyloid fibril production. Over the years, this has been achieved through therapies targeting plasma cells, which include alkylating agents, proteasome inhibitors and immunomodulatory imide drugs (IMiDs),

[a] Divsion of Hematology-Oncology, Tufts Medical Center, 800 Washington Street, Boston, MA 02111, USA; [b] Department of Molecular Medicine, Amyloidosis Research and Treatment Center Foundations, "Istituto di Ricovero e Cura a Carattere Scientifico (IRCCS) Policlinico San Matteo", University of Pavia, Viale Golgi, 19 IT, Pavia 27100, Italy
* Corresponding author.
E-mail address: giovanni.palladini@unipv.it

Hematol Oncol Clin N Am 34 (2020) 1145–1159
https://doi.org/10.1016/j.hoc.2020.08.005
0889-8588/20/© 2020 Elsevier Inc. All rights reserved.

used either alone or in combination together. Therapeutic decision making for patients with newly diagnosed AL amyloidosis relies on a comprehensive approach based on patient's performance status, burden, and genetic characterization of clonal plasma cells and extent of organ involvement.[3] In patients with newly diagnosed AL amyloidosis, melphalan and dexamethasone and cyclophosphamide, bortezomib, and dexamethasone (CyBorD) have 20% to 30% complete response (CR) rates, whereas organ responses are seen in 20% to 40% of patients.[7–9] Most patients are treated upfront with CyBorD or melphalan and dexamethasone; high-dose chemotherapy followed by stem cell rescue is reserved for transplant-eligible patients with a transplant-related mortality rate of less than 5% and a CR rate of up to 40% to 50%.[10,11] Bortezomib-based regimens can also be used after transplant to upgrade patient responses.[12] Long-term survivors with AL amyloidosis are usually patients who have undergone autologous stem cell transplantation, achieving a deep hematologic and organ response.[13] For the vast majority of patients, clonal disease persists despite months of therapy and organ function does not recover.

The profile of an optimal therapy for amyloidosis would constitute an agent with potent antidisease activity but low systemic toxicity. Paul Ehrlich's magic bullet concept forms the inherent basis of developing monoclonal antibodies that target the disease process via an antigen that has a high tumor expression and specificity.[14] Monoclonal antibodies are being used in AL amyloidosis to activate effector cell–mediated actions through their interactions with plasma cell–specific markers or by binding amyloid fibrils. To halt disease progression, first and foremost, a therapy would be considered effective if it can lead to a deep and durable control over the proliferation of the pathologic precursor. In this review, we provide an overview of monoclonal antibodies that are being investigated for AL amyloidosis.

THERAPIES DIRECTED AT PLASMA CELL OR B-CELL CLONE

Monoclonal antibodies have long been in the frontline of treatment for B-cell lymphoma, ever since rituximab became the first monoclonal antibody to be approved for cancer treatment in 1997.[15] In MM, daratumumab, isatuximab (CD38) and elotuzumab (SLAMF7) are approved for treatment in the frontline or relapse/refractory setting.

Daratumumab

Daratumumab is a fully human IgG1 kappa monoclonal antibody directed against transmembrane glycoprotein CD38, which is strongly expressed on both normal and neoplastic plasma cells.[16] CD38 serves many purposes; it functions as an ectoenzyme regulating calcium flux by converting nicotinamide adenine dinucleotide positive to adenosine diphosphate ribose and nicotinic acid adenine dinucleotide phosphate and also serves as a receptor via its interaction with CD31, leading to immune modulation that favors a permissive niche for tumor growth and survival.[17–19]

With daratumumab, the role of CD38 extends beyond a diagnostic marker for plasma cells and brings it into the mainstream therapeutic landscape of MM. Daratumumab includes the killing of plasma cells through antibody-dependent cellular cytotoxicity, antibody-dependent cellular phagocytosis, complement-dependent cytotoxicity, and apoptosis via Fc receptor-mediated crosslinking.[20,21] It was initially approved in 2015 to treat patients with MM who have received at least 3 prior treatments and later the indication for use was expanded to include both transplant-ineligible and -eligible patients with newly diagnosed myeloma. Although daratumumab does have single agent activity in this disease, it is the synergistic combinations with other antimyeloma agents, especially proteasome inhibitors and immunomodulatory drugs (IMiDs) that have transformed the treatment paradigms without significantly altering the toxicity profile.

Initially, a retrospective analysis (**Table 1**) of heavily pretreated patients with AL amyloidosis showed that daratumumab monotherapy led to hematologic responses in 19 out of the 25 patients (CR of 36%, very good partial response [VGPR] 24%). Of interest was the rapid time (median of 4 weeks) taken to achieve deepest hematologic response.[22] Subsequently, other large retrospective experiences with daratumumab in patients with relapsed/refractory AL amyloidosis were published. The Mayo Clinic group reported 40 patients receiving daratumumab as a single agent or combined with bortezomib or IMiDs.[23] Overall hematologic response rate was 78% (CR of 14%) with single agent daratumumab, and 88% (CR of 19%) with daratumumab combinations, and the cardiac response rate was remarkably high (43% and 46% with monotherapy and combinations, respectively).[23] Similarly encouraging results were reported by Chung and coworkers,[24] who treated 72 patients with daratumumab monotherapy and reported high rates of cardiac (55%) and renal (52%) responses. Milani and colleagues[25] reported high rates of renal response (60%) in 72 previously treated patients, 83% of whom achieved a hematologic response (CR of 30%). A few other case series gave similarly promising results.[26,27] The largest retrospective study was performed by the Heidelberg group.[28] A total of 106 patients received single agent daratumumab and 62 were treated with daratumumab, bortezomib, and dexamethasone, achieving a hematologic response in 64% and 66% of cases, respectively. Cardiac and renal responses were reached in 22% and 20% with monotherapy and in 26% and 24% with combination therapy.[27] Interestingly, the Heidelberg investigators observed a shorter hematologic event-free survival in patients with nephrotic syndrome.[27]

More recently, a phase II study of daratumumab monotherapy in 22 patients with relapsed/refractory AL amyloidosis showed clinical effectiveness with a median progression-free survival of 28 months and a favorable safety profile.[29] Daratumumab was given at a dose of 16 mg/kg by intravenous infusion once weekly for weeks 1 to 8, every 2 weeks for weeks 9 to 24, and every 4 weeks thereafter until progression or unacceptable toxicity, for up to 24 months. Nineteen patients (86%) achieved at least a VGPR hematologic response within 4 weeks from the start of treatment. Three of the patients were also MRD-negative ($<10^5$) by multiparametric flow cytometry. High rates of cardiac (50%) and renal (67%) responses were achieved without grade 3 to 4 infusion-related reactions.

A second prospective trial of single agent daratumumab for up to 6 months in 40 previously treated patients was conducted in Europe.[30] Hematologic response rate was 55% (CR of 8%) and, remarkably, responses were reached after a single infusion, whereas patients with no response after 4 doses were unlikely to respond further.[30] Cardiac and renal responses were observed in 25% and 31% of patients, respectively.[30]

The long duration (≤ 7 hours) of the first infusion of daratumumab in naïve patients is a concern when initiating treatment in the outpatient setting. Additionally, a significant proportion of patients with AL amyloidosis will have underlying cardiac involvement and are potentially susceptible to exacerbation of heart failure owing to the high infusion volume (approximately 1000 mL) of the drug. Splitting the first dose of daratumumab over 2 days can help to overcome this limitation.[29] Clinical studies of a subcutaneous formulation of daratumumab are ongoing and showed a favorable safety profile in regards to infusion reactions over the intravenous formulation (13% vs 34%; odds ratio, 0.28; 95% confidence interval [CI], 0.18–0.44; $P<.0001$) in MM, leading to the approval of this formulation by the US Food and Drug Administration for both patients with newly diagnosed and those with relapsed/refractory MM.[31]

Table 1
Daratumumab as monotherapy or in combination with other agents in relapsed/refractory patients

Study	Number of Patients (Prior Therapies)	Hematologic Response	Organ Response (Heart or Kidney)	Median Time to Response (mo)
Monotherapy				
Kaufman et al,[22] 2017	25 (PI 100%, IMiDs 72%, ASCT 16%)	76% (CR 36%, VGPR 24%)	–	1
Khouri et al,[26] 2019	20 (PI: 65%, IMiDs:60, ASCT 65%)	86% (CR 33%, VGPR 53%)	–	1
Roussel et al,[30] 2020	40 (B 32%, IMiDs 59%)	55% (CR 8%, VGPR 40%)	H 25%, K 31%	0.25
Sanchorwala et al,[29] 2020	22 (PI 73%, IMiDs 41%, ASCT 68%)	90% (CR 41%, VGPR 45%)	H 50%, K 67%	0.25
Chung et al,[24] 2020	72 (B 96%, L 44%, P 14%, ASCT 18%)	77% (CR 40%, VGPR 23%)	H 55%, K 52%	1
Combination				
Abeykoon et al,[23] 2019	M: 22	78% (CR 14%, VGPR 64%)	H 43%, K 18%	3
	C: 22 (B 91%, I 11%, Ca 16%, L 57%, P 20%, ASCT 52%)	88% (CR 19%, VGPR 63%)	H 46%, K 36%	2
Godara et al[100]	19 (PI 100%, ASCT 47%, NEOD001 47%)	89% (CR/VGPR)	H 78%, K 67%	1.5
Lecumberri et al,[27] 2020	38 (35 monotherapy) (B 100%, IMiDs 47%, ASCT 40%)	72% (CR 28%, VGPR 36%)	H 37%, K 59%	0.5
Kimmich et al,[28] 200	M: 106 (PI 92%, IMiDs 73%, ASCT 23%)	64% (CR 8%, VGPR 48%)	H 22%, K 20%	–
	C: 62 (B 95%, IMiDs 5%, ASCT 8%)	66% (CR 11%, VGPR 55%)	H 26%, K 24%	
Milani et al[25]	72 (B 94%, L 52%, P 25%, ASCT 24%)	83% (CR 30%, VGPR 29%)	H 29%, K 60%	2

Abbreviations: ASCT, autologous stem cell transplantation; B, bortezomib; C, combination; Ca, carfilzomib; CR, complete response; H, heart; IMiDs, immunomodulatory imide drugs; K, kidney; L, lenalidomide; M, monotherapy; P, pomalidomide; PI, proteasome inhibitor; VGPR, very good partial response.
Data from Refs.[22–30,100]

After the establishment of clinical efficacy and safety of anti-CD38 monotherapy in AL amyloidosis, efforts are underway to study combinations of daratumumab with other antiplasma cell therapies. Hematologic response rate of 96% (VGPR/CR in 83%) was reported with a combination of subcutaneous daratumumab and CyBorD in 28 patients with newly diagnosed AL amyloidosis in the safety run-in of the ANDROMEDA trial (NCT03201965).[32] ANDROMEDA is a phase III open-label clinical trial in which patients were randomized to receive CyBorD with or without subcutaneous daratumumab. Daratumumab was given weekly for the first 8 doses followed by every 2 weeks for the next 8 doses and monthly afterward for up to 2 years, whereas CyBorD was given weekly for six 4-week cycles. Subsequently a total of 388 patients were randomized to receive daratumumab and CyBorD (n = 195) or CyBorD (n = 193) and results presented at the 2020 European Hematology Association meeting showed that the primary end point of a hematologic CR was noted in 53% of the patients receiving daratumumab-CyBorD compared with 18% for CyBorD alone (odds ratio, 5.1; 95% CI, 3.2–8.2; $P<.0001$).[33] The 6-month cardiac (42% vs 22%) and renal (54% vs 27%) response rate was also higher with daratumumab plus CyBorD. This translated into a significant improvement in the major organ deterioration progression-free survival (hazard ratio, 0.58; 95% CI, 0.37–0.93 $P = .02$), which was defined as hematologic progression, end-stage cardiac/renal disease, or death. Overall, the incidence of grade 3 or 4 toxicities was similar (59% in daratumumab plus CyBorD arm and 57% in CyBorD alone) but a higher risk of infections (12% in daratumumab plus CyBorD arm vs 9% with CyBorD), especially pneumonia, was seen in the daratumumab arm.[33] These unprecedented results will pioneer a change in the management, thus establishing a new standard of care for patients with AL amyloidosis.

Treatment with daratumumab is known to increase the risk of both viral and bacterial infections. Infections have been reported in up to 40% to 60% of patients receiving daratumumab.[34,35] As CD38 is also expressed on natural killer (NK) cells, anti-CD38 therapy can deplete the NK cell population and thus impair innate immunity.[36,37] These effects are further amplified by the immune defects associated with plasma cell disorders. Antiviral prophylaxis with acyclovir is recommended to prevent varicella zoster virus reactivation, and patients who develop recurrent infections may require long-term intravenous immunoglobulin maintenance.[35]

Current treatment practices in AL amyloidosis involve varying combination of proteasome inhibitors, alkylating agents, and IMids, but the time to achieve hematologic and organ responses with these regimens is often prolonged. High-dose chemotherapy and autologous stem cell rescue has been successful in improving survival in patients with AL amyloidosis, but only about 20% to 30% of patients with newly diagnosed AL amyloidosis are candidates for stem cell transplantation.[38] Patients who are not candidates for stem cell transplantation have lower long-term survival probabilities and represent a population with an unmet need. The use of daratumumab alone or in combination with other plasma cell–directed therapies in the upfront setting of AL amyloidosis holds the promise for achieving outcomes that parallel those with stem cell transplantation. Most seriously ill patients (Revised Mayo stage IV) with AL amyloidosis do not survive beyond 6 months from their diagnosis and die from cardiac complications.[39] When more effective therapies targeted to rapidly destroy clonal bone marrow disease become available, the outcomes of those with advanced amyloidosis could also improve.

Isatuximab

Isatuximab is a chimeric anti-CD38 antibody that was approved by the US Food and Drug Administration in 2020 for use in MM in combination with pomalidomide and dexamethasone.[40] It targets a different epitope on CD38 and differs in its action from daratumumab through its ability to induce direct cell death.[41] Isatuximab is under clinical investigation in patients with relapsed/refractory AL amyloidosis.[42]

Elotuzumab

Elotuzumab is a humanized IgG1 monoclonal antibody that targets Signaling Lymphocyte Activation Marker Family member 7 (SLAMF7) receptor, which is highly expressed on both normal and neoplastic plasma cells.[43,44] SLAMF7 expression is also seen on NK cells, mature dendritic cells, CD4$^+$ T cells, and B cells. The activity of elotuzumab against plasma cells is mediated through the activation of NK cells directly through the SLAMF7 interaction and antibody-dependent cellular cytotoxicity.[45] This action is further enhanced in the presence of other agents that augment NK cell–mediated cytotoxicity and, therefore, approved in combination with lenalidomide or pomalidomide and dexamethasone.[46,47] No formal clinical studies have been completed with elotuzumab alone or in combination with other agents in AL amyloidosis, although there are case reports on its clinical activity in patients with AL amyloidosis.[48]

Rituximab

CD20 is a cell surface protein that is expressed on B cells until their terminal transformation to plasma cells and serves as a differentiation marker.[49,50] Rituximab is a chimeric monoclonal antibody that targets CD20 and is either used alone or integrated into the chemoimmunotherapy regimen for added synergism for treatment of B-cell neoplasms.[51,52] Rituximab affects proliferation and differentiation of clonal B cells through several mechanisms, predominantly by antibody-dependent cell-mediated cytotoxicity by effector cells, followed by complement-dependent cytotoxicity, and apoptosis.[51,53] CD20 expression is seen invariably on clonal B cells in non-Hodgkin's lymphoma, but its expression is limited to only 10% to 40% of the clonal plasma cells in MM and AL amyloidosis because CD20 expression is lost during B-cell activation and differentiation into plasma cells.[54–56]

The proven efficacy of anti-CD20 therapy seen in non-Hodgkin's lymphoma has not been replicated in MM. Early on, two of the phase II studies conducted to ascertain the role of rituximab in MM showed a lack of meaningful objective responses.[57,58] Subsequently, another phase II study of rituximab monotherapy in 14 patients with MM chosen based on their CD20 expression on plasma cells ($\geq$33%) resulted in only a single patient achieving a durable response (minor response), although short-lasting stable disease was noted in 5 patients (duration of response, 3–12 months).[59] Many reasons have been postulated for lack of anti-CD20 therapeutic efficacy in rituximab, including a relatively lower CD20 expression on plasma cells, the loss of CD20 after initial treatment, and Fc receptor polymorphisms.[60] This lack of clinical efficacy of rituximab seen in MM has led to a dearth of clinical trial interest in AL amyloidosis with anti-CD20 therapies.

Because clinical responses with rituximab in non-Hodgkin's lymphoma are linked with CD20 expression, identifying clonal disease with higher CD20 expression can be potentially predictive of a response with rituximab.[61] The presence of t(11;14) in clonal plasma cells ascribes to a lymphoplasmacytoid subtype and correlates with CD20 expression on clonal plasma cells.[62,63] In contrast with MM, t(11;14) is one of the most common cytogenetic abnormality seen in patients with AL amyloidosis ($\leq$50%).[64,65] This is a distinct group of patients, and bortezomib therapy in these patients is less effective but dedicated studies of treatment regimen containing anti-CD20 antibody are lacking.[66]

About 7% of patients with AL amyloidosis have an underlying IgM clone and have distinct clinicopathological characteristics with more frequent pulmonary and lymph node involvement.[67-71] Eradication of the underlying B cell or a lymphoplasmacytic clone can be achieved by combining rituximab with alkylating agents.[68,72-74] Several treatment regimens have been used for patients with IgM amyloidosis such as bendamustine and rituximab; dexamethasone, rituximab, and cyclophosphamide; and cyclophosphamide, vincristine, and prednisone.[75-77] A retrospective series of 35 pretreated cases of IgM amyloidosis reported clinical responses in 20 patients (57%; 1 CR and 7 VGPR) with a combination of bendamustine (60–100 mg/m^2 on days 1 and 2), prednisone (100 mg on days 1–4), and rituximab (375 mg/m^2 on day 1).[76,78] Combination of rituximab, bortezomib, and bendamustine is also highly effective with durable hematologic responses seen in 7 of 10 patients in a previously published prospective study.[79] Thus, an ideal strategy to target an lymphoplasmacytic clone would include rituximab, a proteasome inhibitor, and an alkylating agent, but complete hematologic remissions are rare and high-dose chemotherapy with stem cell rescue remains the mainstay of treatment for transplant-eligible patients with IgM amyloidosis.[73]

THERAPIES DIRECTED AT AMYLOID AGGREGATES

The process of amyloid formation takes the precursor protein through a series of steps forming oligomers, protofibrils, and eventually amyloid fibrils.[80,81] Amyloid deposits are comprised of insoluble fibrils alongside components such as glycosaminoglycans, apolipoprotein E, and serum amyloid P-component (SAP), a composition that is shared across different types of amyloidosis.[82,83] Over the last 2 decades, monoclonal antibodies that are directed against either the amyloid intermediaries or fibrils or protein cofactors have been in clinical development. By binding their target protein, these antibodies have the potential to limit or regress amyloid deposition.

Dezamizumab (Antiserum Amyloid P-Component Antibody)

SAP belongs to the pentraxin family of glycoproteins and is ubiquitous to all types of amyloidosis. SAP is resistant to proteolysis and its binding to amyloid fibrils protects amyloid deposits from degradation. The importance of SAP in amyloidogenesis has been demonstrated in an SAP knockout murine model, where amyloid formation was deterred relative to the wild-type mice.[84] Dezamizumab is a humanized IgG1 monoclonal that binds the SAP present in amyloid deposits and activates phagocytic clearance of amyloid aggregates. In part A of an open-label phase I study, 15 patients with amyloidosis (8 had AL amyloidosis) initially received a SAP-depleting agent, miridesap, followed by a single dose of dezamizumab, which led to a substantial decrease in the hepatic amyloid burden in 4 patients evaluated by whole body ^{123}I-SAP scintigraphy scan that measures radiolabeled SAP uptake by amyloid deposits.[85,86] Next in the sequence was the part B of this phase I study, which included 23 patients (12 with AL amyloidosis) with systemic amyloidosis and showed varying degree of decrease of amyloid burden in liver (7/9), kidney (7/11), and spleen.[87] Despite an initial encouraging safety profile and evidence of clinical activity, a subsequent phase II trial of anti-SAP antibody in patients with cardiac amyloidosis was terminated for a change in a benefit and risk profile.[88] Further drug development has since been terminated.

Birtamimab (NEOD001)

Birtamimab (NEOD001) is a humanized form of a murine monoclonal antibody (2A4) that binds to an epitope unique to the misfolded light-chains and amyloid fibrils, potentially neutralizing and eliminating the toxic protein deposited in various tissues.[89]

Results from the preclinical studies done in mice bearing subcutaneous AL amyloidoma showed that 2A4 facilitated the clearance of amyloid deposits, possibly through phagocytic opsonization.[90] Later in a phase I study, 27 patients who had received at least 2 previous anti-plasma cell therapies were treated with increasing doses of NEOD001 as monthly infusions without any significant toxicity. Cardiac and renal responses were seen in 57% and 60% of the patients, respectively.[91]

After the initial promise, a phase II study of NEOD001 versus placebo in patients with cardiac AL amyloidosis failed to show an improvement in cardiac responses (39.4% vs 47.6%, respectively).[92] This led to an interim analysis of the then ongoing phase III VITAL trial, which was a double-blind, placebo-controlled study of 260 patients with newly diagnosed AL amyloidosis. A decision to terminate the study was made after the interim analysis failed to show significance in achieving the primary composite end point of all-cause mortality or cardiac hospitalizations (the hazard ratio of 0.84 favored NEOD001 vs placebo).[92] The final safety and efficacy results suggested a lower mortality with NEOD001 compared with placebo, and the hazard ratio was consistent with the interim analysis but lacked statistical significance (hazard ratio, 0.835; 95% CI, 0.5799–1.2011; P = .330).[93] A clinical efficacy signal with NEOD001 was seen in Mayo Stage IV patients, where the median overall survival was not reached compared with 8.3 months for placebo. Improving outcomes in patients with the highest risk of early mortality has long been an area of unmet need in this disease, but validation of these results through a prospective trial will remain unanswered with the termination of NEOD001 drug development.

CAEL-101

CAEL-101 (11-1F4) is an IgG1 chimeric anti–light chain monoclonal antibody with unique properties that allow specific binding to a conformational amyloid-related epitope but not to native immunoglobulin light-chains and leads to removal of amyloid aggregates through phagocytic clearance.[94,95] A radiolabeled form of 11-1F4 is also being developed as an imaging tool to identify amyloid fibrils deposited in the body.[96,97] A phase IA/B dose escalation clinical trial of CAEL-101 was conducted in patients with relapsed or refractory AL amyloidosis who had at least achieved a VGPR with prior anti-plasma cell therapy. Intravenous infusion of the antibody was well tolerated without any dose limiting toxicities and 12 of 18 patients (71%) with cardiac and/or renal involvement achieved an organ response.[98] In addition to the cardiac biomarker response, significant improvement in global longitudinal strain was noted (−15.58 ± −4.14% at screening to −17.37 ± −3.53% at week 12), indicating cardiac remodeling; global longitudinal strain is an independent prognostic factor in amyloidosis.[99] Given these encouraging results, attempts are underway to advance the clinical development of CAEL-101 through further stage clinical trials.

COMBINING MONOCLONAL ANTIBODIES

A two-pronged approach to simultaneously target the plasma cell clone and amyloid fibrils using a combination of monoclonal antibodies might improve the outcomes of patients with AL amyloidosis; however, the clinical evidence is limited. In a retrospective analysis of patients enrolled to the phase III VITAL trial, 7 patients received daratumumab in addition to NEOD001 and all achieved a hematologic response (VGPR or better).[100] Six patients also achieved a cardiac response at a median of 86 days. High rates of hematologic and organ response attained within a short span of time may be indicative of a synergistic interaction between these 2 monoclonal antibodies directed at clonal plasma cells and the ultimate product of their secreted light-chains, the amyloid fibrils.

SUMMARY

Over the past 2 decades, early diagnosis and advancement in anti-plasma cell strategies have resulted in a substantial improvement in survival for patients with AL amyloidosis.[39] Of these treatments, anti-CD38 antibodies have been the most successful and effective in targeting the plasma cell clone. The use of daratumumab in combination with revlimid, bortezomib, and dexamethasone is one such promising example of molecular targeted therapy in plasma cell disorders, which can achieve high response rates by both conventional and minimal residual disease standpoint.[101] Achieving a minimal residual disease response has been associated with improved outcomes in MM and, possibly, in AL amyloidosis.[102,103] Translation of this information into AL amyloidosis has the potential to lead the charge of improving adverse patient outcomes associated with this proteotoxic disease. The undeniable evidence of effectiveness of daratumumab and its combination with other anti-plasma cell therapies in AL amyloidosis has been transformative, leading to high rates of hematologic response and, more important, a rapid pace of achieving it. Patients with advanced stages of amyloidosis need rapid responses to avoid further organ injury and aid functional recovery.[104] The developmental pipeline of antibody-based therapeutics against plasma cell markers (BCMA, CD138, and CD56) will likely provide a robust framework for further therapeutic options in AL amyloidosis.[105–108]

Targeting amyloid fibrils has been challenging and the therapeutic benefit of the investigated agents has been equivocal despite the demonstration of preclinical efficacy. The use of anti-amyloid therapies too late in the disease process and the limitations of trial design may have contributed to the failure of these approaches. Interestingly, an efficacy signal was seen with NEOD001 in stage IV AL amyloidosis and further investigation is warranted. Moreover, clinical studies with CAEL-101 may provide evidence for the efficacy of therapies directed at clearing amyloid aggregates, a hope that is not lost yet!

ACKNOWLEDGMENTS

A. Godara thanks the Division of Hematology-Oncology and John C. Davis Program for Myeloma and Amyloid at Tufts Medical Center.

DISCLOSURE

A. Godara has no competing conflict of interest. GP received an honorarium from Sebia; served on an advisory board for Janssen, and received a travel grant from Celgene.

REFERENCES

1. Kyle RA, Gertz MA. Primary systemic amyloidosis: clinical and laboratory features in 474 cases. Semin Hematol 1995;32(1):45–59.
2. Merlini G, Comenzo RL, Seldin DC, et al. Immunoglobulin light chain amyloidosis. Expert Rev Hematol 2014;7(1):143–56.
3. Palladini G, Merlini G. What is new in diagnosis and management of light chain amyloidosis? Blood 2016;128(2):159–68.
4. Imperlini E, Gnecchi M, Rognoni P, et al. Proteotoxicity in cardiac amyloidosis: amyloidogenic light chains affect the levels of intracellular proteins in human heart cells. Sci Rep 2017;7(1):15661.
5. Gertz MA, Lacy MQ, Dispenzieri A. Amyloidosis: recognition, confirmation, prognosis, and therapy. Mayo Clin Proc 1999;74(5):490–4.

6. Palladini G, Dispenzieri A, Gertz MA, et al. New criteria for response to treatment in immunoglobulin light chain amyloidosis based on free light chain measurement and cardiac biomarkers: impact on survival outcomes. J Clin Oncol 2012;30(36):4541–9.

7. Palladini G, Milani P, Foli A, et al. Oral melphalan and dexamethasone grants extended survival with minimal toxicity in AL amyloidosis: long-term results of a risk-adapted approach. Haematologica 2014;99(4):743–50.

8. Palladini G, Sachchithanantham S, Milani P, et al. A European collaborative study of cyclophosphamide, bortezomib, and dexamethasone in upfront treatment of systemic AL amyloidosis. Blood 2015;126(5):612–5.

9. Manwani R, Cohen O, Sharpley F, et al. A prospective observational study of 915 patients with systemic AL amyloidosis treated with upfront bortezomib. Blood 2019;134(25):2271–80.

10. D'Souza A, Dispenzieri A, Wirk B, et al. Improved outcomes after autologous hematopoietic cell transplantation for light chain amyloidosis: a center for international blood and marrow transplant research study. J Clin Oncol 2015;33(32):3741–9.

11. Merlini G, Dispenzieri A, Sanchorawala V, et al. Systemic immunoglobulin light chain amyloidosis. Nat Rev Dis Primers 2018;4(1):38.

12. Landau H, Smith M, Landry C, et al. Long-term event-free and overall survival after risk-adapted melphalan and SCT for systemic light chain amyloidosis. Leukemia 2017;31(1):136–42.

13. Muchtar E, Gertz MA, Lacy MQ, et al. Ten-year survivors in AL amyloidosis: characteristics and treatment pattern. Br J Haematol 2019;187(5):588–94.

14. Ehrlich P. Address in pathology, on chemotherapy: delivered before the seventeenth international congress of medicine. Br Med J 1913;2(2746):353–9.

15. Grillo-Lopez AJ, White CA, Dallaire BK, et al. Rituximab: the first monoclonal antibody approved for the treatment of lymphoma. Curr Pharm Biotechnol 2000;1(1):1–9.

16. Flores-Montero J, de Tute R, Paiva B, et al. Immunophenotype of normal vs. myeloma plasma cells: toward antibody panel specifications for MRD detection in multiple myeloma. Cytometry B Clin Cytom 2016;90(1):61–72.

17. Deaglio S, Morra M, Mallone R, et al. Human CD38 (ADP-ribosyl cyclase) is a counter-receptor of CD31, an Ig superfamily member. J Immunol 1998;160(1):395–402.

18. Ferrero E, Malavasi F. Human CD38, a leukocyte receptor and ectoenzyme, is a member of a novel eukaryotic gene family of nicotinamide adenine dinucleotide+-converting enzymes: extensive structural homology with the genes for murine bone marrow stromal cell antigen 1 and aplysian ADP-ribosyl cyclase. J Immunol 1997;159(8):3858–65.

19. Lee HC. Structure and enzymatic functions of human CD38. Mol Med 2006;12(11–12):317–23.

20. Wong SW, Comenzo RL. CD38 monoclonal antibody therapies for multiple myeloma. Clin Lymphoma Myeloma Leuk 2015;15(11):635–45.

21. van de Donk N, Richardson PG, Malavasi F. CD38 antibodies in multiple myeloma: back to the future. Blood 2018;131(1):13–29.

22. Kaufman GP, Schrier SL, Lafayette RA, et al. Daratumumab yields rapid and deep hematologic responses in patients with heavily pretreated AL amyloidosis. Blood 2017;130(7):900–2.

23. Abeykoon JP, Zanwar S, Dispenzieri A, et al. Daratumumab-based therapy in patients with heavily-pretreated AL amyloidosis. Leukemia 2019;33(2):531–6.

24. Chung A, Kaufman GP, Sidana S, et al. Organ responses with daratumumab therapy in previously treated AL amyloidosis. Blood Adv 2020;4(3):458–66.
25. Milani P, Fazio F, Basset M, et al. High rate of profound clonal and renal responses with daratumumab treatment in heavily pre-treated patients with light chain (AL) amyloidosis and high bone marrow plasma cell infiltrate. Am J Hematol 2020;95(8):900–5.
26. Khouri J, Kin A, Thapa B, et al. Daratumumab proves safe and highly effective in AL amyloidosis. Br J Haematol 2019;185(2):342–4.
27. Lecumberri R, Krsnik I, Askari E, et al. Treatment with daratumumab in patients with relapsed/refractory AL amyloidosis: a multicentric retrospective study and review of the literature. Amyloid 2020;27(3):163–7.
28. Kimmich CR, Terzer T, Benner A, et al. Daratumumab for systemic AL amyloidosis: prognostic factors and adverse outcome with nephrotic-range albuminuria. Blood 2020;135(18):1517–30.
29. Sanchorawala V, Sarosiek S, Schulman A, et al. Safety, tolerability, and response rates of daratumumab in relapsed AL amyloidosis: results of a phase 2 study. Blood 2020;135(18):1541–7.
30. Roussel M, Merlini G, Chevret S, et al. A prospective phase 2 trial of daratumumab in patients with previously treated systemic light-chain amyloidosis. Blood 2020;135(18):1531–40.
31. Mateos MV, Nahi H, Legiec W, et al. Subcutaneous versus intravenous daratumumab in patients with relapsed or refractory multiple myeloma (COLUMBA): a multicentre, open-label, non-inferiority, randomised, phase 3 trial. Lancet Haematol 2020;7(5):e370–80.
32. Palladini G, Kastritis E, Maurer MS, et al. Daratumumab Plus CyBorD for patients with newly diagnosed AL amyloidosis: safety run-in results of ANDROMEDA. Blood 2020;136(1):71–80.
33. Efstathios Kastritis GP, MC Minnema, AD. Wechalekar, et al. Subcutaneous daratumumab + cyclophosphamide, bortezomib, and dexamethasone (Cybord) in patients with newly diagnosed light chain (AL) amyloidosis: primary results from the phase 3 ANDROMEDA study. 25th EHA Congress. Frankfurt, 2020.
34. Mateos MV, Dimopoulos MA, Cavo M, et al. Daratumumab plus bortezomib, melphalan, and prednisone for untreated myeloma. N Engl J Med 2018;378(6):518–28.
35. Drgona L, Gudiol C, Lanini S, et al. ESCMID Study Group for Infections in Compromised Hosts (ESGICH) consensus document on the safety of targeted and biological therapies: an infectious diseases perspective (agents targeting lymphoid or myeloid cells surface antigens [II]. CD22, CD30, CD33, CD38, CD40, SLAMF-7 and CCR4). Clin Microbiol Infect 2018;24(Suppl 2):S83–94.
36. Nahi H, Chrobok M, Gran C, et al. Infectious complications and NK cell depletion following daratumumab treatment of multiple myeloma. PLoS One 2019;14(2):e0211927.
37. Johnsrud AJ, Johnsrud JJ, Susanibar SA, et al. Infectious and immunological sequelae of daratumumab in multiple myeloma. Br J Haematol 2019;185(1):187–9.
38. Sidiqi MH, Aljama MA, Buadi FK, et al. Stem cell transplantation for light chain amyloidosis: decreased early mortality over time. J Clin Oncol 2018;36(13):1323–9.
39. Muchtar E, Gertz MA, Kumar SK, et al. Improved outcomes for newly diagnosed AL amyloidosis between 2000 and 2014: cracking the glass ceiling of early death. Blood 2017;129(15):2111–9.

40. Attal M, Richardson PG, Rajkumar SV, et al. Isatuximab plus pomalidomide and low-dose dexamethasone versus pomalidomide and low-dose dexamethasone in patients with relapsed and refractory multiple myeloma (ICARIA-MM): a randomised, multicentre, open-label, phase 3 study. Lancet 2019;394(10214): 2096–107.

41. Martin TG, Corzo K, Chiron M, et al. Therapeutic Opportunities with Pharmacological Inhibition of CD38 with Isatuximab. Cells 2019;8(12).

42. S1702 isatuximab in treating patients with relapsed or refractory primary amyloidosis. Available at: https://clinicaltrials.gov/ct2/show/NCT03499808. Accessed September 06, 2020.

43. Boles KS, Mathew PA. Molecular cloning of CS1, a novel human natural killer cell receptor belonging to the CD2 subset of the immunoglobulin superfamily. Immunogenetics 2001;52(3–4):302–7.

44. Tai YT, Soydan E, Song W, et al. CS1 promotes multiple myeloma cell adhesion, clonogenic growth, and tumorigenicity via c-maf-mediated interactions with bone marrow stromal cells. Blood 2009;113(18):4309–18.

45. Campbell KS, Cohen AD, Pazina T. Mechanisms of NK cell activation and clinical activity of the therapeutic SLAMF7 antibody, elotuzumab in multiple myeloma. Front Immunol 2018;9:2551.

46. Ritchie D, Colonna M. Mechanisms of action and clinical development of elotuzumab. Clin Transl Sci 2018;11(3):261–6.

47. Lonial S, Dimopoulos M, Palumbo A, et al. Elotuzumab therapy for relapsed or refractory multiple myeloma. N Engl J Med 2015;373(7):621–31.

48. Iqbal SM, Stecklein K, Sarow J, et al. Elotuzumab in combination with lenalidomide and dexamethasone for treatment-resistant immunoglobulin light chain amyloidosis with multiple myeloma. Clin Lymphoma Myeloma Leuk 2019; 19(1):e33–6.

49. Riley JK, Sliwkowski MX. CD20: a gene in search of a function. Semin Oncol 2000;27(6 Suppl 12):17–24.

50. Banchereau J, Rousset F. Human B lymphocytes: phenotype, proliferation, and differentiation. Adv Immunol 1992;52:125–262.

51. Pierpont TM, Limper CB, Richards KL. Past, present, and future of rituximab-the world's first oncology monoclonal antibody therapy. Front Oncol 2018;8:163.

52. Marcus R, Imrie K, Belch A, et al. CVP chemotherapy plus rituximab compared with CVP as first-line treatment for advanced follicular lymphoma. Blood 2005; 105(4):1417–23.

53. Maloney DG, Smith B, Rose A. Rituximab: mechanism of action and resistance. Semin Oncol 2002;29(1 Suppl 2):2–9.

54. Robillard N, Avet-Loiseau H, Garand R, et al. CD20 is associated with a small mature plasma cell morphology and t(11;14) in multiple myeloma. Blood 2003;102(3):1070–1.

55. Lisenko K, Schonland SO, Jauch A, et al. Flow cytometry-based characterization of underlying clonal B and plasma cells in patients with light chain amyloidosis. Cancer Med 2016;5(7):1464–72.

56. Deshmukh M, Elderfield K, Rahemtulla A, et al. Immunophenotype of neoplastic plasma cells in AL amyloidosis. J Clin Pathol 2009;62(8):724–30.

57. Treon SP, Pilarski LM, Belch AR, et al. CD20-directed serotherapy in patients with multiple myeloma: biologic considerations and therapeutic applications. J Immunother 2002;25(1):72–81.

58. Zojer N, Kirchbacher K, Vesely M, et al. Rituximab treatment provides no clinical benefit in patients with pretreated advanced multiple myeloma. Leuk Lymphoma 2006;47(6):1103–9.

59. Moreau P, Voillat L, Benboukher L, et al. Rituximab in CD20 positive multiple myeloma. Leukemia 2007;21(4):835–6.

60. Kapoor P, Greipp PT, Morice WG, et al. Anti-CD20 monoclonal antibody therapy in multiple myeloma. Br J Haematol 2008;141(2):135–48.

61. Johnson NA, Boyle M, Bashashati A, et al. Diffuse large B-cell lymphoma: reduced CD20 expression is associated with an inferior survival. Blood 2009; 113(16):3773–80.

62. Garand R, Avet-Loiseau H, Accard F, et al. t(11;14) and t(4;14) translocations correlated with mature lymphoplasmacytoid and immature morphology, respectively, in multiple myeloma. Leukemia 2003;17(10):2032–5.

63. Hoyer JD, Hanson CA, Fonseca R, et al. The (11;14)(q13;q32) translocation in multiple myeloma. A morphologic and immunohistochemical study. Am J Clin Pathol 2000;113(6):831–7.

64. Bryce AH, Ketterling RP, Gertz MA, et al. Translocation t(11;14) and survival of patients with light chain (AL) amyloidosis. Haematologica 2009;94(3):380–6.

65. Warsame R, Kumar SK, Gertz MA, et al. Abnormal FISH in patients with immunoglobulin light chain amyloidosis is a risk factor for cardiac involvement and for death. Blood Cancer J 2015;5:e310.

66. Bochtler T, Hegenbart U, Kunz C, et al. Translocation t(11;14) is associated with adverse outcome in patients with newly diagnosed AL amyloidosis when treated with bortezomib-based regimens. J Clin Oncol 2015;33(12):1371–8.

67. Palladini G, Russo P, Bosoni T, et al. AL amyloidosis associated with IgM monoclonal protein: a distinct clinical entity. Clin Lymphoma Myeloma 2009;9(1):80–3.

68. Wechalekar AD, Lachmann HJ, Goodman HJ, et al. AL amyloidosis associated with IgM paraproteinemia: clinical profile and treatment outcome. Blood 2008; 112(10):4009–16.

69. Gertz MA, Kyle RA. Amyloidosis with IgM monoclonal gammopathies. Semin Oncol 2003;30(2):325–8.

70. Gertz MA, Kyle RA, Noel P. Primary systemic amyloidosis: a rare complication of immunoglobulin M monoclonal gammopathies and Waldenstrom's macroglobulinemia. J Clin Oncol 1993;11(5):914–20.

71. Cohen AD, Zhou P, Xiao Q, et al. Systemic AL amyloidosis due to non-Hodgkin's lymphoma: an unusual clinicopathologic association. Br J Haematol 2004; 124(3):309–14.

72. Terrier B, Jaccard A, Harousseau JL, et al. The clinical spectrum of IgM-related amyloidosis: a French nationwide retrospective study of 72 patients. Medicine (Baltimore) 2008;87(2):99–109.

73. Gertz MA, Buadi FK, Hayman SR. IgM amyloidosis: clinical features in therapeutic outcomes. Clin Lymphoma Myeloma Leuk 2011;11(1):146–8.

74. Milani P, Merlini G. Monoclonal IgM-related AL amyloidosis. Best Pract Res Clin Haematol 2016;29(2):241–8.

75. Manwani R, Sachchithanantham S, Mahmood S, et al. Treatment of IgM-associated immunoglobulin light-chain amyloidosis with rituximab-bendamustine. Blood 2018;132(7):761–4.

76. Milani P, Schonland S, Palladini G, et al. Response to bendamustine is associated with a survival advantage in a heavily pretreated patients with AL amyloidosis. Amyloid 2017;24(sup1):56–7.

77. Sidana S, Larson DP, Greipp PT, et al. IgM AL amyloidosis: delineating disease biology and outcomes with clinical, genomic and bone marrow morphological features. Leukemia 2020;34(5):1373–82.
78. Milani P, Schonland S, Merlini G, et al. Treatment of AL amyloidosis with bendamustine: a study of 122 patients. Blood 2018;132(18):1988–91.
79. Palladini G, Foli A, Russo P, et al. Treatment of IgM-associated AL amyloidosis with the combination of rituximab, bortezomib, and dexamethasone. Clin Lymphoma Myeloma Leuk 2011;11(1):143–5.
80. Rambaran RN, Serpell LC. Amyloid fibrils: abnormal protein assembly. Prion 2008;2(3):112–7.
81. Blancas-Mejia LM, Misra P, Ramirez-Alvarado M. Differences in protein concentration dependence for nucleation and elongation in light chain amyloid formation. Biochemistry 2017;56(5):757–66.
82. Ramirez-Alvarado M. Amyloid formation in light chain amyloidosis. Curr Top Med Chem 2012;12(22):2523–33.
83. MacRaild CA, Stewart CR, Mok YF, et al. Non-fibrillar components of amyloid deposits mediate the self-association and tangling of amyloid fibrils. J Biol Chem 2004;279(20):21038–45.
84. Togashi S, Lim SK, Kawano H, et al. Serum amyloid P component enhances induction of murine amyloidosis. Lab Invest 1997;77(5):525–31.
85. Richards DB, Cookson LM, Berges AC, et al. Therapeutic clearance of amyloid by antibodies to serum amyloid P component. N Engl J Med 2015;373(12): 1106–14.
86. Pepys MB, Herbert J, Hutchinson WL, et al. Targeted pharmacological depletion of serum amyloid P component for treatment of human amyloidosis. Nature 2002;417(6886):254–9.
87. Richards DB, Cookson LM, Barton SV, et al. Repeat doses of antibody to serum amyloid P component clear amyloid deposits in patients with systemic amyloidosis. Sci Transl Med 2018;10(422):eaan3128.
88. Multiple treatment session study to assess GSK2398852 administered following and along with GSK2315698. ClinicalTrials.gov identifier: NCT03044353. Available at: https://clinicaltrialsgov/ct2/show/NCT03044353. Accessed September 06, 2020.
89. Wall JS, Kennel SJ, Williams A, et al. AL amyloid imaging and therapy with a monoclonal antibody to a cryptic epitope on amyloid fibrils. PLoS One 2012; 7(12):e52686.
90. Renz M, Torres R, Dolan PJ, et al. 2A4 binds soluble and insoluble light chain aggregates from AL amyloidosis patients and promotes clearance of amyloid deposits by phagocytosis (dagger). Amyloid 2016;23(3):168–77.
91. Gertz MA, Landau H, Comenzo RL, et al. First-in-human phase I/II study of NEOD001 in patients with light chain amyloidosis and persistent organ dysfunction. J Clin Oncol 2016;34(10):1097–103.
92. Release PP. Prothena Discontinues Development Of NEOD001 For AL Amyloidosis. Available at: https://ir.prothena.com/news-releases/news-release-details/prothena-discontinues-development-neod001-al-amyloidosis.
93. Gertz MA, Cohen AD, Comenzo RL, et al. Results of the Phase 3 VITAL Study of NEOD001 (Birtamimab) Plus Standard of Care in Patients with Light Chain (AL) Amyloidosis Suggest Survival Benefit for Mayo Stage IV Patients. Blood 2019; 134(Supplement_1):3166.
94. Hrncic R, Wall J, Wolfenbarger DA, et al. Antibody-mediated resolution of light chain-associated amyloid deposits. Am J Pathol 2000;157(4):1239–46.

95. Solomon A, Weiss DT, Wall JS. Therapeutic potential of chimeric amyloid-reactive monoclonal antibody 11-1F4. Clin Cancer Res 2003;9(10 Pt 2):3831S–8S.
96. Bhatt NKJ, Kim J, Mintz A, et al. ImmunoPET imaging with radiolabeled CAEL-101 for personalizing amyloidosis immunotherapy. J Nucl Med 2019;60(supplement 1):1010.
97. Wall JS, Kennel SJ, Stuckey AC, et al. Radioimmunodetection of amyloid deposits in patients with AL amyloidosis. Blood 2010;116(13):2241–4.
98. Edwards CV, Gould J, Langer AL, et al. Interim analysis of the phase 1a/b study of chimeric fibril-reactive monoclonal antibody 11-1F4 in patients with AL amyloidosis. Amyloid 2017;24(sup1):58–9.
99. Edwards CV, Bhutani D, Mapara M, et al. One year follow up analysis of the phase 1a/b study of chimeric fibril-reactive monoclonal antibody 11-1F4 in patients with AL amyloidosis. Amyloid 2019;26(sup1):115–6.
100. Godara A, Siddiqui NS, Lee LX, et al. Dual monoclonal antibody therapy in patients with systemic AL amyloidosis and cardiac involvement. Clin Lymphoma Myeloma Leuk 2020;20(3):184–9.
101. Voorhees PM, Kaufman JL, Laubach JP, et al. Depth of response to daratumumab (DARA), lenalidomide, bortezomib, and dexamethasone (RVd) Improves over Time in Patients (pts) with Transplant-Eligible Newly Diagnosed Multiple Myeloma (NDMM): Griffin Study Update. Blood 2019;134(Supplement_1):691.
102. Munshi NC, Avet-Loiseau H, Rawstron AC, et al. Association of minimal residual disease with superior survival outcomes in patients with multiple myeloma: a meta-analysis. JAMA Oncol 2017;3(1):28–35.
103. Sidana S, Muchtar E, Sidiqi MH, et al. Impact of minimal residual negativity using next generation flow cytometry on outcomes in light chain amyloidosis. Am J Hematol 2020;95(5):497–502.
104. Manwani R, Foard D, Mahmood S, et al. Rapid hematologic responses improve outcomes in patients with very advanced (stage IIIb) cardiac immunoglobulin light chain amyloidosis. Haematologica 2018;103(4):e165–8.
105. Godara A, Zhou P, Kugelmass A, et al. Presence of soluble and cell-surface B-cell maturation antigen in systemic light-chain amyloidosis and its modulation by gamma-secretase inhibition. Am J Hematol 2020;95(5):E110–3.
106. Lonial S, Lee HC, Badros A, et al. Belantamab mafodotin for relapsed or refractory multiple myeloma (DREAMM-2): a two-arm, randomised, open-label, phase 2 study. Lancet Oncol 2020;21(2):207–21.
107. Jagannath S, Heffner LT Jr, Ailawadhi S, et al. Indatuximab ravtansine (BT062) monotherapy in patients with relapsed and/or refractory multiple myeloma. Clin Lymphoma Myeloma Leuk 2019;19(6):372–80.
108. Chanan-Khan A, Wolf J, Gharibo M, et al. Phase I study of IMGN901, used as monotherapy, in patients with heavily pre-treated CD56-positive multiple myeloma - a preliminary safety and efficacy analysis. Blood 2009;114(22):2883.

Solid Organ Transplantation

Susan Bal, MD[a], Heather J. Landau, MD[b],*

KEYWORDS

- Amyloidosis • Organ transplantation • Cardiomyopathy • ESRD • Directed-donor
- Extended-donor

KEY POINTS

- Hematologic disease control combined with solid organ transplantation can result in long-term survival in selected patients with light chain (AL) amyloidosis and limited other organ involvement.
- Restoration of critical cardiac function with organ transplantation can render patients eligible for effective disease-directed therapies, including high-dose therapy and autologous stem cell transplantation.
- Access to directed-donor organs, exchange programs for renal transplantation, and extended-donor organs for cardiac transplantation improve the availability of organs for patients with AL amyloidosis.
- Disease recurrence in the graft and progression in other organ remains concerns but often can be managed with a variety of effective plasma cell–directed therapies.

INTRODUCTION

Systemic light chain (AL) amyloidosis is caused by clonal plasma cells that produce abnormal immunoglobulins, which misfold into amyloid fibrils and deposit in organs, causing morphologic and physiologic dysfunction. Unfortunately, given its insidious onset and nonspecific symptomatology, diagnosis frequently is delayed, resulting in significant organ compromise at diagnosis in many patients. The severity of organ involvement, especially cardiac involvement, as appraised by cardiac biomarker elevation in AL, drives patient outcomes. Patients with extensive cardiac involvement have an estimated survival less than 6 months.[1–4] Similarly, advanced AL-associated kidney disease can lead to the need for renal replacement therapy (RRT) in up to 50% of patients.[5]

Funding Sources: MSK Cancer Center Supports with Grant/Core Grant (P30 CA008748).
[a] Division of Hematology and Oncology, O'Neal Comprehensive Cancer Center, University of Alabama at Birmingham, 1802 6th Avenue South, Birmingham, AL 35294, USA; [b] Memorial Sloan Kettering Cancer Center, 530 East 74th Street, New York, NY 10021, USA
* Corresponding author.
E-mail address: landauh@mskcc.org
Twitter: @SusanBal9 (S.B.)

Hematol Oncol Clin N Am 34 (2020) 1161–1175
https://doi.org/10.1016/j.hoc.2020.08.006
0889-8588/20/© 2020 Elsevier Inc. All rights reserved.

hemonc.theclinics.com

To date, therapeutic strategies target the clonal plasma cell population. Curtailing the production of toxic light chain can lead to organ responses over time, but the mechanisms by which this occurs remain elusive.[6] The depth of hematologic response predicts the likelihood of organ recovery, and high-dose therapy (HDT) and autologous hematopoietic cell transplantation (AHCT) was the first treatment to result in meaningful responses, including complete hematologic responses (CRs).[7–9] Although only a fraction (20%–25%) of patients are candidates for this approach, HDT/AHCT is associated with the potential for long-term disease control and survival in those eligible.[10] Patients with extensive cardiac or multisystem involvement, however, are not appropriate for this strategy due to prohibitive treatment-related mortality (TRM) in this population.[11] Fortunately, novel agents, such as monoclonal antibodies with more favorable therapeutic indices, are being studied in AL amyloidosis with encouraging results.

In some patients, multisystem involvement, organ failure, and poor performance status at diagnosis preclude any form of therapy, whereas in others, progressive organ dysfunction and failure may occur despite the institution of effective therapy and adequate hematologic disease control. In both instances, solid organ transplantation may extend survival dramatically improve patients' quality of life.[12,13] Yet, the role of solid organ transplantation in AL amyloidosis has not been entirely straightforward and at times has been fraught with numerous challenges. In an era where there is improved efficacy of plasma cell–directed therapies, however, the role of organ transplantation in AL is being redefined. Deep and durable hematologic responses in an increased proportion of patients confers greater opportunity for organ transplantation in these patients.

CHALLENGES

Although solid organ transplantation may be lifesaving, transplantable organs are limited precious gifts, and patients with AL amyloidosis must compete with a large pool of recipients, many of whom have disorders unlikely to relapse. The rarity of the disease results in a lack of robust data among those who have received grafts for this indication, and transplantation physicians are not necessarily familiar with the disease biology. Additionally, the multisystem nature of AL amyloidosis means that several organ systems may be affected at the same time and single organ transplantation may not suffice. Disseminated organ involvement also poses challenges, such as surviving the surgery, tolerating immunosuppression, and potential for progressive dysfunction in nontarget organs which may compromise outcomes. Along with these obstacles, the prospect of disease recurrence within the transplanted organ resulting in graft failure led to limited acceptance of solid organ transplantation as a therapeutic strategy, especially among physicians who are unaccustomed with the disease.

OPPORTUNITIES

Patients presenting with advanced amyloid-driven organ dysfunction may have predominant involvement of a single organ, resulting in high symptom burden and poor performance status. Plasma cell–directed systemic therapy can exacerbate disease-related symptoms, hasten critical organ deterioration, and result in additional toxicity. Patients with advanced organ disease do not have the luxury of time to pursue systemic therapy and await organs to respond, which takes time, if it happens at all. Organ transplantation can restore the function of a failing organ, which is causing the vast majority of symptom burden. Patients' candidacy for systemic therapy is reclaimed, and elimination of amyloidogenic plasma cells after organ transplantation can result in long-term disease control and preservation of graft function.

Alternately, patients with critically compromised organs who receive plasma cell–directed therapy can achieve deep hematologic responses without recovery of organ function. Although it is more likely for patients who achieve a hematologic CR compared with those with less than a CR to improve organ function, a deep hematologic response does not guarantee an organ response. Fewer than 60%% of patients with CR to high-dose melphalan achieved organ responses.[8,14–16] In some patients, with hematologic disease control, organ function stabilizes. Yet, critically compromised amyloid-laden organs may deteriorate despite an optimal hematologic response and patients with amyloid-associated nephropathy are particularly sensitive to other insults, which may lead to end-stage renal disease (ESRD) and the need for RRT. Given the burden of RRT and the availability of directed-donor and exchange programs for renal transplantation, forgoing referral for consideration of transplantation in this setting is a missed opportunity.

CARDIAC TRANSPLANTATION

Systemic therapy for AL amyloidosis in the 1980s resulted in modest hematologic responses and rarely led to organ response.[17] Patients presenting with advanced cardiac involvement had a particularly poor survival and, even with modern therapies, these patients are at high risk for early mortality. Traditional heart failure medications are of limited benefit; use of left ventricular assist devices is fraught with a multitude of challenges, and implantable defibrillators are unable to prevent sudden cardiac death. In such patients, orthotropic heart transplantation (OHT) represents lifesaving therapy.

The first published report of cardiac transplantation in amyloidosis was in 1988. Conner and colleagues[18] reported successful 1-year survival despite early evidence of disease recurrence in the graft by electron microscopy. It appears that even prior to this report, a professor of medicine in the United Kingdom had undergone a successful cardiac transplantation for AL amyloidosis in 1984 and published a personal account in 1994.[19] Subsequently, independent case series showed dismal survival for cardiac transplantation recipients with amyloidosis compared with other common indications for OHT, predominantly secondary to disease progression within the graft. **Table 1** includes a summary of reports of OHT in AL patients.

The first multicenter study by Hosenpud and colleagues[20] in 1991 reported a 4-year overall survival of 39%. Subsequently, Dubrey and colleagues[21] reported 1-year and 5-year survival of 60% and 30%, respectively. Although modestly improved from early abysmal outcomes, the United Network for Organ Sharing database reported on 69 patients receiving OHT with a diagnosis of amyloidosis with 1-year and 5-year survival rates of 76% and 54%, respectively.[22] These numbers continued to compare unfavorably to patients receiving OHT for other conditions with 1-year and 5-year survival rates of 81.6% and 63.8%, respectively. The risk of disease recurrence combined with the overall shortage of donor hearts resulted in virtual cessation of cardiac transplantations for amyloidosis at that time.

Although OHT for amyloidosis was abandoned, the concept of HDT/AHCT in AL amyloidosis was investigated.[7] The use of HDT/AHCT resulted in the deeper hematologic responses, including CRs, improvements in organ function, and consequently improved survival.[8,9] When used in patients with advanced amyloid-related organ disease, however, this approach resulted in the unacceptable rates of TRM.[11]

With the availability of more efficacious albeit more toxic therapy, there was a renewed interest in consideration of OHT followed by HDT/AHCT among patients

Table 1
Outcomes of patients undergoing cardiac transplantation for AL amyloidosis

Authors, Year of Publication	Time Period	Patients	Survival after Organ Transplantation
Hosenpud et al,[20] 1991	NR	8 AHCT = 0	At 4 y 39%
Dubrey et al,[57] 2004	1984–2002	17 AHCT = 3	Median 2.4 y 1 y 59%; 5 y 38% With plasma cell therapy (N = 7): 1 y 71%; 5 y 36% Without plasma cell therapy (N = 10): 1 y 50%; 5 y 20%
Kpodonu et al,[22] 2005	1987–2002	69	1 y 75%; 5 y 54%
Gillmore et al,[23] 2006	1992–2005	5 ASCT = 5	Approximately 8 y 60%
Maurer et al,[24] 2007	1997–2004	10 AHCT = 8	1 y 90%
Lacy et al,[26] 2008	1994–2005	11 AHCT = 11	1 y 82%; 5 y 65% Median survival 6.3 y
Mignot et al,[27] 2008	2001–2006	8 ASCT = 3	1 y 89% 2 y 75%
Kristen et al,[28] 2009	2001–2007	12 AHCT = 5	1 y 83% 3 y 83%
Roig et al,[25] 2009	1984–2008	13 AHCT = 3	1 y 43% 5 y 36%
Dey et al,[29] 2010	2000–2008	9 ASCT = 8	At 4.6 y, 62.5%
Sattianayagam et al,[35] 2010	1984–2009	14 AHCT = 8	1 y 86% 5 y 45%
Gray Gilstrap et al,[30] 2014	2000–2011	18 AHCT = 14	5 y 60%
Davis et al,[36] 2015	2008–2013	9 AHCT = 5	1 y 100%
Grogan et al,[58] 2016	1992–2011	23 ASCT = 13	1 y 77%; 5 y 43% Median 3.5 y

Data from Refs.[20,22–30,35,36,57,58]

with severe heart disease. Several groups reported successful outcomes with this approach. The first reports came from the UK National Amyloidosis Centre (NAC), where the feasibility of sequential OHT followed by HDT/AHCT in select patients without clinically significant extracardiac amyloidosis was established.[23] OHT restored normal functional status, permitting AHCT to be performed with acceptable TRM Rate. Median overall survival was not reached at the time of report with 95 months of follow-up. Two patients died of progressive amyloidosis at 95 months and 37, respectively, months after OHT. The remaining 3 patients were alive and without evidence of amyloidosis at the time of publication.

The following year, Maurer and colleagues[24] reported outcomes of OHT followed by HDT/AHCT using extended-donor criteria organs. These are cardiac allografts not traditionally considered for cardiac transplantation because of advanced donor age, concomitant nonobstructive coronary artery disease or inability to obtain a cardiac catheterization, mild left ventricular hypertrophy, prolonged ischemic time, or positive donor serologies for hepatitis C. Ten patients with AL amyloidosis received an OHT and, of these, 8 were able to proceed with HDT/AHCT. One-year overall survival was 90% in this cohort. Importantly, survival did not differ by standard-donor or extended-donor criteria, and there was no difference in allograft rejection among age-matched and sex-matched controls without amyloid (7% vs 10%, respectively). This pivotal study showed that extended-donor organ OHT was feasible in patients with AL amyloidosis and associated with improved survival compared with patients who were not transplanted. The authors attempted to address the ethical question of using a limited resource, such as cardiac transplantation, for patients with a severe systemic disease but acknowledge that this remains unanswered.

Roig and colleagues[25] evaluated outcomes over a 24-year period from 1984 to 2008. Thirteen patients with AL amyloidosis received OHT. The 5-year survival was disappointing at 34% in this cohort. They included patients, however, treated in the 1980s who did not receive any systemic treatment beyond OHT and these patients died of progressive disease. Two of the 3 patients who did receive HDT/AHCT after OHT lived for 2 years and 10 years, respectively. In the following years, several other groups provided additional evidence to support the sequential approach of OHT followed by HDT/AHCT in select patients with impressive short-term survival and intermediate-term survival exceeding 80% at 1 year.[26–29]

Although sequential cardiac and stem cell transplantation for patients with AL amyloidosis resulted in encouraging outcomes, the number of patients dying while listed remained substantial. The mortality of patients who die while awaiting a heart is significantly higher for patients with amyloidosis compared with patients with other causes of cardiomyopathy.[30] With limited utility of traditional support modalities and progressive organ dysfunction from untreated amyloidosis, despite the use of extended-organ donors, long wait times made death inevitable for many patients.

In the mid-2000s, several novel agents were tested in multiple myeloma and showed remarkable efficacy against the pathologic plasma cells. These agents subsequently were tested in amyloidosis and their safety, tolerability, and efficacy in frail amyloid patients expanded the therapeutic armamentarium for this population.[31–34] Even patients with advanced organ disease who were ineligible for HDT/AHCT due to unacceptable rates of TRM could experience deep responses without HDT/AHCT. The result was that patients with advanced amyloid-related cardiomyopathy could be treated while awaiting a donor heart and then undergo HDT/AHCT if warranted after OHT.

Sattianayagam and colleagues[35] reported outcomes of 14 patients with AL amyloidosis who underwent OHT between 1984 and 2009. Two patients died in the immediate perioperative period and the median survival of the entire cohort was 7.5 years. Five of the 14 patients received therapy prior to OHT, and all achieved partial remission. Eleven of the 14 patients received additional therapy post-OHT, including 8 patients without significant extracardiac organ involvement who underwent HDT/AHCT. The median survival of the patients receiving HDT/AHCT was 9.7 years compared with 3.4 years among those who did not.

Davis and colleagues[36] published the largest single-center series in recent years. Between 2008 and 2013, 9 patients with AL amyloidosis underwent OHT at Stanford University Medical Center. Most patients (8 of 9; 89%) received plasma cell–directed therapy prior to OHT, all of whom received novel agents. Six patients received additional plasma cell–directed therapy after OHT, including 5 who underwent HDT/AHCT. Although the follow-up was short (median follow-up 380 days), the survival in the AL cohort is 100% with no TRM. This series indicates that with prompt institution of effective therapy and control of the underlying disease, improved outcomes are possible. Additionally, in this series, patients resumed disease-directed therapy at a median of 78 days post-OHT, which was well tolerated and without adverse effects on graft function.

Overall, recent series suggest comparable outcomes of cardiac transplantations for amyloid cardiomyopathy and for other nonamyloid indications for OHT. This represents a significant step forward compared with results from older publications. Better patient selection and advances in supportive care are responsible, at least in part, but most important is the rapid and sustained control of the underlying disease. Early diagnosis followed by an evaluation of the extent of extracardiac organ involvement is critical. Once extensive multisystem disease is ruled out and medical management of cardiomyopathy (although limited) is optimized, plasma cell–directed therapy should be instituted alongside listing of patients for organ transplantation. This approach reduces the burden and ongoing insult from circulating toxic light chains and halts further organ injury. After OHT, in patients who have not achieved a hematologic CR or were too sick to receive therapy prior to OHT, additional therapy may be necessary. HDT/AHCT can be considered in those eligible among the several options now available for treatment, including proteasome inhibitors, immunomodulatory agents, or even monoclonal antibodies. Patients require ongoing monitoring for graft rejection and disease progression or recurrence. Both, however, can be managed effectively. In the current era, AL amyloidosis patients who undergo OHT now can enjoy extended survival with a marked improvement in their quality of life.

RENAL TRANSPLANTATION

Kidneys are organs involved most commonly in AL amyloidosis, typically resulting in proteinuria from glomerular deposition. Renal vascular and other organ (ie, autonomic or cardiac) involvement or toxic insult can lead, however, to renal insufficiency, and a significant number of patients require RRT over the course of their disease.[37,38] Treatment of the underlying clonal process can cease ongoing injury from pathologic light chains, and kidneys can improve, especially when the major manifestation is proteinuria. Renal responses frequently are delayed, however, with a median time to response of 10 months, and renal functional impairment rarely reverses.[5,39,40] The need for RRT results in significant morbidity and, ultimately, drives mortality.[5,38] When considering renal transplantation for AL amyloidosis, access to living donor organs makes this situation unique. In the modern era of effective plasma cell clone–directed therapy, patients who achieve adequate hematologic disease control but already have ESRD or are destined to need RRT should be referred to a renal transplantation program as long as they have limited extrarenal involvement. **Table 2** includes a summary of reports of renal transplantation in AL patients.

One of the original series of renal transplantation for amyloidosis was from Pasternack and colleagues,[41] who reported the outcomes of 45 amyloid patients, 3 of whom had AL amyloidosis between 1973 and 1981. The cases were compared with 45 controls with glomerulonephritis also undergoing renal transplantation. In line with other early publications, inferior survival was noted among patients receiving grafts for amyloidosis compared with other indications. Despite similar incidence of graft failure in both groups, patients with amyloidosis were at higher risk of early mortality, presumably in the absence of treatment to control the underlying clonal disease.

In the 1990s, fueled by the increasing use of calcineurin inhibitors and availability of more efficacious therapy for AL amyloidosis, there was a renewed interest in renal

Table 2
Outcomes of patients undergoing renal transplantation for AL amyloidosis

Authors, Year of Publication	Time Period	Patients	Donor	Survival after Renal Transplantation	Graft Survival	Disease Recurrence
Pasternack et al,[41] 1986	1973–1981	45 (ASCT = 0)	Deceased = 45	3 y 51%; controls 79%	3-y GS 38%; controls 45%	9%
Leung et al,[42] 2005	N/A	8 (ASCT = 6)	Living = 8	75% (follow-up 0.7–4.1 y)	GS 75%	12.5%
Sattianayagam et al,[35] 2010	1984–2009	22	Living = 3 Deceased = 19	Median survival from diagnosis 13 y, from transplantation 6.5 y	2 patients experienced graft failure at 0.9 y and 13.1 y	23%
Herrmann et al,[43] 2011	1999–2008	19	Living = 18 Deceased = 1	Median survival from diagnosis and from renal transplantation not reached. With follow-up 3.4 y, OS 79%	At 41.4 mo, follow-up, GS 79%	10.5%
Sathick et al,[44] 2019	1999–2018	16 (ASCT = 16)	Living = 14 Deceased = 2	Median survival from diagnosis 16.5 y	11.3 y	25%
Angel-Korman et al,[45] 2019	1987–2017	49 (ASCT = 39)	Living = 32 Deceased = 10 Unknown = 7	Median survival from diagnosis 15.4 y and from renal transplantation 10.5 y 1-y OS 96% 3-y OS 91% 5-y OS 86%	Median GS 6.5 y 1-y GS 94% 3-y GS 89% 5-y GS 81%	29%
Cohen et al,[59] 2020	2004–2019	40 (evaluable)	Living=20 Deceased=20	Median OS from renal transplantation 9 y	median graft survival was 12.4 y	22.5%

Abbreviations: GS, graft survival; OS, overall survival.
Data from Refs.[35,41–45,59]

transplantation for patients presenting with advanced renal involvement. In 2005, Leung and colleagues[42] reported the Mayo Clinic experience of living donor renal transplantation followed by HDT/AHCT for patients with AL amyloidosis. The investigators hypothesized that restoration of organ function would allow the patients to tolerate HDT targeting the underlying disease, and use of a living donor potentially could shorten the otherwise long wait time for a cadaver kidney. Of the 8 patients who underwent renal transplantation, 6 subsequently had planned HDT/AHCT, 1 died prior to HCT/AHCT, and the other declined HCT/AHCT. With 18 months of follow-up, 6 patients, 5 of whom underwent both planned procedures, were alive without evidence of graft failure.

In 2011, the Mayo group published the long-term outcomes of 19 patients who underwent renal transplantation for AL amyloidosis between 1999 and 2008 (18 living donor and 1 deceased donor).[43] Outcomes were reported based on sequence and intensity of disease-directed therapy. Cohort A included patients receiving renal transplantation followed by AHCT similar to their initial report (n = 8). Patients in cohort B (n = 6) received AHCT followed by renal transplantation. Cohort C included patients who achieved a CR to less intense, nontransplant chemotherapy and subsequently underwent renal transplantation (n = 5). Although the numbers in each group were small, there were no differences in the overall survival between the 3 groups. With 41 months of follow-up, 79% of patients were alive and all had functioning allografts. Disease recurrence within the allograft was rare (N = 2). These data suggest effective therapy to control the underlying disease was critical and the actual sequence of therapy appeared less important. Although the rate of rejection statistically was similar, numerically there were more acute rejection events in cohort A, the group of patients who received renal allografts upfront, before disease-directed therapy. The need to hold immunosuppression (mycophenolate) in order to facilitate engraftment in patients who underwent AHCT may be responsible for this observation. The investigators concluded that it appeared to be more favorable to treat the underlying disease with confirmed response prior to consideration for renal allograft.

Sattianayagam and colleagues[35] reported outcomes of 22 patients (3 living donor and 19 deceased donor) with AL amyloidosis who underwent kidney transplantation between 1984 and 2009 at the UK NAC. With a median follow-up of 4.8 years, the median overall survival was 13 years from time of diagnosis and 6.5 years from renal transplantation. No perioperative deaths were reported. A majority of patients (86%) received plasma cell–directed therapy prior to renal allograft, including 5 patients who received HDT/AHCT; 14/15 evaluable patients achieved a hematologic response. The incidence of graft failure was 9% but none due to recurrence of disease. Of 5 patients who had recurrent amyloidosis, no patient lost the graft. This study provided further evidence to support early treatment of underlying disease to halt progression followed by consideration of renal allograft in those with sustained disease control.

Sathick and colleagues[44] also recently reported outcomes of 16 patients (14 living donor and 2 deceased donor) who underwent kidney transplantation between 1999 and 2018. With median follow-up of 10 years from diagnosis and 3.3 years from renal transplantation, 75% patients were alive. Interestingly, 2 patients were transplanted with progressive disease and remain alive up to 10 years after renal transplantation. Two patients who experienced disease recurrence and ultimately died from progressive disease were alive for 8 years and 11 years, respectively, after renal allograft. These data challenge the notion that all patients require a CR prior to pursuing renal transplantation.

The largest series was recently published from the Amyloidosis Center at Boston University in 2019.[45] They reported the outcomes of 49 patients with AL amyloidosis who underwent kidney transplantation between 1987 and 2017. With follow-up of 7.2 years, median survival was 10.5 years from renal transplantation, and 5-year graft survival was 81%. Patients achieving hematologic response of very good partial response (VGPR) or CR had median time to graft loss of 10.4 years compared with 5.5 years for patients with a partial response or no response. Overall survival from renal transplantation was 11.7 years for those who achieved at least VGPR versus 7 years for less than VGPR. The investigators concluded that deeper responses before renal transplantation were associated with improved outcomes.

Although there are no universally accepted criteria for selecting patients with AL amyloidosis for renal transplantation, based on recently published literature, the overwhelming majority of patients fares favorably. Obtaining rapid and sustained hematologic disease control with efficacious therapies, is associated with the best outcomes. It is not clear, however, that patients who have not achieved VGPR or CR should be denied a renal transplantation when the median survival exceeds 5 years and the morbidity of RRT is significant. Graft failure remains rare overall and disease recurrences can be salvaged effectively with a host of novel therapies that are now available. Furthermore, with the availability of directed-donor kidney transplantations and exchange programs, allocating a renal allograft to an AL amyloidosis patient does not preclude another eligible recipient from receiving an organ.

Lastly, because preemptive renal transplantation was shown to improve patients' outcome while reducing the costs to the health care system, identification of potential living donors, preemptive wait-listing, or both should be considered early in the course of the disease.[13,46]

LIVER TRANSPLANTATION

Similar to patients with extensive cardiac involvement, patients presenting with advanced liver disease have dismal outcomes.[47] Although the median survival of patients with primary hepatic amyloidosis is dismal, at 9 months, those presenting with a cholestatic picture do even worse with survival less than 2 months. Orthotropic liver transplantation (OLT), therefore, can serve as lifesaving therapy. Unfortunately, outcomes of liver transplantation are not as promising as cardiac and renal transplantation. Case reports of liver transplantation for AL amyloidosis date back to 1998 when Sandberg-Gertzén and colleagues[48] reported the first case of successful liver transplantation in this disease. A 61-year-old man was discovered to have amyloidosis after presenting with splenic rupture. He underwent successful decreased donor OLT without any chemotherapy either before or after organ transplantation and remained alive at 18 months' follow-up despite recurrence within the graft. Multiple case reports of OLT became available in the early 2010s. Ueno and colleagues[49] aggregated the data to show a 1-year survival of only 50%.

Sattianayagam and colleagues[35] reported the first cohort of 9 patients with decompensated hepatic AL amyloidosis to undergo OLT at UK NAC between 1984 and 2009. They concluded that the 1-year and 5-year patient survival rates after OLT of 33% and 22%, respectively, of their cohort compared poorly to all-cause OLT survival estimates of 87% and 75%, respectively, in the United States, and of 82% and 71%, respectively, in Europe at the time of this study. Just under half the patients in this report were too sick to receive any plasma cell–directed therapy and succumbed to the illness within the first year. Three patients did undergo HDT/ASCT post-OLT and, of these, 2 patients experienced long-term survival and were alive at the time of censor 12.5 years and 5.7 years, respectively, after OLT. With the dismal outcomes, discussed previously, OLT has been felt to be prohibitive for AL amyloidosis.

More recently, with widespread use of novel agents, Elnegouly and colleagues[50] reported a case of a 52-year-old patient with primary hepatic amyloidosis. He was treated with 1 cycle of bortezomib and dexamethasone after which he developed liver failure requiring urgent organ transplantation. He was able to resume bortezomib and dexamethasone 4 months after OLT and completed 2 cycles and achieved VGPR. He then underwent HDT/ASCT without incident. He was alive at the time of publication with 36 months' follow-up without disease recurrence. Although this is a single case report, it suggests that OLT can be lifesaving in patients with AL-associated acute liver failure and limited extrahepatic organ disease, particularly if restoration of liver function renders a patient eligible for HDT/AHCT.

DISCUSSION

Vital organ failure remains an important cause of morbidity and mortality in AL amyloidosis. Patients presenting with advanced organ dysfunction enter a vicious cycle, where their health status and organ function often precludes therapy and without treatment, they have no chance of tackling the underlying disease. Additionally, even with effective hematologic disease control, organ improvement occurs slowly. Solid organ transplantation in selected patients offers a unique opportunity to replace the diseased organ and restore vital organ function. Disease recurrence in the graft and progression in the nontransplanted organs once resulted in grim attitudes regarding this approach. With the availability of effective treatment to target the underlying disease and improved supportive care, however, the clonal disease can be managed, and the benefits of solid organ transplantation can be appreciated in patients with AL amyloidosis who are living longer.

Referral to centers with experience in the management of this population should be considered. A multidisciplinary team approach often is necessary to address patients' complex pathophysiology and, when solid organ transplantation is considered or has occurred, collaboration between the hematologist and transplant team is essential.

Both before and after organ transplantation, control of pathogenic AL production is imperative and can preserve remaining organ function and prevent deposition of amyloid fibrils in the allograft and progression of disease in other organs. With appropriate patient selection and optimal management of light chains, post-transplant outcomes in this population approach those of patients undergoing solid organ transplantation for nonamyloid indications, at least in the intermediate term. Depth of response prior to solid organ transplantation has been shown to correlate with graft survival of renal allografts.[45] Minimal residual disease (MRD) testing is a prognostic marker for progression-free survival and overall survival in several hematologic malignancies, including multiple myeloma.[51,52] MRD using both flow cytometry, next-generation sequencing approaches, and mass spectrometry–based techniques in AL amyloidosis is being studied.[53,54] Patients achieving MRD negativity have been associated with longer progression-free survival as well as cardiac responses.[55] In the setting of organ transplantation, MRD may emerge as a useful parameter for patient selection as well as for periodic monitoring after solid organ transplantation to make early treatment decisions to institute therapy at disease resurgence and protect the graft.

The importance of learning from experiences of different transplant programs cannot be over-emphasized in a rare disease like AL, especially in an even rarer cohort of patients undergoing solid organ transplantation. Recommendations regarding the management of AL are confounded by the intrinsic heterogeneity of the disease, its overall rarity, and paucity of high quality evidence.[56] Development of a global registry of cases with details of selection criteria and immunosuppressive regimens has the potential to make a significant contribution to the field.[46]

SUMMARY

Early, rapid, and sustained disease control combined with solid organ transplantation can result in long-term survival in selected patients with limited organ involvement. After restoration of organ function, quality of life improves dramatically. Graft failure from recurrent disease is rare and often can be managed with preemptive therapy in patients with biochemical progression. Although depth of hematologic disease prior to organ transplantation is an important predictor of overall survival and organ survival, selected patients who achieve less than CR also may benefit. Access to directed-donor and extended-donor organs improves availability of organs for patients with AL amyloidosis. Both hematologists and transplant physicians must recognize the potential benefits of organ transplantation in this population and consider referring patients for evaluation.

CLINICS CARE POINTS

- Patients with AL amyloidosis and advanced organ involvement may experience vital organ deterioration despite adequate hematologic disease control.
- Patients with amyloid-associated cardiac failure or ESRD who are responding to plasma cell–directed therapies should be considered for organ transplantation.
- Outcomes of cardiac transplantation for patients with cardiac amyloidosis who are transplanted with extended-donor organs are comparable to outcomes of OHT for other indications.
- Directed-donor and exchange programs have increased the availability of organs for patients with AL amyloidosis who can benefit from renal transplantation, justifying allocation and minimizing wait times.
- Overall survival and graft survival after renal transplantation are extended in patients with deeper hematologic responses compared with patients with less than CRs but outcomes are favorable overall.
- Risk of graft and other organ recurrence after solid organ transplantation remain concerns but can be managed with available effective plasma cell–directed therapies.
- Transplantation for advanced amyloid-related liver disease can be lifesaving but often is ineffective.
- Guidelines for solid organ transplantation referral are necessary for more patients with AL amyloidosis to derive the quality of life and survival benefit associated with organ transplantation.

DISCLOSURES/CONFLICTS OF INTERESTS

S. Bal: nothing to disclose; H.J. Landau: received research funding and honoraria from Takeda Pharmaceuticals.

REFERENCES

1. Dispenzieri A, Gertz MA, Kyle RA, et al. Prognostication of survival using cardiac troponins and N-terminal pro-brain natriuretic peptide in patients with primary systemic amyloidosis undergoing peripheral blood stem cell transplantation. Blood 2004;104(6):1881–7.

2. Wechalekar AD, Schonland SO, Kastritis E, et al. A European collaborative study of treatment outcomes in 346 patients with cardiac stage III AL amyloidosis. Blood 2013;121(17):3420–7.

3. Palladini G, Barassi A, Klersy C, et al. The combination of high-sensitivity cardiac troponin T (hs-cTnT) at presentation and changes in N-terminal natriuretic peptide type B (NT-proBNP) after chemotherapy best predicts survival in AL amyloidosis. Blood 2010;116(18):3426–30.

4. Palladini G, Campana C, Klersy C, et al. Serum N-terminal pro–brain natriuretic peptide is a sensitive marker of myocardial dysfunction in AL amyloidosis. Circulation 2003;107(19):2440–5.

5. Palladini G, Hegenbart U, Milani P, et al. A staging system for renal outcome and early markers of renal response to chemotherapy in AL amyloidosis. Blood 2014; 124(15):2325–32.

6. Kaufman GP, Dispenzieri A, Gertz MA, et al. Kinetics of organ response and survival following normalization of the serum free light chain ratio in AL amyloidosis: Response Kinetics in AL Amyloidosis. Am J Hematol 2015;90(3):181–6.

7. Majolino I, Marcenò R, Pecoraro G, et al. High-dose therapy and autologous transplantation in amyloidosis-AL. Haematologica 1993;78(1):68–71.

8. Skinner M, Sanchorawala V, Seldin DC, et al. High-dose melphalan and autologous stem-cell transplantation in patients with AL amyloidosis: an 8-year study. Ann Intern Med 2004;140(2):85.

9. Cibeira MT, Sanchorawala V, Seldin DC, et al. Outcome of AL amyloidosis after high-dose melphalan and autologous stem cell transplantation: long-term results in a series of 421 patients. Blood 2011;118(16):4346–52.

10. Muchtar E, Gertz MA, Lacy MQ, et al. Ten-year survivors in AL amyloidosis: characteristics and treatment pattern. Br J Haematol 2019;187(5):588–94.

11. Gertz M, Lacy M, Dispenzieri A, et al. Troponin T level as an exclusion criterion for stem cell transplantation in light-chain amyloidosis. Leuk Lymphoma 2008;49(1): 36–41.

12. Theodorakakou F, Fotiou D, Dimopoulos MA, et al. Solid organ transplantation in amyloidosis. Acta Haematol 2020;143(4):349–61.

13. Huang Y, Samaniego M. Preemptive kidney transplantation: has it come of age? Néphrol Thér 2012;8(6):428–32.

14. Comenzo RL, Vosburgh E, Simms RW, et al. Dose-intensive melphalan with blood stem cell support for the treatment of AL amyloidosis: one-year follow-up in five patients. Blood 1996;88(7):2801–6.

15. Sanchorawala V, Sun F, Quillen K, et al. Long-term outcome of patients with AL amyloidosis treated with high-dose melphalan and stem cell transplantation: 20-year experience. Blood 2015;126(20):2345–7.

16. Sanchorawala V, Brauneis D, Shelton AC, et al. Induction therapy with bortezomib followed by bortezomib-high dose melphalan and stem cell transplantation for light chain amyloidosis: results of a prospective clinical trial. Biol Blood Marrow Transplant 2015;21(8):1445–51.

17. Palladini G, Russo P, Nuvolone M, et al. Treatment with oral melphalan plus dexamethasone produces long-term remissions in AL amyloidosis. Blood 2007;110(2): 787–8.

18. Conner R, Hosenpud JD, Norman DJ, et al. Heart transplantation for cardiac amyloidosis: successful one-year outcome despite recurrence of the disease. J Heart Transplant 1988;7(2):165–7.

19. Hall R, Hawkins PN. Grand Rounds - Hammersmith Hospital: Cardiac transplantation for AL amyloidosis. BMJ 1994;309(6962):1135–7.

20. Hosenpud JD, DeMarco T, Frazier OH, et al. Progression of systemic disease and reduced long-term survival in patients with cardiac amyloidosis undergoing heart transplantation. Follow-up results of a multicenter survey. Circulation 1991;84(5 Suppl):III338–43.
21. Dubrey S, Simms RW, Skinner M, et al. Recurrence of primary (AL) amyloidosis in a transplanted heart with four-year survival. Am J Cardiol 1995;76(10):739–41.
22. Kpodonu J, Massad MG, Caines A, et al. Outcome of heart transplantation in patients with amyloid cardiomyopathy. J Heart Lung Transplant 2005;24(11): 1763–5.
23. Gillmore JD, Goodman HJ, Lachmann HJ, et al. Sequential heart and autologous stem cell transplantation for systemic AL amyloidosis. Blood 2006;107(3):1227–9.
24. Maurer MS, Raina A, Hesdorffer C, et al. Cardiac transplantation using extended-donor criteria organs for systemic amyloidosis complicated by heart failure. Transplantation 2007;83(5):539–45.
25. Roig E, Almenar L, González-Vílchez F, et al. Outcomes of heart transplantation for cardiac amyloidosis: subanalysis of the spanish registry for heart transplantation. Am J Transplant 2009;9(6):1414–9.
26. Lacy MQ, Dispenzieri A, Hayman SR, et al. Autologous stem cell transplant after heart transplant for light chain (AL) amyloid cardiomyopathy. J Heart Lung Transplant 2008;27(8):823–9.
27. Mignot A, Varnous S, Redonnet M, et al. Heart transplantation in systemic (AL) amyloidosis: A retrospective study of eight French patients. Arch Cardiovasc Dis 2008;101(9):523–32.
28. Kristen AV, Kreusser MM, Blum P, et al. Improved outcomes after heart transplantation for cardiac amyloidosis in the modern era. J Heart Lung Transplant 2018; 37(5):611–8.
29. Dey BR, Chung SS, Spitzer TR, et al. Cardiac transplantation followed by dose-intensive melphalan and autologous stem-cell transplantation for light chain amyloidosis and heart failure. Transplantation 2010;90(8):905–11.
30. Gray Gilstrap L, Niehaus E, Malhotra R, et al. Predictors of survival to orthotopic heart transplant in patients with light chain amyloidosis. J Heart Lung Transplant 2014;33(2):149–56.
31. Dispenzieri A, Lacy MQ, Zeldenrust SR, et al. The activity of lenalidomide with or without dexamethasone in patients with primary systemic amyloidosis. Blood 2007;109(2):465–70.
32. Sanchorawala V, Wright DG, Rosenzweig M, et al. Lenalidomide and dexamethasone in the treatment of AL amyloidosis: results of a phase 2 trial. Blood 2007; 109(2):492–6.
33. Kastritis E, Anagnostopoulos A, Roussou M, et al. Treatment of light chain (AL) amyloidosis with the combination of bortezomib and dexamethasone. Haematologica 2007;92(10):1351–8.
34. Wechalekar AD, Lachmann HJ, Offer M, et al. Efficacy of bortezomib in systemic AL amyloidosis with relapsed/refractory clonal disease. Haematologica 2008; 93(2):295–8.
35. Sattianayagam PT, Gibbs SDJ, Pinney JH, et al. Solid organ transplantation in AL amyloidosis: transplantation in AL amyloidosis. Am J Transplant 2010;10(9): 2124–31.
36. Davis MK, Kale P, Liedtke M, et al. Outcomes after heart transplantation for amyloid cardiomyopathy in the modern era: heart transplant for amyloid cardiomyopathy. Am J Transplant 2015;15(3):650–8.

37. Gertz MA, Leung N, Lacy MQ, et al. Clinical outcome of immunoglobulin light chain amyloidosis affecting the kidney. Nephrol Dial Transplant 2009;24(10): 3132–7.

38. Havasi A, Stern L, Lo S, et al. Validation of new renal staging system in AL amyloidosis treated with high dose melphalan and stem cell transplantation. Am J Hematol 2016;91(10):E458–60.

39. Palladini G, Dispenzieri A, Gertz MA, et al. New criteria for response to treatment in immunoglobulin light chain amyloidosis based on free light chain measurement and cardiac biomarkers: impact on survival outcomes. J Clin Oncol 2012;30(36): 4541–9.

40. Havasi A, Doros G, Sanchorawala V. Predictive value of the new renal response criteria in AL amyloidosis treated with high dose melphalan and stem cell transplantation. Am J Hematol 2018;93(5):E129–32.

41. Pasternack A, Ahonen J, Kuhlbäck B. Renal transplantation in 45 patients with amyloidosis. Transplantation 1986;42(6):598–601.

42. Leung N, Griffin MD, Dispenzieri A, et al. Living donor kidney and autologous stem cell transplantation for primary systemic amyloidosis (AL) with predominant renal involvement. Am J Transplant 2005;5(7):1660–70.

43. Herrmann SMS, Gertz MA, Stegall MD, et al. Long-term outcomes of patients with light chain amyloidosis (AL) after renal transplantation with or without stem cell transplantation. Nephrol Dial Transplant 2011;26(6):2032–6.

44. Sathick IJ, Rosenbaum CA, Gutgarts V, et al. Kidney transplantation in AL Amyloidosis: is it time to maximize access? Br J Haematol 2020;188(3):e1–4.

45. Angel-Korman A, Stern L, Sarosiek S, et al. Long-term outcome of kidney transplantation in AL amyloidosis. Kidney Int 2019;95(2):405–11.

46. Nuvolone M, Merlini G. Improved outcomes for kidney transplantation in AL amyloidosis: impact on practice. Kidney Int 2019;95(2):258–60.

47. Kyle RA, Greipp PR, O'Fallon WM. Primary systemic amyloidosis: multivariate analysis for prognostic factors in 168 cases. Blood 1986;68(1):220–4.

48. Sandberg-Gertzén H, Ericzon B-G, Blomberg B. Primary amyloidosis with spontaneous splenic rupture, cholestasis, and liver failure treated with emergency liver transplantation. Am J Gastroenterol 1998;93(11):2254–6.

49. Ueno A, Katoh N, Aramaki O, et al. Liver transplantation is a potential treatment option for systemic light chain amyloidosis patients with dominant hepatic involvement: a case report and analytical review of the literature. Intern Med 2016;55(12):1585–90.

50. Elnegouly M, Specht K, Zoller H, et al. Liver transplantation followed by autologous stem cell transplantation for acute liver failure caused by AL amyloidosis. Case report and review of the literature. Ann Hepatol 2016;15(4):592–7.

51. Munshi NC, Avet-Loiseau H, Rawstron AC, et al. Association of minimal residual disease with superior survival outcomes in patients with multiple myeloma: a meta-analysis. JAMA Oncol 2017;3(1):28–35.

52. Landgren O, Devlin S, Boulad M, et al. Role of MRD status in relation to clinical outcomes in newly diagnosed multiple myeloma patients: a meta-analysis. Bone Marrow Transplant 2016;51(12):1565–8.

53. Kastritis E, Kostopoulos IV, Terpos E, et al. Evaluation of minimal residual disease using next-generation flow cytometry in patients with AL amyloidosis. Blood Cancer J 2018;8(5):46.

54. Sarosiek S, Sanchorawala V, Fulcinti M, et al. The use of next generation gene sequencing to measure minimal residual disease in patients with AL amyloidosis

and low plasma cell burden: a feasibility study. Blood 2019;134(Supplement_1): 4353.

55. Muchtar E, Dispenzieri A, Jevremovic D, et al. Survival impact of achieving minimal residual negativity by multi-parametric flow cytometry in AL amyloidosis. Amyloid 2020;27(1):13–6.

56. Dispenzieri A, Buadi F, Kumar SK, et al. Treatment of immunoglobulin light chain amyloidosis: mayo stratification of myeloma and risk-adapted therapy (mSMART) consensus statement. Mayo Clin Proc 2015;90(8):1054–81.

57. Dubrey SW, Burke MM, Hawkins PN, et al. Cardiac transplantation for amyloid heart disease: the United Kingdom experience. J Heart Lung Transplant 2004; 23(10):1142–53.

58. Grogan M, Gertz M, McCurdy A, et al. Long term outcomes of cardiac transplant for immunoglobulin light chain amyloidosis: The Mayo Clinic experience. World J Transplant 2016;6(2):380–8.

59. Cohen OC, Law S, Lachmann HJ, et al. The impact and importance of achieving a complete haematological response prior to renal transplantation in AL amyloidosis. Blood Cancer J. 2020;10(5):60.

Supportive Care for Patients with Systemic Light Chain Amyloidosis

Sandy W. Wong, MD[a],*, Teresa Fogaren, AGNP-C[b]

KEYWORDS

- Light chain amyloidosis • Supportive care • Cardiac amyloidosis
- Nephrotic syndrome • Peripheral neuropathy • Factor X deficiency

KEY POINTS

- Supportive care treats the symptoms of amyloid organ involvement, the side effects of the treatment directed at clonal plasma cells, and the psychosocial problems related to the treatment or disease.
- In cardiac amyloidosis, typically loop diuretics and spironolactone are needed to maintain euvolemia but require close monitoring, especially with coexisting renal and autonomic involvement.
- Referral to amyloid centers with a multidisciplinary team is recommended.

INTRODUCTION

Light chain (AL) amyloidosis is a disease in which clonal plasma cells produce misfolded light chains that then deposit in organs and impair their function. Amyloidosis is a multisystem disease, commonly involving the heart, kidneys, and the nervous system. Although antiplasma cell therapy aims to shut down production of the fibrillogenic light chains, supportive care allows for tolerance of clone-directed therapy. Supportive care ameliorates the symptoms of disease, minimizes the side effects of treatment, improves quality of life, and seeks to maintain organ function. In addition, the psychosocial aspect of supportive care addresses the patient's emotional, psychological, and social needs. Owing to the complexities of managing patients with AL amyloidosis, a multidisciplinary team experienced in the treatment of this disease is required to treat these patients successfully.

[a] Hematology/Blood and Marrow Transplantation, Comprehensive Amyloid Program, University of California, 400 Parnassus Avenue, San Francisco, CA 94143, USA; [b] Division of Hematology/Oncology, Tufts Medical Center, 800 Washington Street, Boston, MA 02111, USA
* Corresponding author.
E-mail address: SandyW.Wong@ucsf.edu
Twitter: @SandyWong02111 (S.W.W.)

Hematol Oncol Clin N Am 34 (2020) 1177–1191
https://doi.org/10.1016/j.hoc.2020.08.007
0889-8588/20/© 2020 Elsevier Inc. All rights reserved.

CARDIAC AMYLOIDOSIS

Most patients with newly diagnosed AL amyloidosis have cardiac involvement.[1] In cardiac amyloidosis (CA), amyloid deposits into the ventricular wall result in restrictive cardiomyopathy and cardiac arrhythmias. The goal of supportive treatment is to decrease congestion, minimize symptomatic hypotension, and control cardiac arrhythmias.

Nonpharmacologic management includes fluid and dietary salt restriction. Reading nutrition labels, avoiding additional salt to food, and eating at home should be part of patient education. Recorded weights each morning provide valuable information on fluid status and direct diuretic titrations.

Diuretics are the backbone of fluid management in patients with CA and must be balanced constantly against the risk of worsened renal failure and orthostatic hypotension. Infusions of salt-poor albumin to achieve serum albumin level of greater than 2 g/dL improves intravascular volume and efficacy of diuretics (**Table 1**).[2,3] Loop diuretics in combination with spironolactone are used regularly. Torsemide and bumetanide have greater bioavailability and a longer half-life than furosemide and are preferred in AL amyloidosis. Metolazone may also serve an adjunctive role to augment diuresis. Involvement of the autonomic nervous system (ANS) causes hypotension and necessitates monitoring and dose adjustments of diuretics. Midodrine and compression stockings may be required to control orthostasis. Pleural effusions develop often with advanced heart failure in AL amyloidosis. Aggressive diuresis may be sufficient to alleviate symptoms along with intermittent thoracentesis. Options such as pleurodesis, thorascopy with talc insufflation, or Pleurx tube placement should be explored for recurrent effusions.[4]

Many of the typical drugs used to treat nonamyloid cardiomyopathy are either poorly tolerated or contraindicated in CA. Angiotensin-converting enzyme inhibitors (ACE-I) and angiotensin receptor blockers (ARBs) may cause symptomatic hypotension and further exacerbate renal insufficiency. Verapamil and diltiazem bind to cardiac amyloid fibrils causing heart block and shock and should be avoided.[5] Digoxin also binds to amyloid fibrils and was once considered too toxic to amyloid patients, but now has been found to be safe in low doses with close monitoring.[6] Patients with CA experience physiologic sinus tachycardia to sustain cardiac output. Beta-blockers are difficult for patients with AL amyloidosis to tolerate owing to the blunting of heart rate increases (see **Table 1**). However, low-dose beta-blockers may be used with careful monitoring to control supraventricular arrhythmias.

Atrial fibrillation is the most common arrhythmia in patients with CA.[7] Patients with atrial fibrillation should be on anticoagulation even with a low CHADS2-VASc score owing to the high incidence of atrial thrombi.[8–10] Amiodarone is the preferred antiarrhythmic agent owing to its efficacy in CA with minimal negative inotropic effects (see **Table 1**).[11,12] However, amiodarone can cause thyroid dysfunction and requires careful monitoring of thyroid function.[13] Cardiac ablation for atrial arrhythmias may provide symptomatic relief for select patients.[14]

Complex ventricular arrhythmias are common in patients with AL amyloidosis.[15] However, reduced effectiveness of an implantable cardioverter defibrillator[16–18] owing to electromechanical dissociation casts doubt on the long-term survival benefit of these devices in amyloid patients.[16,19,20] Better patient selection may help to distinguish those who would benefit from an implantable cardioverter defibrillator.[19,21]

Table 1
Supportive care medications in systemic AL amyloidosis

Drug Class	Name	Recommended Dosing Regimen	Safety Notes/Side Effects
Cardiac			
Loop diuretics	Furosemide	Diuretic naïve: oral, IV: Initial: 20–40 mg once then titrate as needed to an effective dose Refractory edema: IV: bolus/intermittent dosing: Initial: Administer 1–2.5 times the total daily oral maintenance dose once Continuous infusion: eGFR ≥30 mL/min/1.73 m²; Initial: 5 mg/h eGFR <30 mL/min/1.73 m²	Correct electrolyte disturbances.
	Bumetanide (preferred)	IV/PO initial: 0.5–1 mg once, then titrate as needed to an effective dose 1–3 times daily Maximum daily dose is 10 mg/d	Higher than usual doses may be required for patients with nephrotic syndrome or renal failure
	Torsemide (preferred)	Heart failure: initial dose 10–20 mg/d increase gradually renal failure: 20 mg/d	Fluid/electrolyte loss Max dose 200 mg/d
Thiazide related	Metolazone	Initial: 2.5–5.0 mg twice weekly to daily	Severe hypokalemia and/or hyponatremia can occur rapidly after the initial doses. Orthostatic hypotension
	Hydrochlorothiazide	25 mg once daily	As needed for weight gain owing to steroids

(continued on next page)

Table 1
(continued)

Drug Class	Name	Recommended Dosing Regimen	Safety Notes/Side Effects
Antiarrhythmic	Amiodarone	IV: initial: 150 mg over 10 min, then 1 mg/min for 6 h, then 0.5 mg/min for 18 h. Continue for a total load of up to 10 g; may finish load with oral dosing. Change to oral maintenance dose when clinically indicated Oral: maintenance dose of 200 mg once daily	Monitor TSH
Antiarrhythmic	Digoxin	Maintenance oral dose: 0.125 mg once daily	Monitor levels carefully. Check levels before the fifth dose.
Renal			
Colloid	Salt-poor human albumin (25%)	25 g IV as needed for albumin ≥2.0	Pruritus, hypervolemia, fever
Alpha-adrenergic agonist	Midodrine	Start 2.5–5.0 mg BID/TID and up titrate to 15 mg TID	Supine hypertension, bladder retention
Nervous system			
Corticosteroid	Fludrocortisone	0.1 mg/d in conjunction with a high-salt diet and adequate fluid intake; may be increased in increments of 0.1 mg per week. Not to exceed 0.3 mg/d.	Fluid retention
Alpha-/beta-agonist	Droxidopa	Oral: initial: 100 mg TID; titrate in increments of 100 mg TID every 24-48 h to symptomatic response (maximum dose: 1800 mg/d).	Upon arising in the morning, at midday, and in the late afternoon ≥3 h before bedtime (to decrease the potential for supine hypertension during sleep). BP check before nighttime dose. Advise patients to elevate the head of bed when resting or sleeping

Acetylcholinesterase inhibitor	Pyridostigmine	Initial dose 30 mg BID/TID gradually increase to 60 mg TID.	Effectiveness enhanced by combining with midodrine 5 mg TID
Anticonvulsant	Gabapentin	100–300 mg 1–TID	Somnolence and dizziness Peripheral edema Dose adjustments for CrCl <49
	Pregabalin	25–150 mg/d once daily or in 2 divided doses	Peripheral edema Dose adjust for renal impairment
Tricyclic antidepressants	Amitriptyline	10 mg once daily at bedtime;	Hypotension, urinary retention
Topical analgesic	Lidoderm patch	1 patch (5% lidocaine) to the area daily for 12 h then remove.	Cautiously with class 1 antiarrhythmic agents
	Capsaicin	OTC- apply to affected areas 3–4 times daily	May cause serious burns. Avoid contact with eyes and mucous membranes
Gastrointestinal			
Dopamine receptor antagonists	Metoclopramide	5–10 mg 2–TID administered before meals	Tardive dyskinesia, QT prolongation
Motilin agonists	Erythromycin	250–500 mg (base) TID before meals	QT prolongation Limit duration of therapy, tachyphylaxis may occur after 4 wk
Bile acid sequestrant	Cholestyramine	4 g once daily; increase by 4 g at weekly intervals in 1–4 divided doses; maximum: 36 g/d	Abnormal hepatic function tests Arthralgia
Antibiotic	Rifaximin	200 mg TID for 3 d	Peripheral edema Anemia Muscle spasm arthralgia
Somatostatin Analog	Octreotide	Short acting: 200–300 μg SQ divided into 2–3 doses/d	Sinus bradycardia hypertension
Coagulation System			

(continued on next page)

Table 1
(continued)

Drug Class	Name	Recommended Dosing Regimen	Safety Notes/Side Effects
Recombinant factor VIIa	Novo 7	30 µg/kg IV every 3–4 h titrated up based on the prothrombin time and partial thromboplastin time	Arterial and venous thromboembolism, hypersensitivity reaction, angina
Activated prothrombin complex concentrate	Factor VIII inhibitor bypassing activity	100–200 units/kg every 12 h until resolution of bleed	Thromboembolism, myocardial infarction, hypersensitivity reaction
Antifibrinolytic	Tranexamic acid	1300 mg PO 1–3 times per day for mucosal bleeds	Thromboembolism, hypersensitivity reaction, stroke

Abbreviations: BID, 2 times per day; BP, blood pressure; CrCl, creatinine clearance; eGFR, estimated glomerular filtration rate; IV, intravenously; OTC, over the counter; PO, by mouth; SQ, subcutaneously; TID, 3 times per day.

RENAL AMYLOIDOSIS

At diagnosis, nearly 70% of patients with systemic AL have renal involvement.[22] Deposition of amyloid in the kidneys commonly involves the glomeruli resulting in nephrotic range proteinuria.[23] Patients often present with lower extremity swelling, pulmonary edema, ascites, or anasarca. Although this fluid shift causes whole body volume overload, patients may be intravascularly volume depleted, complicating the tolerance of diuresis. Most patients with AL also have cardiac or ANS involvement, further contributing to hemodynamic fragility.

The mainstay of treatment for volume overload from proteinuria are loop diuretics, similar to the management of patients with CA, as detailed elsewhere in this article. Diuresis down to dry weight as tolerated is crucial to allow for the administration of antiplasma cell treatment. Treatment regimens for AL amyloidosis require steroids[1,24] for maximum effect and/or prevention of infusion-related reactions.[25] Exposure to steroids over time may cause reaccumulation of fluid; therefore, constant and close monitoring of fluid status is crucial. Patients should keep a weight diary daily and report weight gain of 2 lbs or more over 1 to 2 days to their provider. Patient education on fluid and salt restriction to 1.5 L/d or less and 1500 to 2000 mg/d of sodium, respectively, is necessary to maintain euvolemia. In regard to diet, patients should refrain from high-protein diets, which may cause glomerular hyperfiltration and hyperemia.[26]

ACE-Is and ARBs are well-known for their renal-protective and proteinuria-reducing effects in non-AL kidney disease. However, in patients with AL amyloidosis, the hypotensive effects of these drugs are magnified owing to the heavy reliance on angiotensin to maintain blood pressure (BP).[27] ACE-Is and ARBs are generally contraindicated or if used short-acting ones are preferred at low doses. In the rare situation where the patient remains hypotensive owing to severe nephrosis despite maximal medical management, bilateral renal artery embolization may be used as a last resort.[28]

Unfortunately, despite antiplasma cell treatment, patients with stage 3 AL-related renal disease still have a significant 2-year risk of developing end-stage renal disease.[22] The decision to initiate dialysis should take into account the patient's goals of care, prognosis, and ability to tolerate the procedure. Hypotension from advanced cardiac or ANS involvement may limit the ability to dialyze[29] despite midodrine support especially for hemodialysis compared with peritoneal dialysis. Peritoneal dialysis offers a quality of life advantage over hemodialysis, although it is contraindicated in patients with severe hypoalbuminuria owing peritoneal dialysis-related albumin loss.[30] The most common complication of peritoneal dialysis is peritonitis[29] that can further exacerbate the serum albumin deficit.[31] The pharmacokinetics of antiplasma cell drugs are also less known for patients on peritoneal dialysis. However, there is no difference between hemodialysis and peritoneal dialysis with regard to survival.[29,32] Bleeding diatheses associated with amyloidosis may present an obstacle to the placement of vascular access for hemodialysis. Furthermore, skin fragility owing to vascular and cutaneous deposition may make construction of an arteriovenous fistula not feasible.

AMYLOIDOSIS OF THE NERVOUS SYSTEM

Deposition of amyloid fibers may occur in the peripheral nervous system or ANS, resulting in damage to the blood vessels supplying the nerves or nerve compression. Sixty-five percent of patients with AL amyloidosis develop symptoms of autonomic neuropathy affecting the cardiac, gastrointestinal (GI), and genitourinary systems.[33]

Orthostatic hypotension is a common manifestation of ANS involvement with symptoms of persistent fatigue, lightheadedness on standing, or syncope.[33] On diagnosis of ANS-related orthostatic hypotension, the patient's medications should be reviewed to identify drugs that exacerbate hypotension, such as beta-blockers, diuretics, antihypertensive agents, nitrates, tricyclic ,antidepressants and tamsulosin.[34] The elimination of these drugs or a dose decrease should be attempted to achieve an acceptable BP.

Behavioral modifications are important in improving or preventing symptoms with a focus on fall prevention. Patients should avoid prolonged periods of standing. Male patients should sit while urinating. Slow transitions from supine to sitting to standing are important, especially in the morning, after meals, and after urination or defecation. Waist-high compression stockings at 30 to 40 mm Hg and abdominal binders could be worn to increase venous return to maintain a higher BP.

ANS-related orthostatic hypotension with other amyloid organ involvement is difficult to manage pharmacologically, requiring a delicate balance between fluid status and BP. For ANS-related orthostatic hypotension without volume overload, hydration and increased salt intake is effective, although this is uncommon because most patients have fluid problems. For most patients who have cardiac or renal amyloid and may be volume overloaded, the first line pharmacologic treatment is midodrine (see **Table 1**). Fludrocortisone can be also used, although with caution, owing to fluid retention. Pyridostigmine and droxidopa are newer agents for treatment of ANS-related orthostatic hypotension (see **Table 1**).[35]

Autonomic neuropathy may lead to lower urinary tract dysfunction. Early management of urinary retention should include scheduled voiding and the Crede maneuver to empty the bladder.[36] With progressive retention, scheduled self-catheterization may be required.[36,37] Sildenafil for erectile dysfunction caused by autonomic neuropathy should only be used in patients without ANS-related orthostatic hypotension or advanced CA.

Peripheral nervous system involvement occurs in 17% to 35% of patients with AL amyloidosis.[37] Symptoms often present as symmetric painful paresthesias in the feet. Treatment for painful neuropathy with patients with AL amyloidosis include gabapentin, duloxetine, and venlaxafine (see **Table 1**).[35] Tricyclic antidepressants such as nortriptyline and amitriptyline provide neuropathic pain relief, but can worsen autonomic symptoms and should be used cautiously.[35] Topical agents such as lidocaine patches, ketamine, and capsaicin cream may also be considered.[35]

GASTROINTESTINAL AMYLOIDOSIS

Around 8% of patients with systemic AL amyloidosis have involvement of the GI tract.[38] Amyloid can deposit in the mucosa, muscle, autonomic nerves, and the vasculature of the gut. Dysmotility is the physiologic cause for many GI symptoms. Mucosal bleeding from deposition into the gut vasculature is another important manifestation. Finally, splenic amyloidosis is not common, but may cause morbidity when present.

Dysmotility in the esophagus causes achalasia, esophageal spasms, dysphagia, and/or gastric esophageal reflux disease.[39,40] All dysphagic patients require a swallow evaluation to assess for the presence of aspiration and to undergo swallowing rehabilitation. Dietary modification to thickened liquids and swallowing techniques are usually sufficient to ameliorate most cases of amyloid-related dysphagia.

GI paresis manifests as nausea, abdominal pain, constipation, diarrhea, and, rarely, pseudo-obstruction.[41] Dietary modification should be the front-line treatment in mild cases. Homogenized meals could be tried for easier gut transit compared with solid food.[42] Promotility agents for upper GI gastroparesis include dopamine receptor antagonists[43] and motilin agonists (see **Table 1**). All these agents have modest efficacy, but QT prolongation is a side effect, making it challenging to increase them to an effective dose in patients with CA. Constipation from lower GI gastroparesis is common. Typically, sodium docusate, senna, and fiber supplements are insufficient and an osmotic laxative is regularly added. Treatment of severe fecal impaction consists of manual disimpaction or fluoroscopy-guided stool decompression. Conversely, patients with AL amyloidosis may present with diarrhea. The addition of dietary fiber and antimotility agents are effective for mild cases. Diarrhea may be due to bile acid malabsorption, which is treated with cholestyramine (see **Table 1**). Gastroparesis-induced small intestinal bacterial overgrowth may be treated with long-term rifaximin (see **Table 1**). Patients with chronic diarrhea should be assessed and corrected for mineral and vitamin deficiencies. Last, subcutaneous octreotide is helpful for refractory cases.[44,45] A diverting ostomy to improve the patient's quality of life has also been reported for patients with AL amyloidosis with refractory diarrhea.[46,47]

Patients with systemic AL despite normal coagulation parameters may experience GI bleeding from amyloid deposition in the blood vessels of the gut.[48] Rarely, surgical resection is needed for life-threatening bleeding or mechanical obstruction.[49] Patients with GI deposition are more likely to bleed during stem cell transplantation and should be supported with higher platelet and red blood cell thresholds for transfusion.[50] Splenomegaly from amyloid deposition is rare, although spontaneous rupture has been reported. Emergent splenectomy is the treatment for splenic rupture. Patients with hyposplenism should be vaccinated against encapsulated organisms.[51]

Most patients systemic with AL on presentation suffer from malnutrition,[52,53] which is associated with a poor quality of life[54] and decreased survival.[53] Gastrostomy tubes are usually not helpful in gastroparesis since the motility disorder is present throughout the gut.[55] In select cases, artificial nutrition including total parental nutrition[56] may be offered. Selection of candidates for total parental nutrition should include a careful consideration of the patient's ability to tolerate the volume associated with total parental nutrition, and may not be appropriate for patients with advanced CA.

AMYLOIDOSIS AND THE COAGULATION SYSTEM

Systemic AL amyloidosis can cause 1 or multiple[57,58] coagulation abnormalities, the classic one being an acquired factor X deficiency.[59] The patient needs hemostasis support until the amyloid burden is decreased sufficiently for the factor deficiency to resolve.

In the setting of an acute bleed, we give recombinant factor VIIa titrated based on the prothrombin time and partial thromboplastin time (see **Table 1**).[60,61] For periprocedural bleeding prevention, the patient receives 1 dose of recombinant factor VIIa before the procedure and then continued on treatment. The duration of treatment depends on the extent of the procedure or surgery. Activated prothrombin complex concentrate products like factor VIII inhibitor bypassing activity have also been used to treat[62] bleeding patients or for prophylaxis.[63,64] Recombinant human factor X has been reported to be effective in a limited number of patients.[65] Patients with refractory bleeding despite recombinant factor VIIa and factor VIII inhibitor bypassing activity need a splenectomy, for rapid amyloid burden reduction.[66–68] For mucosal bleeds, tranexamic acid may be used to provide clot stabilization.

SOFT TISSUE AMYLOIDOSIS

Soft tissue deposition in patients with AL amyloidosis is present in close to one-half of all patients.[69] The most common symptoms include submandibular gland enlargement, macroglossia, and carpal tunnel syndrome.[70] Hypothyroidism from amyloid deposition in the thyroid is likely under-recognized and routine screening for serum thyroid-stimulating hormone levels is recommended.[71,72]

The submandibular gland is one of the largest salivary glands and, when affected by amyloid, patients can develop xerostomia.[73,74] Artificial saliva produces short-term lubrication for the mouth and must be used frequently. Chewing sugarless gum or sucking on sialagogues stimulates saliva production. Patients should be counseled to decrease caffeine intake, stop smoking, and stop chewing tobacco, all of which could aggravate xerostomia. Regular dental care to evaluate for caries and dental caries prevention should be part of the patient's treatment plan.

Macroglossia owing to amyloidosis varies in severity. It can cause obstructive sleep apnea and speech abnormalities. Patients should be screened for worsened snoring and undergo a sleep evaluation. In severe cases, it can cause airway obstruction and interfere with swallowing. Surgical management has been reported in limited cases,[75] although owing to postoperative complications, a tracheostomy with gastrostomy tube may be more prudent.

Carpal tunnel syndrome associated with AL amyloidosis leads to neuropathy and loss of function. Supportive care measures include wrist guards, especially at night. Surgical release may be beneficial in select patients.

Cutaneous manifestations of amyloidosis include petechia, purpura, and ecchymoses owing to amyloid infiltration of the blood vessels.[76] Some patients may present with skin bullae or increased skin fragility owing to dermal amyloid deposition.[77] Care must be taken to avoid medical silk tape on the skin of these patients and instead use paper tape. Topical steroids, which could thin out the skin further, should also be avoided.

PSYCHOSOCIAL SUPPORT

Systemic AL amyloidosis is a rare multiorgan disease often diagnosed late in its course.[78] Owing to a late diagnosis, patients frequently suffer great debility requiring assistance with instrumental activities of daily living and, in advanced stages, help with activities of daily living. Treatments for the disease[78] are sometimes difficult to tolerate and worsen their disability.[79] Patients might not be able to work owing to their symptoms and the multiple clinic visits for chemotherapy. They may suffer disconnection from relatives or friends by self-imposed social distancing owing to concern over infection while on chemotherapy, or they may be too symptomatic to continue these social connections. Patients may experience a change in dynamics with their domestic partner or with close friends as they assume the role of caregivers.[80] A fundamental shift in identity occurs with the diagnosis of an incurable disease that carries for many a grim prognosis.[81] With all these issues comes an emotional toll, which could lead to anxiety, depression, sadness, and hopelessness.[78] Patients with AL amyloidosis need help with grieving over the loss of well-being and health. Regular assessments of how patients are coping with amyloidosis and the treatment are crucial to their care. Early referral to psycho-oncology is beneficial to address the psychological burden of their disease.

At diagnosis, providers should discuss the goals of care and advanced directives with the patient and the health care proxy. These topics should be revisited as the patient's condition changes to ensure that medical treatment aligns with the patient's wishes. Timely involvement of palliative care as an integral part of the treating team will aid in the conversations around goals of care and if needed, facilitate a transition to hospice.

Patients with AL amyloidosis not only experience the physical and emotional burden of illness, they also have to endure the financial burden of disease. Patients are often unable to work during treatment yet have increased expenditures for travel to the treatment center, parking, food, and potential overnight stays. Moreover, no drugs approved by the US Food and Drug Administration exist for AL amyloidosis, and current treatments are based on medications approved for multiple myeloma. The cost of treatment may include high copays or deductibles, which may be covered through application for foundation patient funds. A social worker should be enlisted early to identify and address areas of psychosocial need.

CLINICS CARE POINTS

- In CA, use loop diuretics and spironolactone to achieve euvolemia.
- ACE-Is and ARBs are generally contraindicated.
- Patients with atrial fibrillation should be on anticoagulation even with a low CHADS2-VASc score.
- Twenty-five percent salt-poor albumin infusion with furosemide is helpful in diuresing patients with low albumin.
- Patient education on nutrition, a low-salt diet, fluid restriction, daily weights, compression stockings, and fall prevention are part of the management of patients with AL amyloidosis.
- Peripheral neuropathy should be treated in a similar manner to diabetic neuropathy.
- All patients with AL amyloidosis should be evaluated for factor X deficiency.
- All patients with AL amyloidosis should be referred to an amyloid treatment center with a multidisciplinary team.

DISCLOSURE

S.W. Wong receives research funding from Bristol-Myers Squibb, GlaxoSmithKline, Fortis, and Janssen. She also receives consultancy fees from Amgen and serves on the advisory board for Sanofi; T. Fogaren has no disclosures.

REFERENCES

1. Palladini G, Sachchithanantham S, Milani P, et al. A European collaborative study of cyclophosphamide, bortezomib, and dexamethasone in upfront treatment of systemic AL amyloidosis. Blood 2015;126(5):612–5.
2. Comenzo RL. Primary systemic amyloidosis. Curr Treat Options Oncol 2000; 1(1):83–9.
3. Phakdeekitcharoen B, Boonyawat K. The added-up albumin enhances the diuretic effect of furosemide in patients with hypoalbuminemic chronic kidney disease: a randomized controlled study. BMC Nephrol 2012;13(1):92.
4. Berk JL. Pleural effusions in systemic amyloidosis. Curr Opin Pulm Med 2005; 11(4):324–8.
5. Pollak A, Falk RH. Left ventricular systolic dysfunction precipitated by verapamil in cardiac amyloidosis. Chest 1993;104(2):618–20.
6. Muchtar E, Gertz MA, Kumar SK, et al. Digoxin use in systemic light-chain (AL) amyloidosis: contra-indicated or cautious use? Amyloid 2018;25(2):86–92.

7. Longhi S, Quarta CC, Milandri A, et al. Atrial fibrillation in amyloidotic cardiomyopathy: prevalence, incidence, risk factors and prognostic role. Amyloid 2015; 22(3):147–55.

8. Feng D, Syed IS, Martinez M, et al. Intracardiac thrombosis and anticoagulation therapy in cardiac amyloidosis. Circulation 2009;119(18):2490–7.

9. Martinez-Naharro A, Gonzalez-Lopez E, Corovic A, et al. High prevalence of intracardiac thrombi in cardiac amyloidosis. J Am Coll Cardiol 2019;73(13): 1733–4.

10. Feng D, Edwards WD, Oh JK, et al. Intracardiac thrombosis and embolism in patients with cardiac amyloidosis. Circulation 2007;116(21):2420–6.

11. Merlini G, Dispenzieri A, Sanchorawala V, et al. Systemic immunoglobulin light chain amyloidosis. Nat Rev Dis Primers 2018;4(1):38.

12. Rubin J, Maurer MS. Cardiac amyloidosis: overlooked, underappreciated, and treatable. Annu Rev Med 2020;71:203–19.

13. Muchtar E, Blauwet LA, Gertz MA. Restrictive cardiomyopathy: genetics, pathogenesis, clinical manifestations, diagnosis, and therapy. Circ Res 2017;121(7): 819–37.

14. Tan NY, Mohsin Y, Hodge DO, et al. Catheter ablation for atrial arrhythmias in patients with cardiac amyloidosis. J Cardiovasc Electrophysiol 2016;27(10): 1167–73.

15. Palladini G, Malamani G, Co F, et al. Holter monitoring in AL amyloidosis: prognostic implications. Pacing Clin Electrophysiol 2001;24(8):1228–33.

16. Kristen AV, Dengler TJ, Hegenbart U, et al. Prophylactic implantation of cardioverter-defibrillator in patients with severe cardiac amyloidosis and high risk for sudden cardiac death. Heart Rhythm 2008;5(2):235–40.

17. Wright BL, Grace AA, Goodman HJ. Implantation of a cardioverter-defibrillator in a patient with cardiac amyloidosis. Nat Clin Pract Cardiovasc Med 2006;3(2): 110–4 [quiz: 115].

18. Hess EP, White RD. Out-of-hospital cardiac arrest in patients with cardiac amyloidosis: presenting rhythms, management and outcomes in four patients. Resuscitation 2004;60(1):105–11.

19. Rezk T, Whelan CJ, Lachmann HJ, et al. Role of implantable intracardiac defibrillators in patients with cardiac immunoglobulin light chain amyloidosis. Br J Haematol 2018;182(1):145–8.

20. Lin G, Dispenzieri A, Kyle R, et al. Implantable cardioverter defibrillators in patients with cardiac amyloidosis. J Cardiovasc Electrophysiol 2013;24(7):793–8.

21. Varr BC, Zarafshar S, Coakley T, et al. Implantable cardioverter-defibrillator placement in patients with cardiac amyloidosis. Heart Rhythm 2014;11(1):158–62.

22. Palladini G, Hegenbart U, Milani P, et al. A staging system for renal outcome and early markers of renal response to chemotherapy in AL amyloidosis. Blood 2014; 124(15):2325–32.

23. Dember LM. Amyloidosis-associated kidney disease. J Am Soc Nephrol 2006; 17(12):3458–71.

24. Palladini G, Milani P, Foli A, et al. Melphalan and dexamethasone with or without bortezomib in newly diagnosed AL amyloidosis: a matched case–control study on 174 patients. Leukemia 2014;28(12):2311–6.

25. Roussel M, Merlini G, Chevret S, et al. A prospective phase 2 trial of daratumumab in patients with previously treated systemic light-chain amyloidosis. Blood 2020;135(18):1531–40.

26. Friedman AN. High-protein diets: potential effects on the kidney in renal health and disease. Am J Kidney Dis 2004;44(6):950–62.

27. Kapoor P, Thenappan T, Singh E, et al. Cardiac amyloidosis: a practical approach to diagnosis and management. Am J Med 2011;124(11):1006–15.

28. Yeh C-T, Tseng H-S, Liu W-S, et al. Severe proteinuria secondary to amyloidosis requiring bilateral renal artery embolization. Case Rep Nephrol Urol 2012;2(1): 78–82.

29. Moroni G, Banfi G, Montoli A, et al. Chronic dialysis in patients with systemic amyloidosis: the experience in northern Italy. Clin Nephrol 1992;38(2):81–5.

30. Kagan A, Bar-Khayim Y. Role of peritoneal loss of albumin in the hypoalbuminemia of continuous ambulatory peritoneal dialysis patients: relationship to peritoneal transport of solutes. Nephron 1995;71(3):314–20.

31. Krediet RT, Zuyderhoudt FMJ, Boeschoten EW, et al. Peritoneal permeability to proteins in diabetic and non-diabetic continuous ambulatory peritoneal dialysis patients. Nephron 1986;42(2):133–40.

32. Gertz MA. Dialysis support of patients with primary systemic amyloidosis. Arch Intern Med 1992;152(11):2245.

33. Kapoor M, Rossor AM, Jaunmuktane Z, et al. Diagnosis of amyloid neuropathy. Pract Neurol 2019;19(3):250–8.

34. Freeman R, Abuzinadah AR, Gibbons C, et al. Orthostatic hypotension: JACC state-of-the-art review. J Am Coll Cardiol 2018;72(11):1294–309.

35. Kaku M, Berk JL. Neuropathy associated with systemic amyloidosis. Semin Neurol 2019;39(5):578–88.

36. Andrade MJ. Lower urinary tract dysfunction in familial amyloidotic polyneuropathy, Portuguese type. Neurourol Urodyn 2009;28(1):26–32.

37. Burakgazi AZ, Alsowaity B, Burakgazi ZA, et al. Bladder dysfunction in peripheral neuropathies. Muscle Nerve 2012;45(1):2–8.

38. Menke DM, Kyle RA, Fleming CR, et al. Symptomatic gastric amyloidosis in patients with primary systemic amyloidosis. Mayo Clin Proc 1993;68(8):763–7.

39. Rubinow A, Burakoff R, Cohen AS, et al. Esophageal manometry in systemic amyloidosis. A study of 30 patients. Am J Med 1983;75(6):951–6.

40. Battle WM, Rubin MR, Cohen S, et al. Gastrointestinal-motility dysfunction in amyloidosis. N Engl J Med 1979;301(1):24–5.

41. Tada S, Iida M, Yao T, et al. Intestinal pseudo-obstruction in patients with amyloidosis: clinicopathologic differences between chemical types of amyloid protein. Gut 1993;34(10):1412–7.

42. Olausson EA, Storsrud S, Grundin H, et al. A small particle size diet reduces upper gastrointestinal symptoms in patients with diabetic gastroparesis: a randomized controlled trial. Am J Gastroenterol 2014;109(3):375–85.

43. Stevens JE, Jones KL, Rayner CK, et al. Pathophysiology and pharmacotherapy of gastroparesis: current and future perspectives. Expert Opin Pharmacother 2013;14(9):1171–86.

44. Yam LT. Octreotide for diarrhea in amyloidosis. Ann Intern Med 1991;115(7):577.

45. Carvalho M, Alves M, Luis ML. Octreotide–a new treatment for diarrhoea in familial amyloidotic polyneuropathy. J Neurol Neurosurg Psychiatry 1992;55(9):860–1.

46. Gertz MA, Lacy MQ, Dispenzieri A. Therapy for immunoglobulin light chain amyloidosis: the new and the old. Blood Rev 2004;18(1):17–37.

47. Ek BO, Holmlund DE, Sjodin JG, et al. Enterostomy in patients with primary neuropathic amyloidosis. Am J Gastroenterol 1978;70(4):365–70.

48. Yood RA. Bleeding manifestations in 100 patients with amyloidosis. JAMA 1983; 249(10):1322.

49. Rives S, Pera M, Rosiñol L, et al. Primary systemic amyloidosis presenting as a colonic stricture: successful treatment with left hemicolectomy followed by

autologous hematopoietic stem-cell transplantation: report of a case. Dis Colon Rectum 2002;45(9):1263–6.

50. Comenzo RL, Gertz MA. Autologous stem cell transplantation for primary systemic amyloidosis. Blood 2002;99(12):4276–82.

51. Frank JM, Palomino NJ. Primary amyloidosis with diffuse splenic infiltration presenting as fulminant pneumococcal sepsis. Am J Clin Pathol 1987;87(3):405–7.

52. Caccialanza R, Palladini G, Klersy C, et al. Nutritional status of outpatients with systemic immunoglobulin light-chain amyloidosis. Am J Clin Nutr 2006;83(2): 350–4.

53. Sattianayagam PT, Lane T, Fox Z, et al. A prospective study of nutritional status in immunoglobulin light chain amyloidosis. Haematologica 2013;98(1):136–40.

54. Caccialanza R, Palladini G, Klersy C, et al. Nutritional status independently affects quality of life of patients with systemic immunoglobulin light-chain (AL) amyloidosis. Ann Hematol 2012;91(3):399–406.

55. Wixner J, Suhr OB, Anan I. Management of gastrointestinal complications in hereditary transthyretin amyloidosis: a single-center experience over 40 years. Expert Rev Gastroenterol Hepatol 2018;12(1):73–81.

56. Russo M, Vita GL, Stancanelli C, et al. Parenteral nutrition improves nutritional status, autonomic symptoms and quality of life in transthyretin amyloid polyneuropathy. Neuromuscul Disord 2016;26(6):374–7.

57. Ericson S, Shah N, Liberman J, et al. Fatal bleeding due to acquired factor IX and X deficiency: a rare complication of primary amyloidosis; case report and review of the literature. Clin Lymphoma Myeloma Leuk 2014;14(3):e81–6.

58. McPherson RA, Onstad JW, Ugoretz RJ, et al. Coagulopathy in amyloidosis: combined deficiency of factors IX and X. Am J Hematol 1977;3:225–35.

59. Gertz MA, Lacy MQ, Dispenzieri A. Amyloidosis: recognition, confirmation, prognosis, and therapy. Mayo Clin Proc 1999;74(5):490–4.

60. Boggio L, Green D. Recombinant human factor VIIa in the management of amyloid-associated factor X deficiency. Br J Haematol 2001;112(4):1074–5.

61. Thompson CA, Kyle R, Gertz M, et al. Systemic AL amyloidosis with acquired factor X deficiency: a study of perioperative bleeding risk and treatment outcomes in 60 patients. Am J Hematol 2010;85(3):171–3.

62. Takabe K, Holman PR, Herbst KD, et al. Successful perioperative management of factor X deficiency associated with primary amyloidosis. J Gastrointest Surg 2004;8(3):358–62.

63. Veneri D, Giuffrida AC, Bonalumi A, et al. Use of prothrombin complex concentrate for prophylaxis of bleeding in acquired factor X deficiency associated with light-chain amyloidosis. Blood Transfus 2016;14(6):585–6.

64. Litvak A, Kumar A, Wong RJ, et al. Successful perioperative use of prothrombin complex concentrate in the treatment of acquired factor X deficiency in the setting of systemic light-chain (AL) amyloidosis. Am J Hematol 2014;89(12): 1153–4.

65. Mahmood S, Blundell J, Drebes A, et al. Utility of factor X concentrate for the treatment of acquired factor X deficiency in systemic light-chain amyloidosis. Blood 2014;123(18):2899–900.

66. Greipp PR, Kyle RA, Bowie EJ. Factor X deficiency in primary amyloidosis: resolution after splenectomy. N Engl J Med 1979;301(19):1050–1.

67. Rosenstein ED, Itzkowitz SH, Penziner AS, et al. Resolution of factor X deficiency in primary amyloidosis following splenectomy. Arch Intern Med 1983;143(3): 597–9.

68. Bohrer H, Waldherr R, Martin E, et al. Splenectomy in an uraemic patient with acquired factor X deficiency due to AL amyloidosis. Nephrol Dial Transplant 1998; 13(1):190–3.
69. Prokaeva T, Spencer B, Kaut M, et al. Soft tissue, joint, and bone manifestations of AL amyloidosis: clinical presentation, molecular features, and survival. Arthritis Rheum 2007;56(11):3858–68.
70. Muchtar E, Derudas D, Mauermann M, et al. Systemic immunoglobulin light chain amyloidosis–associated myopathy: presentation, diagnostic pitfalls, and outcome. Mayo Clin Proc 2016;91(10):1354–61.
71. Muchtar E, Dean DS, Dispenzieri A, et al. Prevalence and predictors of thyroid functional abnormalities in newly diagnosed AL amyloidosis. J Intern Med 2017;281(6):611–9.
72. Rich MW. Hypothyroidism in association with systemic amyloidosis. Head Neck 1995;17(4):343–5.
73. Myssiorek D, Alvi A, Bhuiya T. Primary salivary gland amyloidosis causing sicca syndrome. Ann Otol Rhinol Laryngol 1992;101(6):487–90.
74. Al-Hashimi I, Drinnan AJ, Uthman AA, et al. Oral amyloidosis: two unusual case presentations. Oral Surg Oral Med Oral Pathol 1987;63(5):586–91.
75. Jacobs P, Sellars S, King HS. Massive macroglossia, amyloidosis and myeloma. Postgrad Med J 1988;64(755):696–8.
76. Eder L, Bitterman H. Amyloid Purpura. N Engl J Med 2007;356(23):2406.
77. Westermark P. Bullous amyloidosis. Arch Dermatol 1981;117(12):782.
78. Lousada I, Comenzo RL, Landau H, et al. Light chain amyloidosis: patient experience survey from the amyloidosis research consortium. Adv Ther 2015;32(10): 920–8.
79. Bayliss M, McCausland KL, Guthrie SD, et al. The burden of amyloid light chain amyloidosis on health-related quality of life. Orphanet J Rare Dis 2017;12(1):15.
80. Lin HM, Seldin D, Hui AM, et al. The patient's perspective on the symptom and everyday life impact of AL amyloidosis. Amyloid 2015;22(4):244–51.
81. Mathieson CM, Stam HJ. Renegotiating identity: cancer narratives. Sociol Health Illn 1995;17(3):283–306.

The Impact of AL Amyloidosis
The Patient Experience

Isabelle Lousada, MA[a],*, Mackenzie Boedicker[b,1]

KEYWORDS

- Amyloidosis • Patient • Voices • Perspective • Experience

KEY POINTS

- There are no Food and Drug Administration–approved therapies for AL amyloidosis. Patients benefit from treatments developed for other plasma cell diseases. Because of the multisystemic nature of the disease patients may experience significant side effects from treatments.
- The heterogeneity of disease presentation and nonspecific symptoms pose significant challenges in obtaining an accurate and timely diagnosis, leading to a long road to diagnosis and high burden of disease for many patients.
- Quality of life of patients with AL amyloidosis is significantly affected by treatment as well as disease. With an increase in expected survival, there is a great unmet need to address quality as well as length of life.

INTRODUCTION

"A great patient experience connects clinical excellence with outcomes. It connects efficiency, quality, behaviors, and mission with caregiver experience and engagement. The patient experience relies on teamwork, communication, shared decision making, empathy, compassion, and human connection. It is also influenced by dignity, respect and humanistic values, as well as the ability and willingness of clinicians to relate to their patients as people, not as a medical condition or a room number." wrote Christy Dempsey on her experience as a nurse of more than 30 years, a breast cancer survivor, and family member of a critically injured police officer.

In years past, the overwhelming urgency has been increasing the short life expectancy of patients with AL amyloidosis. Lack of physician awareness, driven in part by the rarity of the disease, led to a significant number of patients having advanced cardiac disease at the time of diagnosis, and the resulting drop in the Kaplan-Meier curve was for most precipitous.

[a] Amyloidosis Research Consortium, 320 Nevada Street, Suite 210, Newton, MA 02460, USA;
[b] Mackenzie's Mission, Great Falls, Virginia
[1] Present address: 11602 Meadow Ridge Lane, Great Falls, VA 22066.
* Corresponding author.
E-mail address: ilousada@arci.org

Hematol Oncol Clin N Am 34 (2020) 1193–1203
https://doi.org/10.1016/j.hoc.2020.08.003
0889-8588/20/© 2020 Elsevier Inc. All rights reserved.

hemonc.theclinics.com

In the absence of approved therapies for AL amyloidosis, physicians use off-label multiple myeloma therapies that target the abnormal plasma cells responsible for the production of the light chain precursor proteins without consideration for the underlying organ dysfunction in the patient. Thus, these treatments can be associated with significant adverse events, and patients often die before experiencing benefit from them.[1] Recent advances in the myeloma treatment landscape have seen a significant increase in life expectancy in AL amyloidosis for those that survive long enough to gain some benefit from these treatments. The heterogeneous clinical phenotypes of AL amyloidosis, including cardiovascular, renal, neurologic, and gastrointestinal system manifestations, contribute to morbidity and/or mortality. Depending on systems involved, prescribed course, and response to treatment, patients' experiences vary widely as does their quality of life.

Greg's Story

Athlete's Heart. That's what doctors told Greg when he was unable to climb a flight of stairs without pausing to catch his breath. An Olympic medalist and world-record-holding hurdler, Greg's body, was a fine-honed instrument, and despite having the heart of a champion, athlete's heart was a diagnosis that nearly cost him his life.

Symptoms started for Greg 3 years before he was finally correctly diagnosed, a delay that could have been fatal. At first, shortness of breath would affect his workouts. Then, he reported losing muscle and body mass and getting weaker as he lifted weights.

As time went on, Greg got progressively worse. He went from being able to run 6 miles comfortably to not being able to run, from playing basketball to no longer being able to shoot hoops. All of this strengthened his belief that this was, in fact, not athletes' heart and drove him to seek more answers. A second opinion revealed nothing new and confirmed the diagnosis of athlete's heart.

Greg's symptoms continued to progress and affect all aspects of his daily life. When Greg could no longer climb a flight of stairs, he decided to see as many doctors as it would take to find the cause of his rapidly failing health. Three years from the onset of symptoms, and after consulting multiple physicians, Greg was given the diagnosis of multiple myeloma by a cardiologist, who then went on to perform further tests before concluding it was AL amyloidosis.

> Amyloidosis is a very mind-boggling disease because first of all, I've never heard of it, so I went online... the very first thing I read was that amyloidosis is a death sentence... I didn't know what to do from there, didn't know where to go, didn't know what the next steps were, so I called the doctor, and we talked for a minute. He calmed me down and said, no, it is not a death sentence.

Greg underwent a stem cell transplant, and the adverse side effects of the treatment were short-lived. Greg went into full remission and was able to return to work within a short period of time. Despite the success of the treatment, Greg's fatigue and cardiac symptoms persisted and progressed. On several occasions, he passed out and was injured by the falls. Two years after his initial stem cell transplant, Greg was informed that he would need a heart transplant.

Greg is now 2 months post heart transplant, doing well, and regaining his strength. But the financial burden follows him. Between the stem cell and heart transplants, his medical bills are high, but they do not stop there. Frequent follow-ups are critical to maintaining his health and continue to contribute to the financial burden of his medical care.

JOURNEY TO DIAGNOSIS

Clinical presentation of AL amyloidosis can vary widely and depends on the extent and number of organs affected. Initial symptoms at onset are often nonspecific (eg, weight loss, fatigue) and consequently accurate, and early diagnosis is challenging. As the disease progresses, symptoms reflect the organ dysfunction due to amyloid, most commonly the heart and the kidneys.[2]

For many patients, the onset of symptoms is slow and often initially attributed to less serious conditions or even mental health. Some patients describe "knowing something was wrong" but are unable to get their health care provider to look further. Before diagnosis, patients reported multiple symptoms. In a community-based AL amyloidosis patient survey, 32 different symptoms were reported by at least one patient; the most commonly reported symptoms were fatigue, dizziness on standing, feelings of fullness in the stomach when not full, shortness of breath, edema, numbness, cognition problems, pain, tingling or burning in limbs, and sleep problems[3] (**Fig. 1**).

In a patient survey conducted by the Amyloidosis Research Consortium, one-third of patients reported experiencing carpal tunnel syndrome (45 [32.8%]). For 32 (71.1%) of those patients, their carpal tunnel diagnosis preceded their AL amyloidosis diagnosis by more than 2 years. This should be considered an early, red flag symptom of systemic amyloidosis.[4]

Many AL amyloidosis patients exhibit real tenacity in pursuing an accurate diagnosis, seeing multiple specialists as their symptoms progress. Patients consult a broad spectrum of specialists before diagnosis dependent on organ involvement. These include primary care physicians, cardiologists, hematologists, nephrologists, gastroenterologists, pulmonologists, and others (**Fig. 2**).

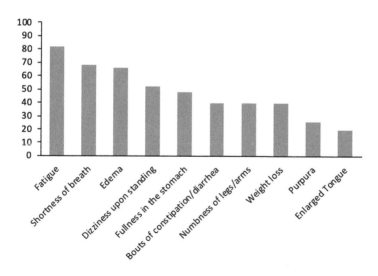

Respondents, % (341 total responses)

Fig. 1. Prevalence of initial symptoms. (*Adapted from* McCausland KL et al.: Health-Related Quality of Life in Patients with AL Amyloidosis: Qualitative Interviews with Physicians and Patients. December 2015. Blood 126(23):4525-4525; with permission.)

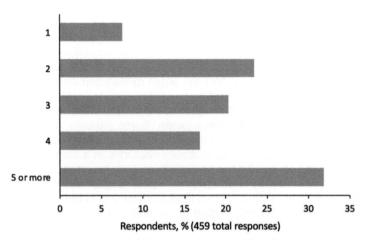

Fig. 2. Number of physicians seen before establishment of diagnosis. (*From* Amyloidosis Research Consortium: The Voice of the Patient. A report from the Amyloidosis Research Consortium, June 2016.)

The challenge of accurate and timely diagnosis of AL amyloidosis was highlighted in a patient-focused survey conducted by the Amyloidosis Research Consortium, which examined the patient journey to diagnosis and treatment (**Fig. 3**).

- Most patients (63%) experience delays in diagnosis of greater than or equal to 6 months.
- 31.8% of respondents in the survey visited 5 or more different physicians before receiving a correct diagnosis.
- Hematologists/oncologists were most likely (34.1%) to make a correct diagnosis; however, for the 443 patients reporting missed diagnosis at one or more

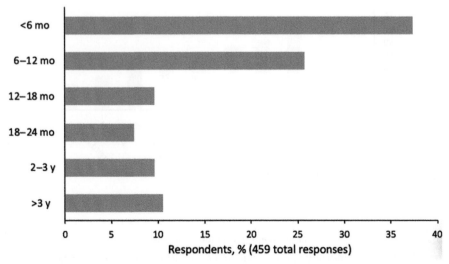

Fig. 3. Time from initial symptoms to diagnosis. (*From* Amyloidosis Research Consortium: The Voice of the Patient. A report from the Amyloidosis Research Consortium, June 2016.)

physician visits, 223 hematologists and 220 cardiologists did not diagnose the condition accurately.

- Patients with cardiac involvement may experience more substantial delays in diagnosis.[1]

With the first Food and Drug Administration (FDA)-approved treatments for ATTR amyloidosis, awareness of all types of amyloidosis has grown significantly among physicians; however, there are still significant challenges in establishing an accurate and timely diagnosis. Delays in diagnosis may lead to irreparable organ damage and are emotionally taxing for patients and caregivers. Nearly all patients who received misdiagnoses (83.3%; n = 50/60) reported undergoing treatment of their misdiagnosed condition, including beta-blockers, calcium channel blockers, or angiotensin-converting enzyme inhibitors, which may contribute to early mortality and worsening of symptoms.[4]

Patients describe the emotional impact of diagnosis, which often includes experiencing fear, anxiety, and depression. Patients also expressed relief at receiving the ultimate diagnosis because of the anxiety and uncertainty they felt beforehand.

PATIENT-FOCUSED DRUG DEVELOPMENT

In 2012, the US FDA established the Patient-Focused Drug Development (PFDD) initiative to more systematically obtain the patient perspective on specific diseases and their currently available treatments. People living with a condition are uniquely positioned to inform the understanding of the therapeutic context for drug development and evaluation. The format is designed to engage patients and elicit their perspectives on 2 topic areas: the most significant symptoms of their condition and the impact of the disease on daily life and their current approaches to treatment.

In 2015 the Amyloidosis Research Consortium held the first externally led PFDD meeting, thus establishing a pathway for foundations and patient advocates in other disease areas to follow suit. What follows are some findings from that meeting, which were shared with the FDA in the form of a Voice of the Patient Report.[5]

This forum provided unique and in-depth insights into patient experiences with AL amyloidosis from diagnosis through treatments, relapse, and remission, as well as participation in clinical trials. As treatment choices increase, the importance of understanding the patient perspective is critical to enhancing shared decision-making whereby "the physician and the patient make health-related decisions collaboratively, based on both the best available evidence and the patient's values, beliefs, and preferences…. Patients and their physicians can exchange information, weigh risks and benefits, and arrive at a therapeutic choice together, aligning care with goals, wishes, and values." says Brad Bott, MBA, CCRP, Director, Oncology Clinical Program, Intermountain Healthcare.[6]

MEETING OVERVIEW

Patients, caretakers, and other patient representatives shared their experiences with amyloidosis and the available treatments, with the FDA. The meeting focused on (1) disease symptoms and the daily impact that mattered the most to patients, (2) patient perspectives on current approaches to treatment, and (3) clinical trial participation. After the meeting, attendees were given a set of follow-up questions on these same topics to collect further information on specific areas that they deemed essential but that were not sufficiently discussed during the day.

Approximately 69 patients (46 patients with AL amyloidosis and 23 with ATTR amyloidosis) and 56 caregivers or family members (43 AL and 13 ATTR caregivers) attended the meeting; several patient advocates were also present. Using the audience response system, a total of 88 patients at the meeting answered questions. Patients in attendance represented a broad spectrum of experiences across the disease. Most of the patients aged between 51 and 70 years, but the age range of patients was from the late 20s to older than 70 years. The disease was in remission in 47% of patients and progressing in 37% of patients.

Patients spoke to a wide variety of experiences that reflect the heterogeneous nature of the disease, varied therapeutic approaches, treatment responses, and the impact on their quality of life.

Karen's Story

"I'm the patient that needs the new treatments and needs them faster. I need them very soon." These are the words Karen softly spoke at the Amyloidosis Patient Focused Drug Development meeting with the FDA in 2015.

Karen was diagnosed with AL amyloidosis in 2014 at the age of 54 years, with significant organ involvement in her heart and kidneys. Within the first year, Karen had to undergo 3 different regimens of treatment to reduce the plasma cell burden. Over the years, Karen has dealt repeatedly with the challenges of managing long and complex courses of treatment, while attempting to maintain her quality of life, as she battles repeated relapses in remission.

Karen describes herself as being completely incapacitated by her AL amyloidosis. She used to be an athlete—doing some form of physical exercise or sport every day—but since being diagnosed, she has struggled to even walk for exercise. Karen describes how it is not just her body that is struggling but it is also her mind. "My brain is fuzzy, I play solitaire now, not as a game, but as brain training to try to keep my brain functioning and understanding and processing, which has made it impossible to return to my work in accounting." During her first year after diagnosis, Karen had more than 122 medical appointments, tests, and procedures; as she describes it, "Amyloidosis is my life." She is unable to take part in family gatherings, "I am either too tired or too sick."

Karen suffers from severe fatigue, shortness of breath, muscle wasting, and weight loss, as well as neuropathy in her limbs; the treatments exacerbate most of these. "My biggest worry… is managing the side effects of the disease and the chemo because often times I can't tell the difference. I don't know if the chemotherapy is making me sick or the disease, and after this 3-month vacation [from treatment], I can kind of tell the chemotherapy has been rough." The anxiety was palpable as Karen contemplated starting another round of treatment, knowing there were few options left for her.

It is clear that this disease has had and continues to have a devastating impact on Karen. The road ahead for treatment looks bleak. She is not eligible for a stem cell transplant because her doctors fear she would not survive the procedure due to her advanced heart failure. But she is not eligible for a heart transplant because her amyloidosis severely involves her kidneys.

Now, her chemotherapy is critical to keeping her alive, making pausing treatment to join and participate in a clinical trial, out of the question. So that leaves her with few choices. "I've already blown through three different therapies. I'm down to some of the worst ones that I have to start now because that's all I have left."

MOST SIGNIFICANT SYMPTOMS OF AL AMYLOIDOSIS

Patients and caregivers described the substantial array of symptoms experienced by patients with AL amyloidosis. Several key themes emerged throughout the day.

Weakness and Fatigue

Fatigue was the most commonly mentioned symptom. Many patients described suffering from extreme weakness and fatigue that prevented their participation in daily activities. *"I am shackled by… a disease that leaves me fatigued and unable to do so many of the things that I enjoy."*

Weight Loss and Muscle Wasting

Weight loss and muscle wasting can result from several facets of the disease and its treatment. Patients with AL amyloidosis may experience macroglossia (enlarged tongue) as a result of amyloid deposition in their tongues, which can affect eating. In addition, early satiety is a symptom experienced by many patients both before and after treatment, and nausea is often associated with treatment.

Peripheral and Autonomic Neuropathy

Neuropathy, both peripheral and autonomic, is a significant symptom of amyloidosis. Often a part of patients' initial clinical presentation, neuropathy can manifest as cardiac arrhythmias and orthostatic hypotension, gastrointestinal problems including intractable diarrhea, carpal tunnel syndrome symptoms, and lower limb neuropathic pain. Autonomic neuropathy has a significant impact on patients.

Heart/Cardiac Involvement

Impaired heart function caused by amyloid deposition can lead to symptoms that include congestive heart failure, severe edema, and shortness of breath. Patients described the impact that cardiac involvement has had on them: "Sadly, I can't run anymore" and "I can't play any longer because my heart can't handle it." Patients shared how cardiac impairment has affected and limited their treatment options: *"Because of my cardiac involvement, it was determined I was not healthy enough to withstand a stem cell transplant."*

SYMPTOMS OF DISEASE VERSUS SIDE EFFECTS OF TREATMENT

Current off-label treatments are not well tolerated. Patients often find it difficult to distinguish between symptoms of the disease and the side effects of treatments. Many patients shared similar experiences, reporting that several of their most debilitating daily symptoms, both in the short term and long term, were primarily a result of treatment rather than the underlying symptoms of their disease. This can affect the perceived benefit of treatment, as well as their ability to complete the prescribed course of treatment. *"I thought I was dying from the disease, but when I stopped the chemo, I started feeling better."*

Common side effects to treatment include:

- Constant diarrhea
- Nausea
- Fatigue
- Difficulty sleeping particularly while taking steroids
- Neuropathy, with severe pain
- Cognitive impairment, can be short term, patients refer to this as "chemo brain"

BURDEN OF DISEASE AND IMPACT ON DAILY LIFE

Patients described a significant burden of AL amyloidosis and treatment on their day-to-day functioning, including affecting their ability to perform activities at work and home and on their mental, emotional, and physical health. Many of these ill effects persisted long after treatment. *"Managing amyloidosis takes a significant amount of time in my daily life."*

Patients' daily activities were affected, including their ability to care for themselves and family members. Patients also described being unable to participate in family gatherings either due to sickness or fatigue. Many physically active patients have had to modify their mode of exercise significantly; some runners described finding walking challenging (**Fig. 4**).

Physical and psychological impairments can also lead to an inability to work. The burden of disease, immunosuppression from treatments, the intensity of doctor visits, and impact on health from both the disease and treatments mean for many patients they can no longer work. Patients describe experiencing anxiety often relating to concerns about need for further treatment.

FINANCIAL CONCERNS

Because of the rarity of AL amyloidosis, patients experience significant challenges both in finding qualified and experienced local providers, in addition to dealing with the complex financial and organizational burden of medical bills and insurance claims. Off-label treatments can cause significant problems for patients dealing with insurance companies for reimbursement and often require multiple insurance appeals. In addition, co-pays and personal expenses associated with traveling to amyloidosis specialty centers for treatments or to participate in clinical trials were identified as a cause for creating significant financial hardships. Financial burden substantially affects treatment decisions for many patients. The financial burden also falls on caregivers; some have had to remain in work or seek employment that has health care benefits to cover treatment costs. *"One of the hardest aspects of this disease is constant uncertainly of treatment-related finances and insurance issues. This is so emotionally taxing; it is like having another disease."*

PSYCHOLOGICAL IMPACT

An underappreciated aspect of AL amyloidosis is the psychological impact it has on both patients and family members from the constant emotional stress resulting from diagnosis. Even with treatment responses, most of the patients experience persistent organ dysfunction and treatment-related side effects and consequently concern about their future. Feeling alone in your disease is common, and support groups and patient

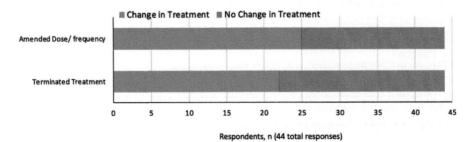

Fig. 4. Patients reporting treatment tolerability. (*From* Amyloidosis Research Consortium: The Voice of the Patient. A report from the Amyloidosis Research Consortium, June 2016.)

foundations can play a role in supporting patients. *"I was recently diagnosed with post-traumatic stress syndrome because of all I went through getting diagnosed..."*

Mackenzie's Story

Mackenzie, a 23-year-old woman at the time of diagnosis, is a rare example of asymptomatic disease presentation in the world of amyloidosis. Her path to diagnosis, treatment, and experience with amyloidosis is very different from the rest. The initial presentation of her disease seemed benign, merely a drop of blood in her saliva. Mackenzie wanted to be a medical professional and knew this was unusual and should be investigated further. A look in the back of her mouth revealed a small lump, which only a week later, was dismissed by a local Ear, Nose, and Throat (ENT) physician as seasonal allergies. Remaining asymptomatic, this answer satisfied her for roughly 12 months before seeking a second opinion from a second ENT. Six months later, a biopsy of the throat lump revealed the presence of amyloid.

She was immediately referred to a hematologist under the suspicion of amyloidosis. Within a week of referral, a full blood workup revealed elevated light chains, and shortly thereafter, a bone marrow biopsy revealed high levels of plasma cells. With hesitation, the physician diagnosed her with amyloidosis. "It was shocking [his uncertainty]; I vividly remember asking him, 'So are we calling it? Do I have amyloidosis?'" With that, she was referred to a center of excellence to confirm the diagnosis and explore treatment options.

Within two weeks, she sat in the office of a highly respected amyloidosis specialist. It was all a whirlwind to her; what seemed to her as a benign throat lump became something that was life-altering. After pouring over the intensive diagnostic testing, with his hands in his hair, the specialist confirmed her worst fears. She had AL amyloidosis. It was a shock to everyone in the room that day. How could a 23-year-old with no organ involvement, have a systemic disease that is usually first diagnosed in people in their sixties? It did not seem possible, but the hardest question was to come—so, what do we do about it?

As a 23-year-old, feeling completely healthy, getting a diagnosis like this was impossible to comprehend. "It came down to trust and believing that the physician sitting across from you not only knows what they are doing but cares about you, and there was never a doubt in my mind that this was the physician for me." At that point, treatment options were presented: a conservative approach of waiting to see how the disease presents itself and begin treatment then or take an aggressive approach and try to eliminate the condition altogether. "We were in uncharted territory; he'd never seen a case like mine, and he made it very clear that whatever option we chose, it was if as if we were going in blind; we had no previous similar patients to go off of."

"Contemplating undergoing a stem cell transplant, a very aggressive treatment option, while feeling completely healthy, was the most difficult decision I'd ever made." But ultimately, her decision was made. She wanted to try to eliminate the disease altogether, as quickly as possible, and the only way to even begin to do so was a stem cell transplant. The next morning, she returned to inform the doctor of her decision, and her transplant was scheduled for two months later.

The treatment itself was grueling—fatigue, nausea, diarrhea, mucositis, loss of appetite, hair loss—but after five weeks, a bone marrow biopsy revealed she had achieved a complete response to therapy and was cleared to return home. "It was exciting for me, it felt like I could live life again without worrying about the disease, but in the back of my mind, I knew that anything was possible. No remission is guaranteed. I just had to live life in the moment." Life quickly returned to normal for Mackenzie, who returned to work full time, feeling great, roughly two months posttransplant.

The durability of the treatment was what surprised her the most. Just 25 months post transplant, her blood work revealed that her light chains had elevated outside the normal range for the first time since her transplant. She returned to her doctor for a full workup and began treatment with Revlimid to get things under control. Over the last several months on treatment, her light chains have remained relatively consistent, not quite back to normal levels, but very close. She continues to feel well while she pursues her dream of becoming a doctor.

> *Looking back, the biggest thing this whole experience has taught me is we still have so much to learn about this disease. No two patients, symptoms, presentations, treatments, or life after are the same. This presents a massive challenge to the medical community. One day, I hope to contribute to that growing base of knowledge.*

SUMMARY

The outlook for AL amyloidosis is improving, in part due to increasing awareness of amyloidosis resulting from the approval of novel treatments for ATTR amyloidosis. Still, more education is needed about "red flags" and common symptoms to expedite diagnosis.

Patients with AL amyloidosis are fragile, complex, and heterogeneous. The breadth of symptoms that patients experience, the burden of disease, as well as the complexities from side effects of treatments, reflect the need for a tailored approach to care.

The expanding treatment options for multiple myeloma used in AL amyloidosis off-label are leading to longer and better outcomes.

In the evolving patient-centered approach to care, the patient is part of the decision-making process. Both the patient and physician need to understand and address the benefits and risks of treatment choices, barriers that may stand in the way (be those physical, emotional, or financial), as well as patient goals of care, to make informed treatment decisions. Digital tools such as My Amyloidosis Pathfinder (see resources) can support and enhance patient/physician communication. Patient support groups (see resources for a comprehensive list) are a valuable resource particularly for patients with rare diseases such as amyloidosis, where patients can feel isolated and accurate; understandable information on their disease may be hard to come by.

DISCLOSURE

The authors have nothing to disclose.

REFERENCES

1. Lousada I, Comenzo R, Landau H, et al. Light chain amyloidosis: patient experience survey from the amyloidosis research consortium. Adv Ther 2015;32(10): 920–8.
2. Merlini G, Wechalekar AD, Palladini G. Systemic light chain amyloidosis: an update for treating physicians. Blood 2013;121:5124–30.
3. McCausland KL, et al. Health-related quality of life in patients with AL amyloidosis: qualitative interviews with physicians and patients. Blood 2015;126(23):4525.

4. Lousada I, Maurer M, Guthrie S, et al. Amyloidosis research consortium cardiac amyloidosis survey: results from patients with AL amyloidosis and their caregivers. J Am Coll Cardiol 2018;71(Issue 11 Supplement). https://doi.org/10.1016/S0735-1097(18)31431-1.
5. Amyloidosis Research Consortium: The Voice of the Patient. A report from the Amyloidosis Research Consortium. June 2016.
6. Thompson G. The patient voice is key to value-based care. Pers Med Oncol 2018;8(7).

Future Perspectives

Angela Dispenzieri, MD[a],*, Giampaolo Merlini, MD[b]

KEYWORDS

- Systemic amyloidosis • Pathogenesis • Early diagnosis • Outcome measures
- Trial design

KEY POINTS

- Further research is necessary to improve our understanding of the structure and biophysics of immunoglobulin light chains and amyloid tropism, formation, and equilibrium.
- Late diagnosis in systemic AL amyloidosis is the biggest impediment to improve patient outcome. Increased awareness, appropriate use of biomarkers and imaging technologies are necessary to overcome this obstacle.
- Innovative trial designs, combined with updated measures of outcome, may accelerate the development of novel drugs and reduce the costs of trials, thus facilitating the access to more effective medicines.

Opportunities and challenges in the field of systemic amyloidosis can be grouped into 4 categories (**Table 1**). First, a deeper understanding of the pathogenesis of the disease is required. Second, a greater awareness of the disease, which will lead to an earlier diagnosis, is imperative. Third, end points for interventional trials are required to convey us to our fourth aspiration, novel therapies for patients with light chain (AL) amyloidosis.

DISEASE PATHOGENESIS

As described in articles elsewhere in this issue, AL amyloidosis is a condition in which clonal light chains both form nonbranching fibrils that deposit in tissues and directly are toxic to organs. The formation of amyloid is a complex process involving the immunoglobulin light chain, protein homeostasis network, extracellular chaperones and matrix components, metal ions, shear forces, and cells.[1] Although there has been considerable progress in the understanding of the disease, there is much to learn about the structure and biophysics of immunoglobulin light chains and about amyloid tropism, formation, and equilibrium.[2,3]

[a] Division of Hematology, Mayo Clinic, 200 First Street SW Rochester, MN 55905, USA;
[b] Amyloidosis Center, Foundation IRCCS Policlinico San Matteo, University of Pavia, Viale Golgi 19, Pavia 27100, Italy
* Corresponding author.
E-mail address: dispenzieri.angela@mayo.edu

Hematol Oncol Clin N Am 34 (2020) 1205–1214
https://doi.org/10.1016/j.hoc.2020.08.009
0889-8588/20/© 2020 Elsevier Inc. All rights reserved.

Table 1	
Opportunities for better outcomes for amyloidosis	
More science to understand pathogenesis	1. Biophysics of light chains and amyloid fibrils
	2. Tissue tropism and damage
	3. Amyloid proteome
	4. Tissue microenvironment
	5. Animal models
Earlier diagnosis	1. Awareness by cardiologists and internists via amyloid transthyretin awareness
	2. Glycosylation by MASS-FIX
	3. Light chain stability assays
	4. *C elegans* toxicity assay
	5. Imaging with small molecules
	6. Use of biomarkers of organ involvement
Trial design	1. Improve hematologic response end points
	2. Improve organ response end points
	3. Novel trial designs including remote monitoring
Novel therapies directed at plasma cells	1. Daratumumab
	2. Venetoclax
	3. BiTE, chimeric antigen receptor T cells, drug–antibody conjugates
Novel therapies directed at light chains and amyloid fibrils	1. Silencers
	2. Stabilizers
	3. Doxycycline
	4. Anti-amyloid antibodies (eg, Cael-001)

Destabilizing somatic mutations in the variable genes of light chains increase the propensity for light chains to aggregate.[4] A greater understanding (and a high-throughput mechanism for screening for) these biophysical properties could lead to earlier diagnosis and potential treatment strategies.[5,6] Akin to the beneficial effect of tafamadis in stabilizing transthyretin tetramers, thereby improving a composite end point of hospitalizations and death,[7] an immunoglobulin stabilizer might help patients with AL amyloidosis.[8]

The mechanisms leading to tissue tropism are not understood in AL amyloidosis. Although there are tendencies for certain immunoglobulin light chains to deposit in a particular organ like IGVL6-57 in the kidney, IGVL1-44 in the heart, and IGKV1-33 in the liver, these associations are imperfect.[9–11] If and whether other parts of the proteome direct the amyloidogenic light chain to a given organ is unknown.[12] The specific interactions between amyloid proteins and the tissue resident cells, and the ensuing proteotoxicity, may play a role in organ targeting and damage.

Ideally, a mammalian model, like a mouse model, would provide insight into amyloid formation and deposition, but such attempts have been without major success. There is a transgenic mouse model in which amyloid like substance can be found in the stomach,[13] but this is far from a true amyloid model. Subcutaneous injection of amyloid fibrils into mice has provided some insight into antibodies that facilitate amyloid removal.[14] Ex vivo systems using explanted human tissue have been informative, but are complex.[15,16] The *Caenorhabditis elegans*[2] and the zebrafish AL amyloidosis models[17,18] may prove to be helpful understand light chain toxicity and to test drugs that stabilize light chains and decrease cellular injury, but may fall short in terms of understanding fibril formation and deposition. Tissue culture models may also prove useful for similar hypotheses.[19–22] Such models may facilitate an understanding of light chain processing, organelle damage, apoptotic pathways, and cellular interactions.

EARLY RECOGNITION OF LIGHT CHAIN AMYLOIDOSIS

Late diagnosis in systemic AL amyloidosis is the biggest risk factor for poor outcomes. The majority of patients with AL amyloidosis present with chemosensitive clonal plasma cells. With modern therapy, a very good partial response or better is expected in nearly two-thirds of patients, assuming they live long enough to achieve it.[23,24] Over the years, patient and physician advocacy groups have tried to educate medical communities about the diagnosis with limited success. As recently as the early 2010s, the median time from symptoms to diagnosis was in the range of 9 to 12 months, and only 20% of diagnoses of amyloidosis were made by cardiologists despite the fact that 80% of AL patients have cardiac involvement (**Fig. 1**).[25]

AL amyloidosis patients will benefit from the increasing numbers of recognized cases of wild-type transthyretin amyloidosis, which is primarily a cardiac disease. Because wild-type transthyretin is found in approximately 3% of patients aged 75 years or older,[26] all cardiologists and internists will have patients with recognized amyloidosis in their practices. As long as a physician has amyloidosis as part of his or her differential diagnosis and the tools to distinguish AL from amyloid transthyretin, we predict that the time from symptoms to a diagnosis of AL amyloidosis will shorten and with that prognosis will improve dramatically. Rates of patients with Mayo 2012 stage IV disease and Mayo 2004 stage IIIb disease will be lower, and early mortality will decrease.[23,27]

Once the diagnosis of AL is considered, making the diagnosis of AL amyloidosis is typically not difficult. Congo red staining of a fat aspirate and a bone marrow biopsy

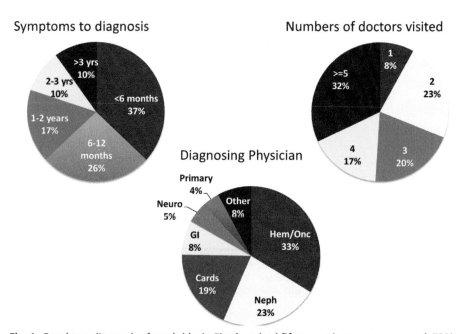

Fig. 1. Road to a diagnosis of amyloidosis. Five hundred fifteen patients were surveyed, 72% of whom had AL amyloidosis; the remainder had hereditary and wild-type transthyretin. Cards, cardiologist; GI, gastroenterologist; Hem/Onc, hematologist/oncologist; Neph, nephrologist; Neuro, neurologist. (*Data from* Lousada I, Comenzo RL, Landau H, Guthrie S, Merlini G. Light Chain Amyloidosis: Patient Experience Survey from the Amyloidosis Research Consortium. Adv Ther. 2015 Oct;32(10):920-8.)

will detect approximately 90% of cases.[28] The typing of the amyloid fibrils by mass spectrometry, immunogold, or immunohistochemistry is straightforward when done by experts to exclude other types of amyloid. For those other 10% to 15% of patients who have a monoclonal protein and symptoms or signs consistent with amyloidosis, a biopsy of the affected organ will typically be required to make the diagnosis.

Why some patients with small monoclonal proteins go on to develop amyloid and others do not has been a major puzzle. Currently, there are no readily available blood assays to diagnose AL amyloidosis. There are, however, some interesting assays that may be available in the not too distant future that measure light chain stability[5] and fibril recruitment.[6] These assays indicate a propensity to form amyloid; however, the diagnosis of amyloidosis requires evidence of organ involvement. This holds true also for the presence of glycosylated light chains on routine MASS-FIX that has been shown to be a potent risk factor for developing AL amyloidosis.[29,30] This finding is more notable for clonal kappa light chains than lambda light chains, and it can serve as a clue for a subset of patients otherwise thought to have monoclonal gammopathy of undetermined significance (MGUS), smoldering myeloma (SMM), or multiple myeloma with unusual symptoms. Furthermore, the restricted repertoire of Ig light chain variable region germline gene use, particularly in those with AL lambda type, may enable identification of AL-related genes expressed by the clones of patients with MGUS, SMM, or multiple myeloma, providing opportunities for early diagnosis of AL or risk of AL.[31] Amyloid imaging using small molecules like florbetapir, florbetaben[32–34] may also someday be able to differentiate an MGUS or SMM case from an early AL amyloidosis case. More research will be required to better understand the sensitivity and specificity of such imaging techniques. The use of sensitive biomarkers of organ involvement, NT-proBNP for heart and proteinuria for kidney, during the follow-up of MGUS and SMM, may allow early diagnosis of AL amyloidosis and trigger timely and optimal therapy.[35]

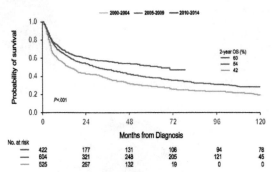

Fig. 2. Improved survival over time: overall survival (OS) for AL amyloidosis by period of diagnosis. (*From* Muchtar E, Gertz MA, Kumar SK, Lacy MQ, Dingli D, Buadi FK, et al. Improved outcomes for newly diagnosed AL amyloidosis between 2000 and 2014: cracking the glass ceiling of early death. Blood. 2017 Apr 13;129(15):2111-9.)

TOOLS FOR BETTER TRIAL DESIGN

Currently, there are no therapies approved by the US Food and Drug Administration (or the European Medicines Agency or other equivalents) for AL amyloidosis. Potential disincentives for pharmaceutical companies not choosing to engage heavily in this field are (1) the frailty of a large percentage of patients; (2) off-label adaption of drugs approved for multiple myeloma; (3) the complexity of the disease; and (4) the small market share.

AL amyloidosis investigators have dealt effectively with the frailty issue by using cardiac biomarkers to identify those patients likely to die in the first 6 months of therapy.[36,37] In most instances, these patients—about 15% to 20% of newly diagnosed patients—are excluded from interventional trials. The second disincentive is a mixed blessing. Investigators are gratified to have myeloma drugs available for patients with AL amyloidosis, but also realize that the absence of controlled trials in this space can lead to late recognition of unexpected toxicities[38–40] in this cohort as well as patchy access to these drugs for their patients.

The third disincentive, that is, the complexity of the disease, is multifaceted and complex in its own right. Both hematologic and organ response (and progression) are relevant in this disease.[41–44] One would think that hematologic response would be straight forward given the experience in multiple myeloma trials with this measure, but hematologic response in AL amyloidosis is more difficult in part due to the fact that one-half of patients—even at diagnosis—have a very low clonal plasma cell burden. Patients need to have sufficient levels of a given hematologic marker to allow for reproducible measurement of improvement. In addition, because the light chain is what drives the disease, clinicians are wary about allowing them to increase for fear of having organ progression driven by small amounts of monoclonal protein.[45,46] The immunoglobulin free light chain ratio is an unstable measure, yet it is part of the complete hematologic response criteria. This situation leaves us with problems along multiple fronts for trial management: trial eligibility (measurable) hematologic (and organ disease); measurement of hematologic (and organ) response; and perhaps, most important, measurement of hematologic (and organ) progression. Minimal residual disease measurement has not made its way into response criteria for patients with AL amyloidosis, but limited data would suggest that it is a good surrogate for progression, although less valuable for overall survival.[47–50] More granular organ response criteria and composite response end points are also works in progress.[44,51] These are among the issues that the amyloidosis community is working on in association with pharmaceutical companies, academia, patient associations, and the US Food and Drug Administration.[52]

The fourth disincentive, the fact that AL amyloidosis is a rare disease, makes accrual challenging owing to long distances to travel to treatment centers. Pharmaceutical companies help by paying for transportation and lodging, but even with these opportunities, travel can be physically difficult for frail patients and increased time away from work for those still employed is also a major challenge. Innovative adaptations for clinical trial patients during the coronavirus disease-19 pandemic may pave the way for future opportunities for patients with rare disease who would like to participate on clinical trials, like video follow-up visits and home infusions.[53,54]

NOVEL THERAPIES FOR LIGHT CHAIN AMYLOIDOSIS

There are 2 potential treatment pathways for patients with AL amyloidosis. The first exploits treatments that are highly effective against the plasma cells that produce the amyloidogenic light chains, the mainstay of AL amyloidosis therapy for nearly 50 years. As described elsewhere, corticosteroids, alkylators, proteasome inhibitors, and immune modulatory drugs have more than tripled the overall survival of patients with AL amyloidosis (**Fig. 2**).[23,24,55–57] Daratumumab has been an important addition to the armamentarium to treat plasma cell disorders in general, and AL amyloidosis specifically. Trials are ongoing to explore the best use of daratumumab in patients with AL amyloidosis.[58,59] The Andromeda Trial is an important phase III randomized such trial testing cyclophosphamide, bortezomib, and dexamethasone with or without daratumumab (NCT03201965).[60] Venetoclax has already been shown to be effective therapy in myeloma patients with up regulated BCL2 and or translocation t(11;14).[61] Case reports have demonstrated similar efficacy among patients with AL.[62] Venetoclax is especially appealing in patients with AL because nearly 50% of them harbor t(11;14).[63,64] Silencing RNAs have been a stunning addition to the treatment armamentarium for amyloid transthyretin amyloidosis.[65,66] Zhou and colleagues[67] have developed a siRNA that reduces lambda light chain production and causes terminal endoplasmic reticulum stress. Light chain stabilizers are also being explored in vitro. In addition, other immunotherapies that are showing promise in multiple myeloma clinical trials will hopefully be offered to patients with AL amyloidosis, including chimeric antigen receptor T cells, bispecific T-cell engager antibodies, and antibody–drug conjugates.[68]

Finally, amyloid-directed therapy is an appealing opportunity. The antibiotic doxycycline has been shown to interfere with amyloid fibril formation[13] and in 2 uncontrolled studies demonstrated improved survival.[69,70] Two prospective studies are on-going (NCT02207556; NCT03474458) to assess the value of this intervention. The NEOD001 compound seemed to be quite promising,[71] but a phase III trial failed to meet its end points (NCT03474458). There is controversy as to whether this failure was related to the compound itself or to the trial design. The GSK drug proved to be too toxic. Another amyloid directed monoclonal antibody is CAEL-101.[72] Phase III trials are to begin in 2020.

The future of AL amyloidosis is bright. If 3 drugs to treat amyloid transthyretin amyloidosis could be approved by the US Food and Drug Administration in 2018 and 2019,[7,65,66] the same should be achievable for patients with AL amyloidosis.

DISCLOSURE

A. Dispenzieri - Trial support: Takeda, Celgene, Pfizer, Alnylam, Caelum. Consultancy: Akcea, Janssen, Prothena. G. Merlini has nothing to disclosure.

FUNDING

G. Merlini is supported by grants from the Italian Ministry of Health (Ricerca Finalizzata, grant RF-2013-02355259 and GR-2018-12368387), the CARIPLO Foundation (grant 2013-0964 and 2018-0257), the Amyloidosis Foundation, the "Associazione Italiana per la Ricerca sul Cancro–Special Program Molecular Clinical Oncology 5 per mille" (grant 9965) and by an Accelerator Award from the Cancer Research UK, the Fundación Científica – Asociación Española Contra el Cáncer and the Associazione Italiana Ricerca sul Cancro.

REFERENCES

1. Merlini G. AL amyloidosis: from molecular mechanisms to targeted therapies. Hematology Am Soc Hematol Educ Program 2017;2017(1):1–12.
2. Diomede L, Rognoni P, Lavatelli F, et al. A Caenorhabditis elegans-based assay recognizes immunoglobulin light chains causing heart amyloidosis. Blood 2014; 123(23):3543–52.
3. Marin-Argany M, Lin Y, Misra P, et al. Cell damage in light chain amyloidosis: fibril internalization, toxicity and cell-mediated seeding. J Biol Chem 2016;291(38): 19813–25.

4. Misra P, Blancas-Mejia LM, Ramirez-Alvarado M. Mechanistic insights into the early events in the aggregation of immunoglobulin light chains. Biochemistry 2019;58(29):3155–68.

5. Rennella E, Morgan GJ, Kelly JW, et al. Role of domain interactions in the aggregation of full-length immunoglobulin light chains. Proc Natl Acad Sci U S A 2019; 116(3):854–63.

6. Martin EB, Williams A, Wooliver C, et al. Differential recruitment efficacy of patient-derived amyloidogenic and myeloma light chain proteins by synthetic fibrils-A metric for predicting amyloid propensity. PLoS One 2017;12(3):e0174152.

7. Maurer MS, Schwartz JH, Gundapaneni B, et al. Tatamidis Treatment for Patients with Transthyretin Amyloid Cardiomyopathy. N Engl J Med 2018;379(11): 1007–16.

8. Morgan GJ, Yan NL, Mortenson DE, et al. Stabilization of amyloidogenic immunoglobulin light chains by small molecules. Proc Natl Acad Sci U S A 2019;116(17): 8360–9.

9. Kourelis TV, Dasari S, Theis JD, et al. Clarifying immunoglobulin gene usage in systemic and localized immunoglobulin light-chain amyloidosis by mass spectrometry. Blood 2017;129(3):299–306.

10. Perfetti V, Palladini G, Casarini S, et al. The repertoire of lambda light chains causing predominant amyloid heart involvement and identification of a preferentially involved germline gene, IGLV1-44. Blood 2012;119(1):144–50.

11. Comenzo RL, Zhang Y, Martinez C, et al. The tropism of organ involvement in primary systemic amyloidosis: contributions of Ig V(L) germ line gene use and clonal plasma cell burden. Blood 2001;98(3):714–20.

12. Kourelis T, Dasari S, Fayyaz AU, et al. A Proteomic Atlas of Cardiac Amyloidosis. Blood 2019;134:1790.

13. Ward JE, Ren R, Toraldo G, et al. Doxycycline reduces fibril formation in a transgenic mouse model of AL amyloidosis. Blood 2011;118(25):6610–7.

14. Wall JS, Kennel SJ, Paulus M, et al. Radioimaging of light chain amyloid with a fibril-reactive monoclonal antibody. J Nucl Med 2006;47(12):2016–24.

15. Vora M, Kevil CG, Herrera GA. Contribution of human smooth muscle cells to amyloid angiopathy in AL (light-chain) amyloidosis. Ultrastruct Pathol 2017;41(5): 358–68.

16. Teng J, Turbat-Herrera EA, Herrera GA. Extrusion of amyloid fibrils to the extracellular space in experimental mesangial AL-amyloidosis: transmission and scanning electron microscopy studies and correlation with renal biopsy observations. Ultrastruct Pathol 2014;38(2):104–15.

17. Mishra S, Guan J, Plovie E, et al. Human amyloidogenic light chain proteins result in cardiac dysfunction, cell death, and early mortality in zebrafish. Am J Physiol Heart Circ Physiol 2013;305(1):H95–103.

18. Mishra S, Joshi S, Ward JE, et al. Zebrafish model of amyloid light chain cardiotoxicity: regeneration versus degeneration. Am J Physiol Heart Circ Physiol 2019; 316(5):H1158–66.

19. Levinson RT, Olatoye OO, Randles EG, et al. Role of mutations in the cellular internalization of amyloidogenic light chains into cardiomyocytes. Sci Rep 2013;3: 1278.

20. Imperlini E, Gnecchi M, Rognoni P, et al. Proteotoxicity in cardiac amyloidosis: amyloidogenic light chains affect the levels of intracellular proteins in human heart cells. Sci Rep 2017;7(1):15661.

21. Monis GF, Schultz C, Ren R, et al. Role of endocytic inhibitory drugs on internalization of amyloidogenic light chains by cardiac fibroblasts. Am J Pathol 2006; 169(6):1939–52.

22. Lin Y, Marin-Argany M, Dick CJ, et al. Mesenchymal stromal cells protect human cardiomyocytes from amyloid fibril damage. Cytotherapy 2017;19(12):1426–37.

23. Muchtar E, Gertz MA, Kumar SK, et al. Improved outcomes for newly diagnosed AL amyloidosis between 2000 and 2014: cracking the glass ceiling of early death. Blood 2017;129(15):2111–9.

24. Manwani R, Cohen O, Sharpley F, et al. A prospective observational study of 915 patients with systemic AL amyloidosis treated with upfront bortezomib. Blood 2019;134(25):2271–80.

25. Lousada I, Comenzo RL, Landau H, et al. Light chain amyloidosis: patient experience survey from the amyloidosis research consortium. Adv Ther 2015;32(10): 920–8.

26. Mohamed-Salem L, Santos-Mateo JJ, Sanchez-Serna J, et al. Prevalence of wild type ATTR assessed as myocardial uptake in bone scan in the elderly population. Int J Cardiol 2018;270:192–6.

27. Manwani R, Foard D, Mahmood S, et al. Rapid hematologic responses improve outcomes in patients with very advanced (stage IIIb) cardiac immunoglobulin light chain amyloidosis. Haematologica 2018;103(4):e165–8.

28. Gertz MA. Immunoglobulin light chain amyloidosis: 2020 update on diagnosis, prognosis, and treatment. Am J Hematol 2020;95(7):848–60.

29. Milani P, Murray DL, Barnidge DR, et al. The utility of MASS-FIX to detect and monitor monoclonal proteins in the clinic. Am J Hematol 2017;92(8):772–9.

30. Kumar S, Murray D, Dasari S, et al. Assay to rapidly screen for immunoglobulin light chain glycosylation: a potential path to earlier AL diagnosis for a subset of patients. Leukemia 2019;33(1):254–7.

31. Zhou P, Kugelmass A, Toskic D, et al. Seeking light-chain amyloidosis very early: the SAVE trial—identifying clonal lambda light chain genes in patients with MGUS or smoldering multiple myeloma. J Clin Oncol 2019;37(15_suppl):8010.

32. Ehman EC, El-Sady MS, Kijewski MF, et al. Early detection of multiorgan light chain (AL) Amyloidosis by Whole Body (18)F-florbetapir PET/CT. J Nucl Med 2019;60(9):1234–9.

33. Kircher M, Ihne S, Brumberg J, et al. Detection of cardiac amyloidosis with (18)F-Florbetaben-PET/CT in comparison to echocardiography, cardiac MRI and DPD-scintigraphy. Eur J Nucl Med Mol Imaging 2019;46(7):1407–16.

34. Wall JS, Martin EB, Richey T, et al. Preclinical validation of the heparin-reactive peptide p5+14 as a molecular imaging agent for visceral amyloidosis. Molecules 2015;20(5):7657–82.

35. Palladini G, Basset M, Milani P, et al. Biomarker-based screening of organ dysfunction in patients with MGUS allows early diagnosis of AL amyloidosis. Blood 2017;130:1670 [abstract].

36. Dispenzieri A, Gertz MA, Kyle RA, et al. Serum cardiac troponins and N-terminal pro-brain natriuretic peptide: a staging system for primary systemic amyloidosis. J Clin Oncol 2004;22(18):3751–7.

37. Wechalekar AD, Schonland SO, Kastritis E, et al. A European collaborative study of treatment outcomes in 346 patients with cardiac stage III AL amyloidosis. Blood 2013;121(17):3420–7.

38. Dispenzieri A, Dingli D, Kumar SK, et al. Discordance between serum cardiac biomarker and immunoglobulin-free light-chain response in patients with

immunoglobulin light-chain amyloidosis treated with immune modulatory drugs. Am J Hematol 2010;85(10):757–9.

39. Batts ED, Sanchorawala V, Hegerfeldt Y, et al. Azotemia associated with use of lenalidomide in plasma cell dyscrasias. Leuk Lymphoma 2008;49(6):1108–15.

40. Palladini G, Perfetti V, Perlini S, et al. The combination of thalidomide and intermediate-dose dexamethasone is an effective but toxic treatment for patients with primary amyloidosis (AL). Blood 2005;105(7):2949–51.

41. Gertz MA, Comenzo R, Falk RH, et al. Definition of organ involvement and treatment response in immunoglobulin light chain amyloidosis (AL): a consensus opinion from the 10th International Symposium on Amyloid and Amyloidosis, Tours, France, 18-22 April 2004. Am J Hematol 2005;79(4):319–28.

42. Palladini G, Dispenzieri A, Gertz MA, et al. New criteria for response to treatment in immunoglobulin light chain amyloidosis based on free light chain measurement and cardiac biomarkers: impact on survival outcomes. J Clin Oncol 2012;30(36): 4541–9.

43. Comenzo RL, Reece D, Palladini G, et al. Consensus guidelines for the conduct and reporting of clinical trials in systemic light-chain (AL) amyloidosis. Leukemia 2012;26:2317–25.

44. Sidana S, Milani P, Binder M, et al. A validated composite organ and hematologic response model for early assessment of treatment outcomes in light chain amyloidosis. Blood Cancer J 2020;10(4):41.

45. Milani P, Gertz MA, Merlini G, et al. Attitudes about when and how to treat patients with AL amyloidosis: an international survey. Amyloid 2017;24(4):213–6.

46. Palladini G, Milani P, Foli A, et al. Presentation and outcome with second-line treatment in AL amyloidosis previously sensitive to nontransplant therapies. Blood 2018;131(5):525–32.

47. Staron A, Burks EJ, Lee JC, et al. Assessment of minimal residual disease using multiparametric flow cytometry in patients with AL amyloidosis. Blood Adv 2020; 4(5):880–4.

48. Sidana S, Muchtar E, Sidiqi MH, et al. Impact of minimal residual negativity using next generation flow cytometry on outcomes in light chain amyloidosis. Am J Hematol 2020;95(5):497–502.

49. Palladini G, Massa M, Basset M, et al. Persistence of minimal residual disease by multiparameter flow cytometry can hinder recovery of organ damage in patients with AL amyloidosis otherwise in complete response. Blood 2016;128(22):3261.

50. Muchtar E, Dispenzieri A, Jevremovic D, et al. Survival impact of achieving minimal residual negativity by multi-parametric flow cytometry in AL amyloidosis. Amyloid 2020;27(1):13–6.

51. Muchtar E, Dispenzieri A, Leung N, et al. Depth of organ response in AL amyloidosis is associated with improved survival: grading the organ response criteria. Leukemia 2018;32(10):2240–9.

52. Panelists TiAF. The Amyloidosis Forum: a public private partnership to advance drug development in AL amyloidosis. Orphanet Journal of Rare Disease 2020. [Epub ahead of print].

53. Pollard VT, Ryan MW, Geetter FS, et al. FDA offers guidance on clinical trials during COVID-19 Pandemic. The National Law Review 2020;X(84).

54. Shah T. FAQs On FDA Guidance For Clinical Trials During The COVID-19 Pandemic. imarc research. 2020. Available at: https://www.imarcresearch.com/blog/fda-guidance-covid-19. Accessed April 8, 2020.

55. Kyle RA, Gertz MA, Greipp PR, et al. A trial of three regimens for primary amyloidosis: colchicine alone, melphalan and prednisone, and melphalan, prednisone, and colchicine. N Engl J Med 1997;336(17):1202–7.

56. Skinner M, Anderson J, Simms R, et al. Treatment of 100 patients with primary amyloidosis: a randomized trial of melphalan, prednisone, and colchicine versus colchicine only. Am J Med 1996;100(3):290–8.

57. Kumar SK, Gertz MA, Lacy MQ, et al. Recent improvements in survival in primary systemic amyloidosis and the importance of an early mortality risk score. Mayo Clin Proc 2011;86(1):12–8.

58. Sanchorawala V, Sarosiek S, Schulman A, et al. Safety, tolerability, and response rates of daratumumab in relapsed al amyloidosis: results of a phase II study. Blood 2020;135(18):1541–7.

59. Roussel M, Merlini G, Chevret S, et al. A prospective phase II of daratumumab in previously treated systemic light chain amyloidosis (AL) patients. Blood 2020; 135(18):1531–40.

60. Palladini G, Kastritis E, Maurer MS, et al. Daratumumab Plus CyBorD for patients with newly diagnosed AL amyloidosis: safety run-in results of ANDROMEDA. Blood 2020;136(1):71–80.

61. Moreau P, Chanan-Khan A, Roberts AW, et al. Promising efficacy and acceptable safety of venetoclax plus bortezomib and dexamethasone in relapsed/refractory MM. Blood 2017;130(22):2392–400.

62. Leung N, Thome SD, Dispenzieri A. Venetoclax induced a complete response in a patient with immunoglobulin light chain amyloidosis plateaued on cyclophosphamide, bortezomib and dexamethasone. Haematologica 2018;103(3):e135–7.

63. Warsame R, Kumar SK, Gertz MA, et al. Abnormal FISH in patients with immunoglobulin light chain amyloidosis is a risk factor for cardiac involvement and for death. Blood Cancer J 2015;5:e310.

64. Bochtler T, Hegenbart U, Kunz C, et al. Translocation t(11;14) Is associated with adverse outcome in patients with newly diagnosed AL amyloidosis when treated with bortezomib-based regimens. J Clin Oncol 2015;33(12):1371–8.

65. Adams D, Gonzalez-Duarte A, O'Riordan WD, et al. Patisiran, an RNAi therapeutic, for hereditary transthyretin amyloidosis. N Engl J Med 2018;379(1):11–21.

66. Benson MD, Waddington-Cruz M, Berk JL, et al. Inotersen treatment for patients with hereditary transthyretin amyloidosis. N Engl J Med 2018;379(1):22–31.

67. Zhou P, Ma X, Iyer L, et al. One siRNA pool targeting the lambda constant region stops lambda light-chain production and causes terminal endoplasmic reticulum stress. Blood 2014;123(22):3440–51.

68. Soekojo CY, Ooi M, de Mel S, et al. Immunotherapy in multiple myeloma. Cells 2020;9(3):292–8.

69. Kumar SK, Dispenzieri A, Lacy MQ, et al. Doxycycline used as post transplant antibacterial prophylaxis improves survival in patients with light chain amyloidosis undergoing autologous stem cell transplantation. ASH Annual Meeting Abstracts 2012;120(21):3138.

70. Wechalekar AD, Whelan C. Encouraging impact of doxycycline on early mortality in cardiac light chain (AL) amyloidosis. Blood Cancer J 2017;7(3):e546.

71. Gertz MA, Landau H, Comenzo RL, et al. First-in-human phase I/II Study of NEOD001 in patients with light chain amyloidosis and persistent organ dysfunction. J Clin Oncol 2016;34(10):1097–103.

72. Edwards CV, Bhutani D, Mapara M, et al. One year follow up analysis of the phase 1a/b study of chimeric fibril-reactive monoclonal antibody 11-1F4 in patients with AL amyloidosis. Amyloid 2019;26(sup1):115–6.

Moving?

Make sure your subscription moves with you!

To notify us of your new address, find your **Clinics Account Number** (located on your mailing label above your name), and contact customer service at:

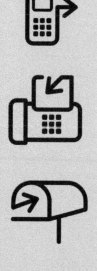

Email: journalscustomerservice-usa@elsevier.com

800-654-2452 (subscribers in the U.S. & Canada)
314-447-8871 (subscribers outside of the U.S. & Canada)

Fax number: 314-447-8029

Elsevier Health Sciences Division
Subscription Customer Service
3251 Riverport Lane
Maryland Heights, MO 63043

*To ensure uninterrupted delivery of your subscription, please notify us at least 4 weeks in advance of move.

ELSEVIER